The

WEIGHT WATCHERS
COMPLETE
COOKBOOK &
PROGRAM BASICS

◆

MACMILLAN ◆ U.S.A.

Since 1963, Weight Watchers has grown from a handful of people to millions of enrollments annually. Today, Weight Watchers is the recognized leading name in safe and sensible weight control. Weight Watchers members are a diverse group from youths, 10 years old and over, to senior citizens, attending meetings virtually around the globe.

Growing numbers of people purchase and enjoy our popular expanding line of convenience foods, best-selling cookbooks, personal calendar planners, and audio and video tapes. Weight loss and weight management results vary by individual, but we recommend that you attend Weight Watchers meetings, follow the Weight Watchers Food Plan, and participate in regular physical activity. For the Weight Watchers meeting nearest you, call 1-800-651-6000.

Our thanks to the recipe developers and testers who were instrumental in creating this book: Beth Allen, Catherine Chatham, Jean Galton, Catherine Garvey, Sandra Gluck, Luli Gray, Tamara Holt, Joel Jason, Phyllis Kohn, Kristine Napier, M. P. H., R.D., Linda Ann Rosensweig, and Marianne Zanzarella; and to Nutrition Consultant Lynne S. Hill, M.S., R.D., L.D. Photography by Martin Jacobs; Prop Styling by Linda Johnson; Food Styling by William Smith.

Charts on pages 188, 204 and 214 courtesy of the National Live Stock and Meat Board.

Cover photo: Whole-Wheat Pizza Dough with Tomato-Basil Topping, page 69

MACMILLAN GENERAL REFERENCE
A Prentice Hall Macmillan Company
15 Columbus Circle
New York, NY 10023

A Macmillan General Reference Book

MACMILLAN is a registered trademark of Macmillan, Inc.
WEIGHT WATCHERS is the registered trademark of Weight Watchers International, Inc.

Library of Congress Cataloging-in-Publication Data
The Weight Watchers complete cookbook & program basics.
    p. cm.
  Includes index.
  ISBN 0-671-88184-1 : $25.00
  1. Reducing diets. I. Weight Watchers International.
RM222.2.W312 1994
613.2'5—dc20   94-15686
                                   CIP

Manufactured in the United States of America

10 9 8 7 6 5 4 3 2

CONTENTS

CHAPTER ONE

WEIGHT WATCHERS FROM THE BEGINNING

Weight Watchers is one of the largest and most trusted weight-loss companies. In addition, Weight Watchers offers a comprehensive approach to weight loss and weight control, combining a sensible, easy-to-follow Food Plan, an Activity Plan, and Behavior Modification and Maintenance Plans, coupled with encouragement and support.

Developed with the guidance and supervision of respected medical, nutrition, exercise physiology and psychology professionals, the Weight Watchers Program represents the most current and scientifically designed approach to weight loss and control known today.

In this country, obesity is one of the most widespread health problems. It has been widely recognized that overweight is linked to increased risk of heart disease, diabetes, high blood pressure, stroke, gallbladder disease and some types of cancer. Fortunately, even a moderate weight loss of 10 to 15 pounds can help reduce these health risks.

HOW THE WEIGHT WATCHERS FOOD PLAN WORKS

Losing weight is about more than just a diet. In order to accomplish a goal of losing weight, you will need behavioral skills, new and wiser eating skills and a program that puts you in control. In a comprehensive approach to weight loss, Weight Watchers employs four unique strategies:

1 ◆ *Decreasing Caloric Intake*

Through a healthy eating plan that meets the nutritional recommendations of many major health organizations in North America, including the USDA Food Guide Pyramid and Canada's Food Guide to Healthy Eating (also known as Rainbow), the plan is high in complex carbohydrates, moderate in protein and low in fat.

Its design suggests eating a wide variety of foods in amounts appropriate for a safe rate of weight loss, approximately 1 to 2 pounds per week, with possible larger losses occurring in the first three weeks.

2 ◆ *Increasing Caloric Output*

Research has well established that exercise increases the likelihood that a weight-reducing diet will succeed. In addition, the advantages derived from increased physical activity extend to physiological, psychological and social benefits. By taking time to be more active, you are, in many ways, taking charge of your life, improving your self-image and strengthening your commitment to good health and weight control. It may be surprising to learn that even small changes in your normal activity can impact your weight over time. Consider that a 30-minute walk, four times a week, can burn approximately 10 pounds of fat in a year! The Weight Watchers Activity Plan includes low-to-moderate aerobic activities designed to help enhance weight loss and weight control. Exercises for stretching, firming and toning are also provided.

3 ◆ *Reshaping Behavior*

In order to accomplish the goal of weight loss and maintenance, overweight individuals must develop strong motivation. Weight Watchers, employing behavior modification and cognitive restructuring techniques, helps people learn positive attitudes and strategies for dealing with weight-loss challenges. The self-reinforcement of dealing successfully with obstacles enhances motivation and confirms the wisdom of making long-term lifestyle changes.

4 ◆ *Group Support: Nothing Helps More Than a Weight Watchers Meeting!*

Although many people are concerned about eating right and losing weight, the stress of daily living, pressures of work and family obligations and lack of time often get in the way of positive actions. By sharing these concerns with caring leaders and a supportive group, it becomes easier to learn skills and tactics to take better care of yourself. You learn how to stop eating on the run or overeating from stress, anxiety or boredom and to make time for increased activity. Hearing how others deal with bad eating habits, stay on track during the holidays or on vacation, have a good time at parties, deal with leftovers or handle diet saboteurs will reinforce your own ability to cope and succeed in these common situations.

WHAT CAN I EAT?

While the foods you choose cannot themselves guarantee good health or weight loss, eating the right kinds of foods in appropriate amounts improves your health and helps you to lose weight.

Eat a Variety of Foods

Break out of the same breakfast-lunch-dinner choices each day and try some new foods. Just one new recipe from this book each week will add interest and variety to your meals, help avoid menu boredom and expand your food repertoire. And, since no single food can supply all the nutrients your body requires, eating a variety of foods from all the food groups is important. The Weight Watchers Food Plan includes foods from six different groups. Make it a point to choose different foods from these lists every day.

Concentrate on Carbohydrates

Carbohydrates, the major source of energy on the Food Plan, are supplied by fruits, vegetables and grains, which are also a good source of vitamins, minerals and fiber. A good rule to follow is that 50 to 60 percent of your daily calories should come from foods that supply carbohydrates. Two chapters in this book provide 69 recipes featuring pasta, grains, rice, potatoes and beans, all excellent sources of complex carbohydrates. In addition, throughout the book, there are delicious ideas for appetizers, soups, entrées, side dishes and desserts featuring fruits, vegetables and grains, making it easy for you to incorporate them into every meal.

Choose a Low-in-Fat Diet

Leading health authorities recommend a diet reduced in total fat, saturated fat and cholesterol, one that provides no more than 30 percent of calories from fat and less than 10 percent from saturated fat, the type found in animal products and certain vegetable oils. See page 28 for a discussion of fat.

The Weight Watchers Food Plan automatically ensures that this recommendation is fulfilled. All you need to do is follow the Daily Totals and Weekly Limits of the Basic Food

Plan to meet these nutritional guidelines. The health benefits of restricting fat intake include reduced risk of heart disease and certain types of cancer.

Eat Appropriately to Maintain a Healthy Body Weight

Weighing either too much or too little has been found to pose a health risk, but merely counting calories will not guarantee good nutrition. You need to choose the right balance of foods, rich in complex carbohydrates, fiber, vitamins and minerals while low in fat and cholesterol. Following the balanced eating plan offered by Weight Watchers that includes such a variety of nutritious foods will help you to learn how to shed those extra pounds, practice good eating habits and lower your risk for certain diseases.

WEIGHT WATCHERS BASIC FOOD PLAN FOR WOMEN

The Weight Watchers Food Plan is based on a Selection System from six Food Lists. By following this plan and choosing a wide variety of foods from these lists, you will be enjoying a nutritious diet and learning how to plan balanced meals that meet the recommended dietary guidelines for good health. All the recipes in this book provide Weight Watchers Selection™ Information as well as nutritional analysis for calories and six nutrients. In Chapter Two, Eating for Health and Nutrition (page 27), these nutrients and their role in your diet and health are explained.

Youths (females under 16 and males under 19) should add these Selections to the Basic Food Plan they are following: 1 Milk, 1 Fat, 1 Fruit, 2 Proteins and 2 Breads.

Men should add these Selections to the Basic Food Plan they are following: 1 Fat, 1 Fruit, 2 Proteins and 2 Breads.

In addition to the Basic Food Lists, the Weight Watchers Food Plan includes these "extras": A weekly bonus of up to 14 Personal Selections may be made from any of the Milk, Fruit, Protein or Bread Lists.

Up to 700 Optional Calories may be added each week to further enhance the flavor of recipes and meals. A Combination List includes foods made up of more than one Food List item, and the Expanded Food List extends the Combination List by providing Selection Information on foods as they are generally consumed (i.e., in combination with one another).

BASIC FOOD PLAN FOR WOMEN

Food List	Selections/Day	What They Provide
Milk	2	Low-fat milk and dairy products provide the essential nutrients vitamins A and D and calcium. Low-fat dairy products provide the desired nutrients of whole-milk products, with much less fat and fewer calories.
Fat	3	The fats on this list are primarily unsaturated and act as carriers for the fat-soluble vitamins A, D, E and K. They are vital for the body to function properly and add a feeling of fullness after meals.
Fruit	2	Fruits supply carotenoids, vitamin C, potassium and fiber. There are more than 50 fruits and a dozen juices to choose from on the Fruit List. For maximum fiber and a greater feeling of fullness, eat fruits in their whole form.
Vegetables	3 (or more)	Vegetables are low in calories, dense in nutrients and fiber. Health professionals now also believe that they play a significant role in disease prevention. The Weight Watchers Vegetable List offers a wide variety of choices; visit it often!
Protein*	4	The body needs protein to make and repair tissue and to regulate body fluids and transport nutrients and oxygen in and out of cells. The foods on this list come from plant and animal sources that are rich in protein and also provide iron, zinc, several B vitamins and other nutrients important for good health.
Bread	5	Whole-grain and enriched breads, cereals, rice and pasta provide B vitamins, iron and fiber. Many satisfying grain-based meals are provided in this book.

*It is recommended that those Protein Selections that are higher in saturated fat be limited to 16 Selections per week. Whole eggs and organ meats are limited to four Selections per week.

WEIGHT WATCHERS FOOD LISTS

MILK (M): ONE SELECTION =

Buttermilk, skim, nonfat *or* 1%, 1 cup
Dairy shake, reduced-calorie, 1 packet
Milk, evaporated skimmed, $\frac{1}{2}$ cup
Milk, instant nonfat dry, $\frac{1}{3}$ cup powder
Milk, skim, nonfat *or* 1%, 1 cup
Yogurt, nonfat, aspartame-sweetened,
    1 cup
Yogurt, nonfat, plain, $\frac{3}{4}$ cup (12 tbsp)

FAT (FA): ONE SELECTION =

Avocado, $\frac{1}{8}$ medium (1 oz)
Margarine, liquid vegetable oil, 1 tsp
Margarine, reduced-calorie, 2 tsp
Mayonnaise, 1 tsp
Mayonnaise, reduced-calorie, 2 tsp
Olives, 10 small *or* 6 large (1 oz)
Peanut butter, 1 tsp
Salad dressing, regular, any type, $\frac{1}{2}$ tbsp
    ($1\frac{1}{2}$ tsp)
Tartar sauce, $\frac{1}{2}$ tbsp ($1\frac{1}{2}$ tsp)
Vegetable oil, 1 tsp

Note: Weights are for item as purchased (e.g., with peel, pits, etc.).

PROTEIN (P): ONE SELECTION =

Meat, Fish and Poultry (*cooked weight*)

*Beef, lamb and pork (except cuts listed
    below), 1 oz
Beef, lamb and pork (loin, round and leg
    cuts), 1 oz

Deli meat, 1 oz
Deli meat, lean (up to 2 grams fat per oz),
    $1\frac{1}{2}$ oz
Fish (salmon, mackerel, anchovy, sardine,
    herring), 1 oz
Fish and shellfish (except those listed
    above), 2 oz
Game, 1 oz
Ground meat *or* poultry, lean (10% or less
    fat), 1 oz
Ham, 1 oz
**Organ meat (e.g., liver, kidney, tongue),
    1 oz
Poultry, without skin (e.g., chicken, duck,
    turkey), 1 oz
*Processed meat (e.g., bologna, frank-
    furters, salami, sausage, wursts), 1 oz
Veal, 1 oz

Cheeses

Cottage, low-fat (1% *or* 2%), $\frac{1}{3}$ cup
Cottage, nonfat, $\frac{1}{2}$ cup
Cottage, regular (4%), $\frac{1}{4}$ cup
Hard *or* semisoft, $\frac{3}{4}$ oz
*Hard *or* semisoft, nonfat, $1\frac{1}{2}$ oz
Pot, $\frac{1}{3}$ cup
*Process cheese slices, 1 slice
Process cheese slices, low-fat *or* nonfat,
    2 slices
Ricotta, part-skim, $\frac{1}{4}$ cup

Other

**Egg, 1
Egg substitute, $\frac{1}{4}$ cup

Egg whites, 3

Legumes (dry beans, lentils *or* peas), 2 oz
    cooked *or* $\frac{3}{4}$ oz uncooked

Tofu, firm, 2 oz

Tofu, soft, 3 oz

*Eat no more than 16 Selections per week of these foods.
**Eat no more than 4 Selections per week of these foods.

VEGETABLES (V): ONE SELECTION ($\frac{1}{2}$ CUP) =
(except as indicated)

Artichokes

Asparagus

Beans, green *or* wax

Beets

Broccoli

Brussels sprouts

Cabbage

Carrots

Cauliflower

Celery

Cucumbers

Eggplant

Endive

Escarole

Greens—beet, chard, kale, mustard, etc.

Hearts of palm (palmetto)

Jerusalem artichokes (sunchokes)

Jicama

Leeks

Lettuce

Mushrooms

Okra

Onions

Peppers

Pickles, unsweetened

Pimientos

Pumpkin

Radishes

Rhubarb

Sauerkraut

Scallions

Snow peas (Chinese pea pods)

Spaghetti squash

Spinach

Sprouts, alfalfa *or* bean

Summer squash

Tomato *or* mixed vegetable juice

Tomato paste, 2 tbsp

Tomato purée *or* sauce, $\frac{1}{4}$ cup

Tomatoes

Tomatoes, dried (not packed in oil),
    2 halves

Turnips

Watercress

Zucchini

BREAD (B): ONE SELECTION =

Breads

Bagel, $\frac{1}{2}$ small (1 oz)

Bread, any type, 1 slice (1 oz)

Bread, reduced-calorie, 2 slices (2 oz)

Bread crumbs, dried, 3 tbsp ($\frac{3}{4}$ oz)

English muffin, $\frac{1}{2}$ (1 oz)

Frankfurter roll, $\frac{1}{2}$ (1 oz)

Hamburger roll, $\frac{1}{2}$ (1 oz)

Pita, 1 small *or* $\frac{1}{2}$ large (1 oz)

Roll, any type, 1 small (1 oz)

Taco *or* tostada shell, 2 (1 oz)

Tortilla, any type, 1 (6" diameter)

Grains

Barley, $\frac{1}{2}$ cup cooked *or* $\frac{3}{4}$ oz uncooked

Bulgur, $\frac{1}{2}$ cup cooked *or* 1 oz uncooked

Cellophane noodles, $\frac{1}{2}$ cup cooked *or* $\frac{3}{4}$ oz uncooked

Cereal, cold, not presweetened, $\frac{3}{4}$ oz

Cereal, hot, $\frac{1}{2}$ cup cooked *or* $\frac{3}{4}$ oz uncooked

Cornmeal, $\frac{1}{2}$ cup cooked *or* 2 tbsp ($\frac{3}{4}$ oz) uncooked

Couscous (semolina), $\frac{1}{2}$ cup cooked *or* 1 oz uncooked

Flour, 3 tbsp ($\frac{3}{4}$ oz)

Hominy grits, $\frac{1}{2}$ cup cooked *or* $\frac{3}{4}$ oz uncooked

Pasta (macaroni, noodles, spaghetti, etc.), $\frac{1}{2}$ cup cooked *or* $\frac{3}{4}$ oz uncooked

Popcorn, plain, 2 cups oil-popped *or* 3 cups hot-air-popped

Pretzels, $\frac{3}{4}$ oz

Rice, $\frac{1}{2}$ cup cooked *or* 1 oz uncooked

Rice cakes, any type, 2 ($\frac{3}{4}$ oz)

Wheat germ, unsweetened, 3 tbsp ($\frac{3}{4}$ oz)

Crackers

Breadsticks, $\frac{3}{4}$ oz

Crispbreads *or* flatbreads, $\frac{3}{4}$ oz

Fat-free crackers, 7 ($\frac{3}{4}$ oz)

Graham crackers, 3 ($2\frac{1}{2}$" squares) *or* 3 tbsp crumbs

Matzo, $\frac{3}{4}$ board ($\frac{3}{4}$ oz)

Melba toast, 6 rounds *or* 4 slices ($\frac{3}{4}$ oz)

Saltines, 6

Starchy Vegetables *(amounts listed are both cooked and uncooked unless otherwise indicated)*

Corn, kernels *or* cream-style, $\frac{1}{2}$ cup

Corn on the cob, 1 small ear (5")

Legumes (dry beans, lentils *or* peas), 2 oz cooked *or* $\frac{3}{4}$ oz uncooked

Lima beans, green, $\frac{1}{2}$ cup

Parsnips, $\frac{1}{2}$ cup

Peas, green, $\frac{1}{2}$ cup

Plantain, peeled, 3 oz *or* $\frac{1}{2}$ cup slices

Potato, sweet, 3 oz cooked *or* 4 oz uncooked

Potato, white, 4 oz cooked *or* 5 oz uncooked

Potato flakes, $\frac{3}{4}$ oz uncooked

Water chestnuts, $\frac{3}{4}$ cup (4 oz)

Winter squash, 1 cup *or* 7 oz cooked

Yam, 3 oz cooked *or* 4 oz uncooked

FRUIT (FR): ONE SELECTION =

Apple, 1 small (4 oz)

Applesauce, $\frac{1}{2}$ cup

Apricots, fresh, 3 medium (4 oz)

Banana, $\frac{1}{2}$ medium (3 oz)

Berries

    Blackberries, $\frac{3}{4}$ cup (4 oz)

    Blueberries, $\frac{3}{4}$ cup (4 oz)

    Boysenberries, $\frac{3}{4}$ cup (4 oz)

    Cranberries, 1 cup (4 oz)

    Loganberries, $\frac{3}{4}$ cup (4 oz)

    Raspberries, $\frac{3}{4}$ cup (4 oz)

    Strawberries, 1 cup (6 oz)

Cantaloupe, $\frac{1}{4}$ small (8 oz) *or* 1 cup

Cherries, 12 large (3 oz)

Currants, fresh, $\frac{3}{4}$ cup (3 oz)

Dates, fresh, 2 ($\frac{3}{4}$ oz)

Dried fruit

    Apple slices, 3 ($\frac{3}{4}$ oz)

    Apricots, 6 halves ($\frac{3}{4}$ oz)

Currants, 2 tbsp ($\frac{3}{4}$ oz)

Dates, 2 ($\frac{3}{4}$ oz)

Fig, 1 large ($\frac{3}{4}$ oz)

Mixed dried fruit, $\frac{3}{4}$ oz

Prunes, 2 large *or* 3 medium ($\frac{3}{4}$ oz)

Raisins, 2 tbsp ($\frac{3}{4}$ oz)

Fig, fresh, 1 large (2 oz)

Fruit salad, $\frac{1}{2}$ cup

Grapefruit, $\frac{1}{2}$ medium (8 oz)

Grapefruit sections, $\frac{1}{2}$ cup

Grapes, 20 small *or* 12 large (3 oz)

Honeydew melon, 2" wedge (8 oz) *or* 1 cup

Juices

Apple juice *or* cider, $\frac{1}{2}$ cup (4 fl oz)

Combined fruit juices, any type, $\frac{1}{3}$ cup (3 fl oz)

Cranberry juice cocktail, low-calorie, 1 cup (8 fl oz)

Cranberry juice cocktail, reguiar, $\frac{1}{3}$ cup (3 fl oz)

Grapefruit juice, $\frac{1}{2}$ cup (4 fl oz)

Grape juice, $\frac{1}{3}$ cup (3 fl oz)

Nectar, any type, $\frac{1}{3}$ cup (3 fl oz)

Orange-grapefruit juice, $\frac{1}{2}$ cup (4 fl oz)

Orange juice, $\frac{1}{2}$ cup (4 fl oz)

Pineapple juice, $\frac{1}{3}$ cup (3 fl oz)

Prune juice, $\frac{1}{3}$ cup (3 fl oz)

Kiwi fruit, 1 medium (4 oz)

Mandarin orange, 1 large (6 oz)

Mango, $\frac{1}{2}$ small (4 oz)

Nectarine, 1 small (4 oz)

Orange, 1 small (6 oz)

Orange sections, $\frac{1}{2}$ cup

Papaya, $\frac{1}{2}$ medium (8 oz) *or* 1 cup

Peach, 1 medium (6 oz)

Pear, 1 small *or* $\frac{1}{2}$ large (6 oz)

Persimmon, $\frac{1}{2}$ medium (3 oz)

Pineapple, $\frac{1}{8}$ medium (6 oz)

Plums, 1 large *or* 2 small (4 oz)

Spreadable fruit, 1 tbsp

Tangerine, 1 large (6 oz)

Watermelon, 2" × 3" wedge (11 oz) *or* 1 cup

Note: Weights are for item as purchased (e.g., with peel, pits, etc.).

OPTIONAL CALORIES (C)

Bacon bits, imitation, 1 tsp ....10 C

Beer, 12 fl oz...................................155 C

Beer, light, 12 fl oz..........................100 C

Bouillon, 1 cube *or* 1 tsp.....................10C

Broth and seasoning mix, instant, 1 packet *or* $\frac{3}{4}$ cup prepared ....10 C

Broth *or* consommé, canned *or* homemade, $\frac{1}{2}$ cup ....10 C

Butter, 1 tsp ....35 C

Butter, whipped, 1 tsp ....25 C

Cheese, hard, grated, 1 tsp ....10 C

Chocolate, any type, 1 oz................150 C

Cocoa, unsweetened, 1 tsp...................5 C

Coconut, shredded, 1 tsp....................5 C

Cookies, any type, 1 large (3") *or* 2 small (1 oz) ....150 C

Cornstarch *or* flour, 1 tsp ....10 C

Cream, light, 1 tbsp..........................30 C

Cream cheese, 1 tbsp ....50 C

Cream cheese, whipped *or* light, 1 tbsp......................................30 C

Cream cheese, nonfat, 1 tbsp ....15 C

Creamer, nondairy, 1 tbsp liquid *or* 2 tsp powder...................20 C

Fruit butter, any type, 1 tsp...............10 C

Gelatin, fruit-flavored, ½ cup
    prepared.....................................80 C

Gum, chewing, 1 stick *or* piece ....10 C

Half-and-half, 1 tbsp.......................20 C

Honey, 1 tsp................................20 C

Ice Cream, ½ cup ....200 C

Jams, jellies *or* preserves, 1 tsp ....15 C

Ketchup, 2 tsp...............................10 C

Liquor (gin, rum, scotch, tequila,
    vodka *or* whiskey), 1½ fl oz ....120 C

Neufchâtel cheese, 1 tbsp..................35 C

Relish, any type, 1 tsp.......................5 C

Salad dressing, fat-free (except Italian),
    1 tbsp..................................20 C

Salad dressing, fat-free Italian,
    1 tbsp...................................5 C

Sauces:
    barbecue, chili, cocktail, steak *or*
        teriyaki, 1 tbsp ....20 C
    sweet & sour, 1 tbsp ....10 C

Seeds (poppy, caraway, pumpkin,
    sesame, sunflower), 1 tsp ....15 C

Sherbet *or* sorbet, ½ cup ....125 C

Sour cream:
    regular, 1 tbsp...........................25 C
    light, 1 tbsp.................................20 C
    nonfat, 1 tbsp.............................10 C

Sugar *or* syrup, 1 tsp ....15 C

Whipped cream *or* whipped
    topping, 2 tbsp..........................25 C

Wine *or* champagne, 4 fl oz.............100 C

Wine, light, 4 fl oz.........................50 C

Wine cooler, 12 fl oz.....................200 C

Wine spritzer, 8 fl oz.....................100 C

Food Plan Selections

1 Milk Selection .... 90 C

1 Fat Selection .... 40 C

1 Fruit Selection .... 60 C

1 Protein Selection .... 60 C

1 Bread Selection .... 80 C

The numbers listed above are *averages*. Some Selections within each Food List will be higher in calories and others will be lower than the averages indicated.

Note: Foods not found on the Food Lists may be taken as Optional Calories as long as *calories per serving* are provided on the label.

ADDITIONAL ITEMS
(use in reasonable amounts)

Beverages

Water, mineral water

Club soda, seltzer

Coffee

Diet soda

Tea

Seasonings/Condiments

Baking powder

Baking soda

Capers

Extracts, flavorings

Gelatin, unflavored

Herbs

Horseradish

Hot sauce (pepper sauce)

Lemon juice

Lime juice (no sugar added)

Mustard

Nonstick cooking
   or baking spray
Salsa, taco sauce
Soy sauce
Spices
Sugar substitutes
Vinegar
Worcestershire sauce

COMBINATION FOODS

Baked beans, without meat, canned
   ½ cup ....1 P, ½ V, 40 C
Barbecued chicken, with skin,
   1 breast *or* leg and
   thigh..........................1 FA, 3 P, 100 C
Beef*, chicken *or* pork* with
   Chinese vegetables,
   1 cup ....1½ V, 3 FA, 2 P, 35 C
Biscuit, any type, 1
   (2" diameter) ....1 FA, ¾ B
Chicken salad, ½ cup..........¼ V, 3 FA, 2 P
Coleslaw, ½ cup .... 1 V, 2 FA
Crackers, ½ oz....................½ FA, ½ B
Croissant, plain, 1 ¾ oz ....1 B, 35 C
Croutons, packaged, ¼ cup
   (½ oz) ....½ FA, ½ B
Fish, packed in oil, drained (except those
   listed below)
   2 oz .... 1 FA, 1P

Fish, packed in oil, drained
   (salmon, mackerel, anchovy,
   sardine, herring), 1 oz..........½ FA, 1 P
Hamburger* on bun, fast food,
   1 small..............................1½ P, 2 B
Lobster, shrimp *or* tuna salad,
   ½ cup ....¼ V, 3 FA, 1 P
Milk *or* buttermilk (2%),
   1 cup ....1 M, 30 C
Milk *or* buttermilk, whole,
   1 cup ....1 M, 50 C
Muffin, any type, 1 large
   (4 oz).........2 FA, ¼ P (egg), ¾ B, 25 C
Peanut butter, 1 tbsp ....1 FA, 1 P
Pizza, cheese*, large, thin-crust,
   1 slice (⅛ of 14" pie) .....½ V, 2 P, 1½ B
Popcorn, microwave, plain,
   butter *or* cheese flavor,
   2 cups popped ....1 B, 40 C
Pudding, reduced-calorie,
   made with skim, nonfat
   or 1% milk, ½ cup ....½ M, 30 C
Yogurt, frozen, low-fat,
   4 fl oz ....¼ M, 100 C
Yogurt *or* dietary dessert,
   frozen, nonfat, 4 fl oz.........¼ M, 75 C
Yogurt, frozen, nonfat,
   sugar-free, 4 fl oz ....¼ M, 50 C
Yogurt, low-fat, plain, ¾ cup
   (12 tbsp) ....1 M, 10 C

*Check Protein List for limits.

MENU 1, DAY 1

Breakfast
Strawberries, $\frac{1}{2}$ cup
Hot toasted wheat cereal, $\frac{3}{4}$ cup
Skim milk, 1 cup
Coffee or tea (optional)

Lunch
Mushroom Hamburgers, 1 serving (see page 194)
Hamburger roll, 1 (2 ounces)
Dilled Carrots, 1 serving (see page 104)
Tomato slices on lettuce leaves
Diet cola with lemon

Dinner
Roast turkey, 2 ounces
Raisin and Sage Bread Stuffing, 1 serving (see page 181)
"Creamed" Spinach, 1 serving (see page 113)
Tossed salad with 1 tablespoon fat-free ranch dressing
Nectarine-Cherry Tart, 1 serving (see page 326)
Decaffeinated coffee or tea (optional)

Snack
Pretzels, $\frac{3}{4}$ ounce
Reduced-calorie chocolate dairy shake, 1 serving

MENU 1, DAY 2

Breakfast
Orange-grapefruit juice, 1 cup
Sour Cream Blueberry-Lemon Pancakes, 1 serving (see page 78)
Skim milk, $\frac{1}{2}$ cup
Coffee or tea (optional)

Lunch
Mixed vegetable juice, $\frac{1}{2}$ cup, with celery stick stirrer
Cornmeal-cheese Soufflé, 1 serving (see page 280)
Crispbreads, $\frac{3}{4}$ ounces
Chicory with Mustard and Caper Dressing, 1 serving (see page 124)
Sugar-free raspberry gelatin, $\frac{1}{2}$ cup
Iced tea

Dinner
Beef Kabobs with Moroccan Spices, 1 serving (see page 198)
Couscous with Lime-Ginger Sauce, 1 serving (see page 278)
Steamed whole green beans
Cucumber slices on lettuce leaves with balsamic vinegar
Reduced-calorie vanilla pudding, $\frac{1}{2}$ cup, with 3 graham crackers
Decaffeinated coffee or tea (optional)

Snack
Oil-popped popcorn, $1\frac{1}{2}$ cups
Skim milk, $\frac{1}{2}$ cup

MENU 1, DAY 3

Breakfast
Honeydew chunks, 1 cup
Whole-wheat bread, 2 slices, toasted, with 2 slices process nonfat
cheese
Skim milk, 1 cup
Coffee or tea (optional)

Lunch
Lentil and Swiss Chard Soup, 1 serving (see page 85)
Oyster crackers, 1 ounce
Whole mushrooms on lettuce leaves with 1 serving Italian Dressing
(see page 136)
Baked Plums, 1 serving (see page 336)
Diet lemon-lime soda

Dinner
Baked Trout with Tomato and Chervil, 1 serving (see page 243)
Herbed Instant Brown Rice, 1 serving (see page 285)
Creole-Style Okra, 1 serving (see page 109)
Torn green and red leaf lettuce with 1 tablespoon fat-free blue cheese
dressing
Aspartame-sweetened nonfat vanilla yogurt, 1 cup
Decaffeinated coffee or tea (optional)

Snack
Sweet Potato Chips, 1 serving (see page 309)
Diet root beer

Menu 1, Day 4

Breakfast
Papaya, 1 cup
Sweet Brown Bread, 1 serving (see page 77)
Reduced-calorie margarine, 1 teaspoon
Skim milk, 1 cup
Coffee or tea (optional)

Lunch
Cooked Virginia ham, $1\frac{1}{2}$ ounces, with lettuce leaves, tomato slices
and mustard on 2 slices rye bread
Zucchini-Carrot Salad with Cumin Dressing, 1 serving (see page 125)
Peach, 1 medium
Berry-flavored sparkling mineral water

Dinner
Green and yellow bell pepper strips with 1 serving Spiced Red Bean
Dip (see page 52)
Chicken with Apples and Cider, 1 serving (see page 147)
Steamed chopped broccoli with 2 ounces sliced water chestnuts
Cappuccino Custard, 1 serving (see page 334)
Decaffeinated coffee or tea (optional)

Snack
Bran flakes cereal, $\frac{3}{4}$ ounce, with 1 tablespoon raisins
Skim milk, $\frac{1}{2}$ cup

MENU 1, DAY 5

Breakfast
Kiwi fruit, 1 medium, sliced
Bagel, 1 small (2 ounces)
Peanut butter, 2 teaspoons
Reduced-calorie strawberry spread, 1 teaspoon
Skim milk, 1 cup
Coffee or tea (optional)

Lunch
Process low-fat cheese, 2 slices, and sliced red onion on 2 slices
pumpernickel bread, broiled
Lemon-Dilled Pasta Salad, 1 serving (see page 276)
Celery and carrot sticks
Apple, 1 small
Diet black cherry soda

Dinner
Honey-Mustard Pork Chops, 1 serving (see page 209)
Baked Potatoes with Sour Cream, 1 serving (see page 310)
Mushroom and Red Bell Pepper Sauté, 1 serving (see page 111)
Endive and romaine salad with 1 tablespoon Herbed Vinegar
(see page 352)
Broiled Pecan Pineapple, 1 serving (see page 336)
Decaffeinated coffee or tea (optional)

Snack
Aspartame-sweetened nonfat lemon yogurt, 1 cup, with $\frac{1}{4}$ cup canned
crushed pineapple

Menu 1, Day 6

Breakfast
Low-calorie cranberry juice cocktail, $\frac{1}{2}$ cup
Frittata, 1 serving (see page 353)
English muffin, $\frac{1}{2}$ (1 ounce), toasted
Reduced-calorie margarine, 1 teaspoon
Skim milk, 1 cup
Coffee or tea (optional)

Lunch
Water-packed tuna, 2 ounces, with chopped celery and onion and $1\frac{1}{2}$
teaspoons reduced-calorie mayonnaise on lettuce leaves
Marinated Three-Bean Salad, 1 serving (see page 130)
Italian Bread, 1 serving (see page 61)
Fresh fruit salad, $\frac{1}{2}$ cup
Diet grape ginger ale

Dinner
Cod with Spaghetti, 1 serving (see page 222)
Oven-Roasted Leeks and Fennel Parmesan, 1 serving (see page 107)
Chicory and cherry tomato salad with 1 tablespoon fat-free Italian
dressing
Cantaloupe, $\frac{1}{4}$ small
Decaffeinated coffee or tea (optional)

Snack
Sticky Buns, 1 serving (see page 73)
Skim milk, 1 cup

MENU 1, DAY 7

Breakfast

Banana, $\frac{1}{2}$ medium
Hot oatmeal, $\frac{1}{2}$ cup, with 1 teaspoon brown sugar and ground cinnamon
Skim milk, 1 cup
Coffee or tea (optional)

Lunch

Chicken-Tomato Chowder, 1 serving (see page 154)
Spinach and mushroom salad with fresh lemon juice
Roll, 1 ounce
Reduced-calorie margarine, 1 teaspoon
Grapes, 20 small
Diet citrus soda

Dinner

Orange-Crumbed Baked Chicken Thighs, 1 serving (see page 157)
Rosemary-Zucchini Pasta, 1 serving (see page 268)
Red and green bell pepper rings on lettuce leaves with 1 teaspoon vegetable oil and red wine vinegar
Vanilla Layer Cake with Chocolate-Ginger Frosting, 1 serving (see page 314)
Decaffeinated coffee or tea (optional)

Snack

Rice cake, 1, with $1\frac{1}{2}$ teaspoons apricot spreadable fruit
Skim milk, 1 cup

MENU 2, DAY 1

Breakfast
Pink grapefruit, ½ medium
English muffin, 1 (2 ounces), toasted
Pear butter, 2 teaspoons
Skim milk, 1 cup
Coffee or tea (optional)

Lunch
Chicken Pita Pizzas, 1 serving (see page 166)
Torn bibb lettuce and sliced red onion with 1 serving Honey-Mustard
Dressing (see page 137)
Apricots, 3 medium
Sparkling mineral water with lime wedge

Dinner
Lamb Chops with Tomato-Dill Salsa, 1 serving (see page 203)
Lyonnaise Potatoes, 1 serving (see page 303)
Romaine and cherry tomato salad with 1 serving Italian Dressing
(see page 136) and 1 serving Croutons (see page 357)
Aspartame-sweetened nonfat strawberry-banana yogurt, 1 cup
Decaffeinated coffee or tea (optional)

Snack
Hot-air-popped popcorn, 3 cups
Diet cherry cola

MENU 2, DAY 2

Breakfast
Blueberries, ¾ cup
Egg, 1, scrambled in 1 teaspoon reduced-calorie margarine
Hash Brown Potatoes, 1 serving (see page 304)
Reduced-calorie honey-bran bread, 1 slice, toasted, with 1½ teaspoons
reduced-calorie margarine
Skim milk, 1 cup
Coffee or tea (optional)

Lunch
Low-fat cottage cheese, ⅔ cup, with ¼ cup canned peach slices and
5 small grapes on lettuce leaves
Cucumbers and Bow-Tie Pasta in Sour Cream–Chive Dressing,
1 serving (see page 275)
Reduced-calorie butterscotch pudding, ½ cup
Diet cream soda

Dinner
Greek Kabobs with Turbot, 1 serving (see page 248)
Grilled eggplant and yellow squash
Shredded green cabbage and carrot with 1 teaspoon vegetable oil and
1 tablespoon Herbed Vinegar (see page 352)
Chocolate Layer Cake, 1 serving (see page 312)
Decaffeinated coffee or tea (optional)

Snack
Irish Soda Bread, 1 serving (see page 77)
Skim milk, ½ cup

MENU 2, DAY 3

Breakfast
Honeydew melon, 2" wedge
Whole-Wheat Sourdough Date Bread, 1 serving (see page 59)
Reduced-calorie margarine, 2 teaspoons
Aspartame-sweetened nonfat peach yogurt, 1 cup
Coffee or tea (optional)

Lunch
Low-sodium beef bouillon, $\frac{3}{4}$ cup
Roast Beef Salad with Arugula, 1 serving (see page 200)
Sesame breadsticks, $1\frac{1}{2}$ ounces
Plums, 2 small
Iced herbal tea

Dinner
Chicken with Spinach and Noodles, 1 serving (see page 148)
Roasted Zucchini Provençale, 1 serving (see page 118)
Torn red leaf lettuce and alfalfa sprouts with 1 serving Pesto Dressing
(see page 137)
Sugar-free cherry gelatin, $\frac{1}{2}$ cup
Decaffeinated coffee or tea (optional)

Snack
Graham crackers, 3
Skim milk, 1 cup

MENU 2, DAY 4

Breakfast
Banana, $\frac{1}{2}$ medium
Cornflakes, $\frac{3}{4}$ ounce
Skim milk, 1 cup
Reduced-calorie wheat bread, 1 slice, toasted
Reduced-calorie grape spread, 1 teaspoon
Coffee or tea (optional)

Lunch
Four Cheese Macaroni, 1 serving (see page 272)
Celery and cucumber sticks
Tossed salad with $1\frac{1}{2}$ teaspoons Thousand Island dressing
Cherries, 12 large
Diet ginger ale

Dinner
Pumpkin Soup with Cinnamon Toast Triangles, 1 serving (see page 93)
Baked ham, 2 ounces
Roasted Sweet Potatoes, 1 serving (see page 306)
Honey-Glazed Carrots, 1 serving (see page 104)
Sliced tomato and green bell pepper rings with balsamic vinegar
Fresh fruit salad, $\frac{1}{2}$ cup
Decaffeinated coffee or tea (optional)

Snack
Potato Chips, 1 serving (see page 309)
Diet coffee soda with $\frac{1}{2}$ cup skim milk

MENU 2, DAY 5

Breakfast
Low-calorie cranberry juice cocktail, $\frac{3}{4}$ cup
Bagel, 1 small (2 ounces)
Reduced-calorie margarine, 2 teaspoons
Skim milk, $\frac{1}{2}$ cup
Coffee or tea (optional)

Lunch
Warm Chicken Salad with Roasted Red Pepper Dressing, 1 serving
(see page 162)
Onion flatbreads, $1\frac{1}{2}$ ounces
Whole mushrooms and radishes with 1 serving Creamy Garlic and
Chive Dressing (see page 138)
Tangerine, 1 large
Club soda

Dinner
Broiled halibut, 3 ounces
5 ounces cooked new potatoes
Steamed broccoli and cauliflower florets with 1 serving Herbed Cheese
Sauce (see page 343)
Belgian endive with 1 teaspoon vegetable oil and fresh lemon juice
Aspartame-sweetened nonfat black cherry yogurt, 1 cup
Decaffeinated coffee or tea (optional)

Snack
Apple-Oatmeal Cookies, 1 serving (see page 330)
Sugar-free hot cocoa, 1 serving

MENU 2, DAY 6

Breakfast
Orange sections, ½ cup
Toasted Oatmeal Bread, 1 serving (see page 65)
Reduced-calorie margarine, 1 teaspoon
Aspartame-sweetened nonfat blueberry yogurt, 1 cup
Skim milk, ½ cup
Coffee or tea (optional)

Lunch
Herbed Split Pea Soup, 1 serving (see page 84)
Semolina roll, 2 ounces
Reduced-calorie margarine, 1 teaspoon
Iceberg lettuce wedge with 1 tablespoon fat-free Italian dressing
Toasted Coconut Custard, 1 serving (see page 334)
Diet cherry-lemon soda

Dinner
Beef Stir-Fry with Mixed Vegetables, 1 serving (see page 199)
Steamed rice, ½ cup
Chinese Noodles in Sesame-Soy Sauce, 1 serving (see page 270)
Steamed snow peas
Pineapple, ⅛ medium
Decaffeinated coffee or tea (optional)

Snack
Taco chips, 1 ounce
Salsa, 1 serving (see page 345)

MENU 2, DAY 7

Breakfast
Cantaloupe, ¼ small
Hot rice cereal, ½ cup, with 1 teaspoon honey
Melba toast, 3 slices
Reduced-calorie raspberry spread, 2 teaspoons
Skim milk, 1 cup
Coffee or tea (optional)

Lunch
Southwestern Black Bean Salad, 1 serving (see page 291)
Fat-free crackers, 7
Carrot and zucchini sticks
Aspartame-sweetened nonfat mixed fruit yogurt, 1 cup
Iced coffee

Dinner
Mushroom-Stuffed Turkey Breast, 1 serving (see page 170)
Orzo with Garlic-Gingered Spring Vegetables, 1 serving (see page 269)
Mixed green salad with 1 serving "Russian" dressing (see page 136)
Applesauce, ½ cup
Decaffeinated coffee or tea (optional)

Snack
Pretzels, 1½ ounces
Diet black cherry soda

We hope that you have enjoyed these menu plans. These menus and the holiday menus on pages 364–413 fit the Weight Watchers Basic Food Plan for Women. To make them even easier to use and to learn how to plan your own meals, we suggest that you attend Weight Watchers meetings. There, guided by a sharing and caring leader and staff, you will find support, advice and motivation from people who understand and can help you learn new, healthy eating habits and ways to manage challenges and who can inspire you to reach your personal goals.

◆

EATING FOR NUTRITION AND HEALTH

Food is your body's energy source for the essential nutrients that fuel it and maintain health. By learning healthy eating habits, incorporating them into your life and becoming more physically active, you may reap many long-term health and psychological benefits.

In order to achieve a healthy body weight, your caloric output must exceed your caloric intake; in order to maintain a healthy body weight, caloric output must equal caloric intake. Energy output is enhanced by physical activity, which helps control body weight while improving body shape and muscle tone.

Caloric intake is regulated by the amount and type of foods you eat. There are three elements in food that provide energy: protein, fat and carbohydrates. Protein and carbohydrates each provide 4 calories per gram, while fat provides 9 calories per gram. Controlling the amount of fat you consume is one of the best ways to manage the energy input side of the equation.

Each recipe in this book has been analyzed for its nutritional contribution of protein, fat, carbohydrate, sodium, cholesterol, dietary fiber and calories. Each of these nutrients provides special components of your diet and has recommended guidelines for daily intake.

Protein: 15 to 20 Percent of Daily Caloric Intake

Often called the body's building blocks because they maintain and build body tissues, proteins are broken down during digestion into subunits called amino acids. Although there are about 22 amino acids used by the body, eight are considered essential and must be obtained from food.

Protein-rich foods, while providing several essential ingredients, are often a significant source of fat and the major source of saturated fat in the foods we eat. Therefore, the Weight Watchers Food Plan balances these apparently conflicting components by emphasizing lower fat choices, such as lean meats, low-fat dairy products and legumes (dried beans).

Fat: Less than 30 Percent of Total Dietary Intake; Less than 10 percent from Saturated Fat

While you do need some dietary fat to provide essential fatty acids and to act as a carrier for certain fat-soluble vitamins (A, D, E and K), fat is the most concentrated source of calories in the diet. And, since fat takes a longer time to be digested and absorbed into your bloodstream, a meal containing fat does help you to feel full and satisfied after eating. So the object is not to eliminate fat entirely but to reduce your consumption to the right amount and the right type, something the Weight Watchers program is designed to ensure. All fat found in food is a combination of three types: saturated, monounsaturated and polyunsaturated, and all three contain the same number of calories. Saturated fats, such as butter, are solid at room temperature. Unsaturated fats (including monounsaturated and polyunsaturated fats) are generally considered to be healthier than saturated, and are found primarily in liquid vegetable oils and most margarines.

Tips for Lowering Your Fat Consumption

When shopping:

Choose lean cuts of meat: top round, top loin, round tip, sirloin, tenderloin, eye of round.

Choose ground meats (e.g., beef, turkey) that are labeled as having 10 percent or less fat.

Choose skim, low-fat or nonfat dairy products.

Read labels. All labels are required to provide the grams of fat, calories from fat and grams of saturated fat in a serving of the product.

Choose margarine that lists water or liquid vegetable oil as the first or second ingredient.

When cooking:

Use nonstick cookware or spray cookware with nonstick cooking spray.

Trim all visible fat from meat and remove skin from poultry before eating.

Broil higher-fat meats on a rack over a pan.

When eating out:

Find out how foods are prepared; make special requests if necessary.

Ask for fish broiled with lemon juice or flavored broth.

Have sauces and gravies served on the side or not at all.

Use reduced-calorie or reduced-fat salad dressings.

Choose whole-grain bread or rolls and then ask for the basket to be removed; enjoy your selection without butter or margarine.

Order fresh fruit, sorbet or low-fat frozen yogurt for dessert.

CARBOHYDRATES: 50 TO 60 PERCENT OF DAILY CALORIC INTAKE

There are two categories of carbohydrates: simple and complex. Simple carbohydrates are found in granulated or brown sugar, honey and syrups, fruits and milk. Foods that have simple carbohydrates and no other nutritional value are found on the Optional Calories Food List. Complex carbohydrates include breads, starchy vegetables, whole grains, cereals, pastas, dried beans (legumes) and vegetables. In addition to providing energy, complex carbohydrates are the major source of dietary fiber in the diet, adding bulk for a feeling of fullness and playing a part in the prevention of certain diseases.

SODIUM: UP TO 3,000 MG A DAY FOR HEALTHY INDIVIDUALS

Sodium's main function is to regulate the amount of fluid in the body, which helps maintain blood pressure. It is also necessary for muscle contraction, nerve impulses, transporting nutrients and maintaining cells. Only a small amount of sodium is required by the body to function and most people consume more than they need, generally in the form of processed food. One teaspoon of salt contains 2,300 mg of sodium, nearly the entire recommended limit for a day! And, since sodium controls your fluid balance, consuming too much may cause bloating and temporary weight gain due to water retention.

Tips for Lowering Your Sodium Consumption

When shopping:

Check ingredients for words like salt, sodium, soda and soy sauce; if any of these words appears as one of the first three ingredients, the product is probably high in sodium. For example, monosodium glutamate is a common food additive that contains a large amount of salt.

Make *fresh* fruits, vegetables and dried beans your first choice. If unavailable, look for low-sodium, low-in-salt, no-salt-added canned or frozen foods. When buying frozen vegetables, pick plain instead of sauced varieties.

Seek out unsalted snacks like popcorn, pretzels, crackers or chips or season your snacks with herbs and spices.

When cooking:

Do not add salt to cooking water, such as for grains and pastas, even if directions indicate that you should.

Experiment with reducing or eliminating the salt in recipes; in most cases you can cut back gradually until you don't even notice that the salt is gone.

Season foods with herbs, spices, fresh lemon and lime juice, butter-flavored granules, vinegar and low-sodium varieties of soy sauce, Worcestershire sauce and mustard.

For fish: try parsley, dillweed, dry mustard, lemon pepper or paprika.

For poultry: try oregano, tarragon, garlic powder, thyme or sage.

For meat and game: try onion, garlic, rosemary or pepper.

For vegetables and grains: try basil, lemon, thyme or chives.

When eating out:

Ask for your food to be prepared without salt or, especially in a Chinese restaurant, without monosodium glutamate (MSG).

Have sauces served on the side or not at all.

Instead of prepared soups or appetizers, start with a tossed salad dressed with a lemon wedge or balsamic vinegar or bring your own dressing.

CHOLESTEROL: LIMIT TO 300 MILLIGRAMS PER DAY

Cholesterol is a fat-like substance that is an essential part of all living cells. It is used by your body to manufacture cell membranes, make vitamin D and some hormones and produce digestive juices. Your body obtains cholesterol from two sources: the liver, which produces serum (blood) cholesterol; and foods of animal origin, such as meat, poultry, fish, shellfish, organ meats, egg yolks and dairy products, known as dietary cholesterol. Plant foods such as fruits, vegetables, grains, nuts, dried beans and peas and vegetable oils do not contain cholesterol.

However, some saturated fats, found in both animal and plant foods, are the main culprits in elevating blood-cholesterol levels. These fats, while found primarily in beef, pork, lamb and whole-milk dairy products, are also found in shortenings, coconut oil, cocoa butter, and palm and palm-kernel oils. Known as "tropical oils," these fats are often ingredients in cookies, crackers and snack foods, so read those labels carefully!

SAMPLE LIST OF CHOLESTEROL CONTENT OF COMMON FOODS

Food	Amount	MG Cholesterol
Apple	1 small	0
Bread	1 ounce	0
Lettuce	½ cup	0
Margarine	1 teaspoon	0
Pasta	½ cup*	0
Peanuts	½ ounce	0
Mayonnaise	1 teaspoon	3
Skim milk	1 cup	4
Butter	1 teaspoon	15
Lobster	1 ounce*	21
Flounder	1 ounce*	23
Chicken, skinless	1 ounce*	24
Beef, lean	1 ounce*	25
Pork, lean	1 ounce*	26
Beef hot dog	2 ounces	29
Cheddar cheese	1 ounce	30
Vanilla ice cream	½ cup	30
Whole milk	1 cup	33
Shrimp	1 ounce*	55
Beef liver	1 ounce*	136
Egg	1 large	213

*cooked portion

DIETARY FIBER

The good news is that fiber (grandma called it roughage) in and of itself has no calories. The bad news is that most people don't get enough of it. Found only in plant foods, fiber is the nondigestible part of carbohydrates and comes in two parts.

Soluble fiber slows down the absorption of food in the stomach, creating a feeling of fullness. It is also associated with reducing blood cholesterol and maintaining stable blood sugar levels. The best sources of soluble fiber are oats, dried beans, lentils, peas, fresh fruits and vegetables. Introduce these foods to your diet gradually over a period of several weeks so that your digestive tract can become comfortable with the changes that will occur.

Insoluble fiber speeds the movement of food through the stomach and is associated with reducing the risk of some forms of cancer. The best sources of insoluble fiber are whole-grain breads, dried beans, cereals, pasta and brown rice.

WATER

You may not think of water as an indispensable nutrient, but without drinking water, humans can survive only a few days. Water is the most abundant substance in the body and performs many functions, including regulating body temperature, assisting in the digestive process and transporting nutrients and waste products to and from body cells.

Your body loses water every minute and needs daily replenishing. Weight Watchers recommends drinking six to eight 8-ounce glasses of water every day. For people exercising for a long time or in hot climates, this will also reduce the risk of dehydration.

Clear, cool tap water from a safe water supply is the easiest and least expensive way to fill up your glass. Bottled water, mineral water, sugar-free seltzer and club soda are other options (if you're watching your sodium, check the club soda label; it could have as much as 75 mg of sodium in 12 ounces). You may also drink up to half the recommended daily amount as milk, juice or caffeine-free diet soda (be sure to count the milk and juice as part of your Daily Totals). Caffeinated beverages are not good substitutes for water since they act as diuretics, causing you to lose more water than you would naturally.

VITAMINS

Vitamins are natural organic substances (from both plant and animal sources) required by the body in small amounts. Thirteen vitamins are essential for normal body growth and maintenance. These are categorized as *fat soluble* or *water soluble*. The fat-soluble vitamins, A, D, E and K, are able to be stored by the body. The water-solubles, C and eight B vitamins, cannot be readily stored, so they must be consumed more frequently. The following chart will help you to understand the function of these vitamins and highlight good food sources for them.

◆ **Vitamin A:** Maintains healthy skin, hair and gums; prevents night blindness; as precursor Vitamin A, beta carotene may help prevent some types of cancer.
Found in: Carrots, dark green leafy vegetables, tomatoes, pumpkins, apricots, cantaloupes, mangoes, sweet potatoes, milk and liver

◆ **B Vitamins:** Convert food to energy; promote normal digestion; aid in appetite and nerve function.
Found in: Meat, liver, poultry and fish; dried beans, lentils and peas; cheese; milk and yogurt; grains and enriched breads and cereals

◆ **Vitamin C:** Helps resist infection; heals wounds; maintains healthy gums.
Found in: Oranges, strawberries, grapefruits, papayas, tangerines; broccoli, bell peppers, tomatoes, dark green leafy vegetables; white and sweet potatoes

◆ **Vitamin D:** Maintains bones.
Found in: Fortified milk, fortified margarine and eggs

◆ **Vitamin E:** Defends the body against potentially harmful oxidations.
Found in: Vegetable oils and margarines; wheat germ; nuts; green leafy vegetables

◆ **Vitamin K:** Aids in the formation of proteins that regulate blood clotting.
Found in: Green leafy vegetables

MINERALS

Minerals are inorganic substances derived from nonliving sources. There are many essential minerals. A few key minerals include the macrominerals calcium, potassium and sodium, which the body needs in relatively large amounts. Trace minerals include iron, zinc and iodine. Although your body needs only small amounts of trace minerals, they do perform important functions, and one of the reasons that Weight Watchers recommends eating a wide variety of foods is to ensure getting these trace minerals. (The roles and food sources for the macromineral sodium begin on page 29.)

CALCIUM

The essential nutrient for building strong teeth and healthy bones, calcium also aids in normal blood clotting and muscle contraction (including the heart muscle). Adequate calcium intake is considered vital in the prevention of osteoporosis.

Found in: Milk, buttermilk, yogurt; hard, semisoft and soft cheese; firm tofu with calcium added; canned salmon with bones, sardines; dried beans, lentils and peas; oysters, shrimp; dark green leafy vegetables, broccoli

POTASSIUM

Contributes to the transmission of nerve impulses, muscle contraction and the maintenance of normal blood pressure.

Found in: Fruits, vegetables, fresh meat and milk

TRACE MINERALS

◆ **Iron:** Aids in the formation of blood cells. Absorption of iron can be enhanced by including a food high in Vitamin C at the same meal.
Found in: Beef, poultry, fish, dried beans, lentils, peas, tofu, eggs, organ meats and liver, dark leafy vegetables, asparagus, artichokes, broccoli, whole-grain and enriched bread, iron-fortified cereals, dried fruits (apricots, dates, figs, prunes, raisins)

◆ **Zinc:** Aids in achievement of normal body height, the maturation of sex glands, normal hair and nail growth and wound healing. Also helps maintain a healthy immune system.
Found in: Seafood (especially oysters), meat, milk, cheese, eggs, wheat germ

◆ **Iodine:** Helps regulate metabolism, prevent goiter
Found in: Seafoods and seaweed, yeast breads, dairy products, iodized salt

Vegetable Saté (page 43)

CHAPTER THREE

APPETIZERS

BRAISED STUFFED ARTICHOKES

Artichokes are a wonderful first course; they're pretty, taste great and take a long time to eat! This recipe is especially savory, using your own homemade seasoned croutons.

MAKES 4 SERVINGS

4 medium artichokes (about 12 ounces each)
2 ounces Croutons (see page 357)
2 cups chicken broth
$\frac{1}{3}$ cup + 2 teaspoons fresh lemon juice
$\frac{1}{4}$ cup chopped fresh parsley
2 garlic cloves, minced

1. With large stainless-steel knife, cut off stem end of each artichoke flush with base so that artichokes will stand upright; remove and discard center leaves and choke. With scissors, trim 1" from the top of each leaf. In food processor or blender, grind croutons into coarse crumbs.

2. Preheat oven to 400°F.

3. In medium bowl, combine crouton crumbs, $\frac{1}{2}$ cup of the broth, 2 tablespoons of the juice, the parsley and garlic; stir to mix well. Spoon one-fourth of the bread mixture into the heart of each artichoke.

4. In large nonstick skillet, combine the remaining $1\frac{1}{2}$ cups broth and the remaining $\frac{1}{4}$ cup juice; bring to a simmer and remove from heat. Arrange stuffed artichokes upright in skillet; cover with foil. Bake 40–45 minutes, or until artichokes are tender.

5. To serve, spoon pan juices evenly over each artichoke.

EACH SERVING PROVIDES: 1 Vegetable, $\frac{1}{2}$ Bread, 10 Optional Calories
PER SERVING: 128 Calories, 7 g Protein, 1 g Fat, 25 g Carbohydrate, 700 mg Sodium, 0 mg Cholesterol, 8 g Dietary Fiber

ASPARAGUS WITH SHERRY-WINE VINAIGRETTE

MAKES 4 SERVINGS

3 cups diagonally sliced asparagus spears (2" pieces)
2 tablespoons sherry-wine vinegar
1 tablespoon + 1 teaspoon sesame oil
1 teaspoon granulated sugar
$\frac{1}{4}$ teaspoon salt
8 Boston lettuce leaves
2 tablespoons chopped fresh chives
2 teaspoons sesame seeds, toasted

1. In large pot of boiling water, cook asparagus 2 minutes; drain. Rinse under cold running water; drain well and dry with paper towels. Set aside.

2. In large bowl, whisk together vinegar, 1 tablespoon + 1 teaspoon water, the oil, sugar and salt; add cooked asparagus. Toss to mix well.

3. To serve, line 4 plates with 2 lettuce leaves each; top each with one-fourth of the asparagus mixture. Sprinkle each with one-fourth of the chives and sesame seeds.

EACH SERVING PROVIDES: 1 Fat, $1\frac{3}{4}$ Vegetables, 10 Optional Calories
PER SERVING: 77 Calories, 3 g Protein, 6 g Fat, 6 g Carbohydrate, 139 mg Sodium, 0 mg Cholesterol, 1 g Dietary Fiber

BAKED BEETS WITH SOUR CREAM

MAKES 4 SERVINGS

8 medium beets
$\frac{1}{4}$ cup plain nonfat yogurt
3 tablespoons light sour cream
3 tablespoons cider vinegar
1 tablespoon whole-grain prepared mustard
$\frac{1}{2}$ teaspoon salt
$\frac{1}{8}$ teaspoon ground allspice
2 small Granny Smith apples (about 4 ounces each), cored and diced
4 ounces cooked all-purpose potato, pared and diced
8 romaine lettuce leaves

1. Preheat oven to 425°F. Cut a 24" sheet of foil.

2. Thoroughly wash beets; cut stems and leaves 1" above beet crowns. Arrange beets on foil; securely seal ends to make a tight packet. Transfer packet to baking sheet. Bake 1½ hours, until beets are soft when pierced by a knife. Unwrap; let stand until cool enough to handle. Slip off skins; cut each beet into 8 wedges.

3. Meanwhile, in large bowl, combine yogurt, sour cream, vinegar, mustard, salt and allspice; stir in baked beets, apples and potato.

4. To serve, line 4 plates with 2 lettuce leaves each. Arrange one-fourth of the beet mixture on each plate.

EACH SERVING (about 1¼ cups) PROVIDES: ½ Fruit, 2½ Vegetables, ¼ Bread , 25 Optional Calories
PER SERVING: 141 Calories, 4 g Protein, 1 g Fat, 30 g Carbohydrate, 432 mg Sodium, 3 mg Cholesterol, 3 g Dietary Fiber

BROCCOLI WITH CAESAR DRESSING

This is adapted from the classic Caesar dressing, but without the oil and egg. Instead, tofu thinned with chicken broth serves as the base of the dressing. It is also good as a salad dressing for greens.

MAKES 4 SERVINGS

24 broccoli spears, trimmed
3 ounces soft tofu
$\frac{1}{4}$ cup chicken or vegetable broth
2 anchovy fillets
1 garlic clove
1 teaspoon Dijon-style mustard
1 teaspoon fresh lemon juice

1. In large pot of boiling water, cook broccoli just until tender, about 4 minutes; drain in colander. Rinse under cold running water 1 minute; drain well.

2. In food processor or blender, combine tofu, broth, anchovies, garlic, mustard and juice; purée until smooth.

3. To serve, on each of 4 plates arrange 6 broccoli spears; spoon one-fourth of the dressing on each plate.

EACH SERVING PROVIDES: 3 Vegetables, ¼ Protein, 5 Optional Calories
PER SERVING: 68 Calories, 7 g Protein, 2 g Fat, 10 g Carbohydrate, 220 mg Sodium, 1 mg Cholesterol, 5 g Dietary Fiber

SNOW PEAS WITH HONEY-GINGER DRESSING

MAKES 4 SERVINGS

3 cups snow peas, stem ends and strings removed
1 tablespoon + 2 teaspoons soy sauce
1 tablespoon + 2 teaspoons honey
1 tablespoon + 1 teaspoon grated fresh ginger root
2 teaspoons peanut oil
1½ teaspoons Dijon-style mustard
1¼ teaspoons rice-wine vinegar
½ cup julienned radishes
2½ cups alfalfa sprouts

1. In large pot of boiling water, cook snow peas 1 minute; drain. Rinse under cold running water; drain thoroughly and dry.

2. In medium bowl, whisk soy sauce, honey, ginger, 1 tablespoon water, oil, mustard and vinegar; add snow peas and radishes. Toss gently to mix well. Refrigerate, covered with plastic wrap, 1 hour.

3. To serve, on each of 4 plates, arrange one-fourth of the sprouts; spoon one-fourth of the snow pea mixture over sprouts.

EACH SERVING PROVIDES: ½ Fat, 3 Vegetables, 25 Optional Calories
PER SERVING: 108 Calories, 4 g Protein, 3 g Fat, 18 g Carbohydrate, 496 mg Sodium, 0 mg Cholesterol, 4 g Dietary Fiber

RED ONION PIZZAS

An Italian favorite with a Greek accent, these little pizzas are built on pita crusts with tangy toppings.

MAKES 4 SERVINGS

2 teaspoons olive oil
3 cups thinly sliced red onions
2 teaspoons red wine vinegar
1 teaspoon julienned orange zest
1 cup thinly sliced zucchini
4 small pitas (1 ounce each)
3 ounces crumbled feta cheese
1 tablespoon + 1 teaspoon chopped fresh cilantro

1. In large nonstick skillet, heat 1 teaspoon of the oil and ¼ cup water; add onions. Cook over low heat, covered, 30 minutes. Stir in vinegar and orange zest; cook, uncovered, 10 minutes, or until all liquid is absorbed.

2. Preheat oven to 400°F. Spray baking sheet with nonstick cooking spray.

3. In small bowl, combine zucchini, 1 tablespoon water and the remaining teaspoon of oil; toss to coat.

4. Arrange pitas on prepared baking sheet; top each with one-fourth of the zucchini slices and bake 8 minutes. Spoon one-fourth of the cooked onions on each pita; bake 6 minutes. Sprinkle each pita with one-fourth of the feta cheese and cilantro; bake 2 minutes.

EACH SERVING (1 pizza) PROVIDES: ½ Fat, 2 Vegetables, 1 Protein, 1 Bread
PER SERVING: 210 Calories, 8 g Protein, 8 g Fat, 29 g Carbohydrate, 403 mg Sodium, 19 mg Cholesterol, 3 g Dietary Fiber

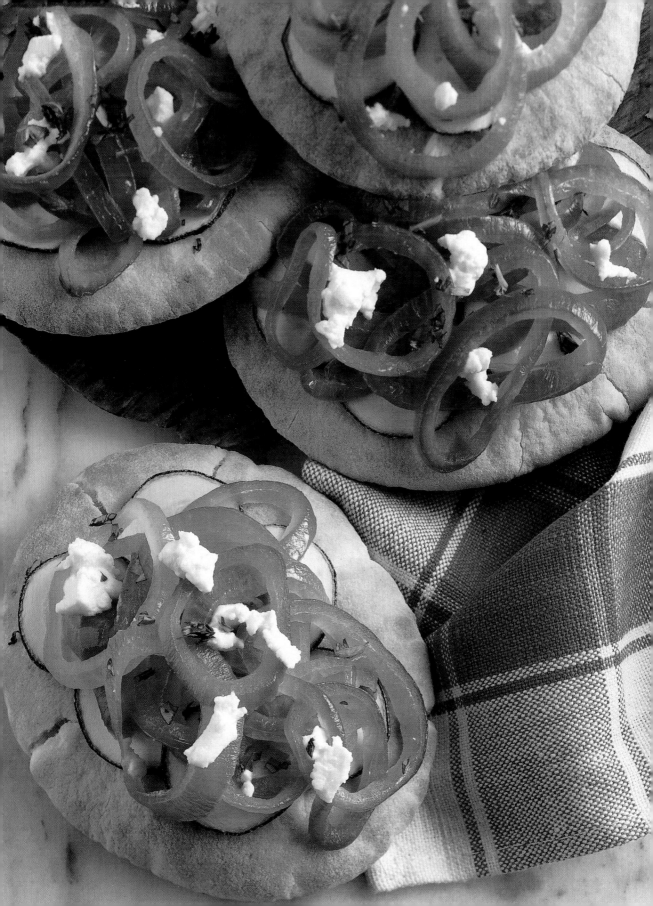

GREEN BEANS IN TOMATO VINAIGRETTE

MAKES 4 SERVINGS

$3\frac{1}{4}$ cups cut green beans (2" pieces)
1 teaspoon olive oil
3 garlic cloves, minced
$\frac{1}{2}$ cup chicken or vegetable broth
$\frac{1}{2}$ cup canned crushed tomatoes
$\frac{1}{4}$ cup mixed vegetable juice
1 tablespoon red wine vinegar
1 teaspoon minced fresh oregano, or $\frac{1}{2}$ teaspoon dried leaves
1 teaspoon minced fresh marjoram, or $\frac{1}{2}$ teaspoon dried leaves
$\frac{1}{2}$ teaspoon salt
$\frac{1}{4}$ teaspoon freshly ground black pepper
$\frac{1}{4}$ teaspoon granulated sugar

1. In large pot of boiling water, cook green beans 4 minutes, until tender-crisp; drain. Rinse under cold running water 1 minute; drain well. Set aside.

2. In large nonstick skillet, heat oil; add garlic. Cook over low heat, stirring frequently, 1 minute. Stir in broth, tomatoes, vegetable juice, vinegar, oregano, marjoram, salt, pepper and sugar; bring to a boil. Reduce heat to low; simmer 5 minutes.

3. Transfer tomato mixture to large bowl. Add green beans; toss to mix well. Marinate 1 hour at room temperature before serving.

EACH SERVING PROVIDES: $\frac{1}{4}$ Fat, 2 Vegetables, 5 Optional Calories
PER SERVING: 56 Calories, 3 g Protein, 1 g Fat, 10 g Carbohydrate, 507 mg Sodium, 0 mg Cholesterol, 2 g Dietary Fiber

LEEKS AND FENNEL IN ORANGE VINAIGRETTE

MAKES 4 SERVINGS

4 thoroughly washed medium leeks (white portion and some green)
2 cups thinly sliced fennel
3 garlic cloves
1 tablespoon + 1 teaspoon olive oil
$\frac{1}{4}$ teaspoon dried sage leaves
$\frac{1}{2}$ cup fresh orange juice
2 tablespoons balsamic vinegar
$\frac{1}{2}$ teaspoon granulated sugar
$\frac{1}{2}$ teaspoon salt

1. Preheat oven to 400°F. Cut a 24" sheet of foil.

2. Arrange leeks, fennel and garlic on half of the sheet of foil; sprinkle with 2 teaspoons of the oil and the sage. Fold the remaining foil over the vegetable mixture; securely seal ends to make a tight packet. Transfer packet to baking sheet; bake 15 minutes, turning once halfway through baking.

3. Meanwhile, in small skillet, cook orange juice over high heat until reduced to $\frac{1}{4}$ cup, about 5 minutes. Remove from heat; add remaining oil, vinegar, sugar and salt. Stir until sugar is dissolved.

4. Carefully transfer baked leek mixture from foil to shallow bowl, pouring any cooking juices over leeks. Pour reduced orange juice mixture over leeks; refrigerate, covered with plastic wrap, 3 hours, or until thoroughly chilled.

EACH SERVING PROVIDES: 1 Fat, $\frac{1}{4}$ Fruit, 2 Vegetables, 2 Optional Calories
PER SERVING: 101 Calories, 2 g Protein, 5 g Fat, 14 g Carbohydrate, 339 mg Sodium, 0 mg Cholesterol, 1 g Dietary Fiber

MUSHROOM TURNOVERS

MAKES 4 SERVINGS

1 teaspoon unsalted stick margarine
$\frac{1}{2}$ cup chicken or vegetable broth
3 tablespoons minced shallots
4 cups thinly sliced mushrooms
1 tablespoon dry sherry
$\frac{1}{2}$ teaspoon salt
$\frac{1}{8}$ teaspoon freshly ground black pepper
1 tablespoon all-purpose flour
$\frac{1}{4}$ cup skim milk
2 tablespoons light sour cream
1 tablespoon chopped fresh mint
4 ounces (about 6 sheets) thawed frozen phyllo
   dough (12 × 17" each)*

1. In large nonstick skillet, melt margarine over low heat; add $\frac{1}{4}$ cup of the broth and the shallots. Cook, stirring frequently, 4 minutes. Add mushrooms and the remaining $\frac{1}{4}$ cup broth; cook, covered, 5 minutes, or until mushrooms are tender and most of the liquid has evaporated. Add sherry; stir to combine. Sprinkle with salt and pepper; cook 1 minute.

2. Sprinkle flour over mushroom mixture; stir quickly to combine. Cook, stirring constantly, 1 minute; stir in milk. Simmer, stirring occasionally, 4–5 minutes. Remove from heat; stir in sour cream and mint. Set aside; let cool.

3. Preheat oven to 400°F. Spray nonstick baking sheet with nonstick cooking spray.

4. Spray clean work surface with nonstick cooking spray. Arrange 3 sheets of the phyllo dough side by side on prepared work surface. Layer 1 more sheet of phyllo dough on each of the 3 sheets, making 3 stacks of 2 sheets each. Cut each stack into 4 equal strips, $4\frac{1}{4}$ × 12" each. Spray surface of each strip with nonstick cooking spray.

5. Spoon $\frac{1}{12}$ of the mushroom mixture onto the narrow end of 1 strip; fold left corner of strip diagonally over filling, making a triangle. Fold triangle up, then to the right, keeping triangular shape. Continue folding, alternating from left to right, until entire strip is folded, ending with a triangle. Repeat procedure, with remaining mushroom mixture and phyllo dough strips, making 11 more turnovers.

6. Arrange turnovers on prepared baking sheet; bake 10–15 minutes, until golden. Serve immediately.

*Phyllo dough must be thawed in refrigerator for at least 8 hours.

EACH SERVING (3 turnovers) PROVIDES: $\frac{1}{4}$ Fat, 2 Vegetables, 1 Bread, 30 Optional Calories
PER SERVING: 152 Calories, 5 g Protein, 4 g Fat, 23 g Carbohydrate, 563 mg Sodium, 2 mg Cholesterol, 1 g Dietary Fiber

◆

HEARTS OF PALM WITH LEMON DRESSING

MAKES 4 SERVINGS

2 tablespoons fresh lemon juice
1 tablespoon chopped fresh dill
2 teaspoons olive oil
1 garlic clove, minced
$\frac{1}{8}$ teaspoon granulated sugar
One 14-ounce can drained hearts of palm, rinsed,
   dried and cut into 1" rounds (about 2 cups)

In medium bowl, whisk lemon juice, dill, oil, garlic and sugar; add hearts of palm and toss to mix well.

EACH SERVING PROVIDES: $\frac{1}{2}$ Fat, 1 Vegetable
PER SERVING: 42 Calories, 2 g Protein, 2 g Fat, 5 g Carbohydrate, 1 mg Sodium, 0 mg Cholesterol, 0 g Dietary Fiber

CHEESE-STUFFED CELERY

MAKES 4 SERVINGS

4 medium celery stalks (about 6" each), cut
   diagonally into thirds
²⁄₃ cup low-fat cottage cheese
¼ cup firmly packed fresh basil leaves
2 garlic cloves
⅛ teaspoon salt

1. With paring knife, slice a thin sliver off the
curved side of each celery stalk so that it lays flat.
In small bowl, cover celery with ice water; soak 30
minutes. Drain; dry well.

2. In mini food processor or blender, combine cottage cheese, basil, garlic and salt; purée 1
minute, until smooth and creamy. Fill each celery
stalk with one-fourth of the cheese mixture.

3. To serve, on each of four serving plates,
arrange three filled celery stalks.

EACH SERVING (3 pieces) PROVIDES: ½ Vegetable, ½ Protein
PER SERVING: 38 Calories, 5 g Protein, 0 g Fat, 4 g Carbohydrate,
250 mg Sodium, 2 mg Cholesterol, 0 g Dietary Fiber

MUSHROOM STEW

*An especially hearty dish, in which the mushrooms add
a meaty flavor.*

MAKES 4 SERVINGS

2 teaspoons olive oil
4 garlic cloves, minced
2 cups sliced shiitake or white button mushrooms
²⁄₃ cup chicken or vegetable broth
2 cups sliced mushrooms
¼ cup canned crushed tomatoes
¼ teaspoon dried marjoram leaves
¼ teaspoon salt
⅛ teaspoon freshly ground black pepper
2 tablespoons chopped fresh basil

1. In large nonstick skillet heat oil; add garlic.
Cook over medium heat, stirring frequently, 1
minute. Add shiitake mushrooms and broth;
cook, covered, 3 minutes. Stir in mushrooms;
cook, covered, 4 minutes, until mushrooms are
almost tender.

2. Stir in tomatoes, marjoram, salt and pepper; cook 4 minutes. Stir in basil and serve.

EACH SERVING PROVIDES: ½ Fat, 2 Vegetables, 5 Optional Calories
PER SERVING: 51 Calories, 2 g Protein, 3 g Fat, 5 g Carbohydrate,
328 mg Sodium, 0 mg Cholesterol, 1 g Dietary Fiber

Vegetable Appetizers

◆

*Vegetables are a great low-fat, low-calorie way to start a meal. Fresh and crisp or lightly steamed and spiced,
their brilliant colors and textures make them an appealing and nontraditional first course. In addition to
the recipes in this chapter, you might want to peruse the Vegetables and Salads chapter for other ideas.
Instead of pasta, try Spaghetti Squash (page 114); Broiled Eggplant (page 108) or Broiled Tomatoes (page
115) would be nice before grilled meat or seafood. Dilled Carrots (page 104) are a perfect starter for
steamed or poached fish, while Herb-Stuffed Artichokes (page 102) are a good choice to precede a roasted
chicken. Winter Greens with Balsamic Vinaigrette (page 122) marry well with a steaming bowl of soup,
and the slightly bitter edge of Chicory with Mustard and Caper Dressing (page 124) would nicely offset a
savory stew.*

SAVORY PUMPKIN PIE

Unlike the Thanksgiving version, herbs and cheese flavor this pumpkin filling in a crisp phyllo crust.

MAKES 4 SERVINGS

1 tablespoon + 1 teaspoon olive oil
1 garlic clove
½ teaspoon sage leaves
4 ounces (about 6 sheets) thawed frozen phyllo
    dough (12 × 17" each)*
1 cup canned pumpkin purée
¾ ounce grated Parmesan cheese
1 egg
1 egg white
¼ teaspoon salt
⅛ teaspoon freshly ground black pepper
⅛ teaspoon freshly grated nutmeg

1. Preheat oven to 400°F.

2. In small skillet heat oil; add garlic and sage. Cook over low heat, stirring frequently, until fragrant, about 4 minutes. Strain and discard solids.

3. To prepare crust, in bottom of a 9" pie plate, arrange phyllo dough, 1 sheet at a time, rotating sheets so they completely cover sides of the plate. Brush last sheet evenly with 2 teaspoons of the prepared garlic oil.

4. To prepare filling, in medium bowl, combine pumpkin, Parmesan cheese, egg, egg white, salt, pepper and nutmeg; stir to mix well. Spoon filling into prepared crust; brush top with the remaining 2 teaspoons garlic oil.

5. Bake 10 minutes; reduce heat to 350°F and continue to bake for 30 minutes or just until set. To serve, cut into 4 equal wedges.

*Phyllo dough must be thawed in the refrigerator for at least 8 hours or overnight.

EACH SERVING PROVIDES: 1 Fat, ½ Vegetable, ½ Protein, 1 Bread, 5 Optional Calories
PER SERVING: 194 Calories, 7 g Protein, 9 g Fat, 21 g Carbohydrate, 404 mg Sodium, 57 mg Cholesterol, 1 g Dietary Fiber

VEGETABLE SATÉ

An all-vegetable version of the Indonesian specialty that's become so popular. Serve this as a first course in the living room with drinks or pass the little skewers at your next party with sauce on the side.

MAKES 4 SERVINGS

1 medium zucchini, cut into 8 wedges
1 medium red bell pepper, cut into 8 wedges
1 small onion, cut into 8 wedges
2 teaspoons creamy peanut butter
2 teaspoons reduced-sodium soy sauce
2 teaspoons honey
¼ teaspoon lemon juice
1 clove garlic
⅛ teaspoon ground ginger

1. Onto each of eight small wooden skewers, thread 1 piece each of the zucchini, bell pepper and onion. Arrange threaded skewers in shallow baking dish; pour in enough water to cover vegetables; set aside for 30 minutes.

2. Preheat broiler. Line baking sheet with heavy-duty foil.

3. In mini food processor or blender, combine peanut butter, soy sauce, honey, lemon juice, garlic and ginger; purée until smooth. Add 2 tablespoons water; purée until well combined.

4. Arrange skewers on prepared baking sheet; broil 4" from source of heat, turning frequently, about 8 minutes, until vegetables are tender and lightly browned.

5. To serve, onto each of 4 plates spoon 1 tablespoon of the peanut sauce; arrange 2 skewers on each plate.

EACH SERVING (2 skewers) PROVIDES: ½ Fat, 1¼ Vegetables, 10 Optional Calories
PER SERVING: 46 Calories, 2 g Protein, 1 g Fat, 8 g Carbohydrate, 115 mg Sodium, 0 mg Cholesterol, 1 g Dietary Fiber

SAMOSAS

These vegetable-filled pastry pockets have their origins in the creative vegetarian cooking of India. They also make a nice supper with a bowl of soup.

MAKES 4 SERVINGS

1 cup minus 1 tablespoon all-purpose flour
2 teaspoons granulated sugar
$\frac{1}{2}$ teaspoon salt
$\frac{1}{4}$ teaspoon paprika
2 tablespoons + 2 teaspoons margarine, chilled
    and cut up
3 tablespoons low-fat cottage cheese
3 tablespoons plain nonfat yogurt
$\frac{1}{2}$ cup chicken broth
2 tablespoons thinly sliced scallions
$\frac{1}{4}$ teaspoon curry powder
1 cup coarsely chopped cauliflower florets
$\frac{1}{4}$ cup thawed frozen peas
2 ounces cooked new potatoes, pared and coarsely
    chopped

1. In large bowl, combine $\frac{3}{4}$ cup of the flour, the sugar, $\frac{1}{4}$ teaspoon of the salt and the paprika. With pastry blender or 2 knives, cut in margarine until mixture resembles coarse crumbs. Add cottage cheese and yogurt; stir until mixture forms soft ball. Gather dough into a ball; wrap in plastic wrap. Refrigerate several hours or overnight.

2. In large nonstick skillet, combine broth, scallions, the remaining $\frac{1}{4}$ teaspoon salt and the curry; cook over medium heat 2 minutes. Add cauliflower; cook, covered, 2 minutes. Stir in peas and potatoes; cook, covered, 3 minutes, or until cauliflower is tender. Let cool to room temperature.

3. Preheat oven to 400°F. Spray baking sheet with nonstick cooking spray.

4. Sprinkle clean work surface with the remaining 3 tablespoons of flour; roll dough into a 12" circle. With a 4" biscuit cutter, cut out 4 circles. Reroll scraps of dough; continue cutting until all dough has been used, making a total of 8 circles.

5. Spoon about $\frac{1}{4}$ cup filling onto bottom half of each round, leaving a $\frac{1}{4}$" border. With a pastry brush, moisten bottom half of the border

with water; fold top half of circle over filling to enclose. With fingers or tines of a fork, press edges together to seal.

6. Arrange samosas on prepared baking sheet; bake 20 minutes, or until crisp and golden brown. Serve immediately.

EACH SERVING (2 samosas) PROVIDES: 2 Fats, $\frac{1}{2}$ Vegetable, $1\frac{1}{2}$ Breads, 30 Optional Calories
PER SERVING: 227 Calories, 7 g Protein, 9 g Fat, 31 g Carbohydrate, 553 mg Sodium, 1 mg Cholesterol, 2 g Dietary Fiber

◆

FRESH TOMATO MINI PIZZAS

MAKES 4 SERVINGS

2 large plum tomatoes, thinly sliced lengthwise
    (reserve juices)
$\frac{1}{4}$ teaspoon salt
2 tablespoons + 1 teaspoon chopped fresh basil
2 garlic cloves, minced
2 teaspoons olive oil
4 small pitas (1 ounce each)
$1\frac{1}{2}$ ounces shredded reduced-fat mozzarella cheese

1. Preheat oven to 400°F. Spray baking sheet with nonstick cooking spray.

2. In small bowl, combine tomatoes and salt; toss to mix well. Stir in basil, garlic and oil; set aside.

3. Arrange pitas on prepared baking sheet. Arrange one-fourth of the tomato mixture on each pita; spoon one-fourth of the reserved tomato juices on each. Bake 8 minutes, or until the tomatoes are hot and softened.

4. Sprinkle each pizza with one-fourth of the cheese; bake 3 minutes, or until cheese is bubbly.

EACH SERVING PROVIDES: $\frac{1}{2}$ Fat, $\frac{1}{2}$ Vegetable, $\frac{1}{2}$ Protein, 1 Bread
PER SERVING: 131 Calories, 6 g Protein, 4 g Fat, 18 g Carbohydrate, 346 mg Sodium, 4 mg Cholesterol, 1 g Dietary Fiber

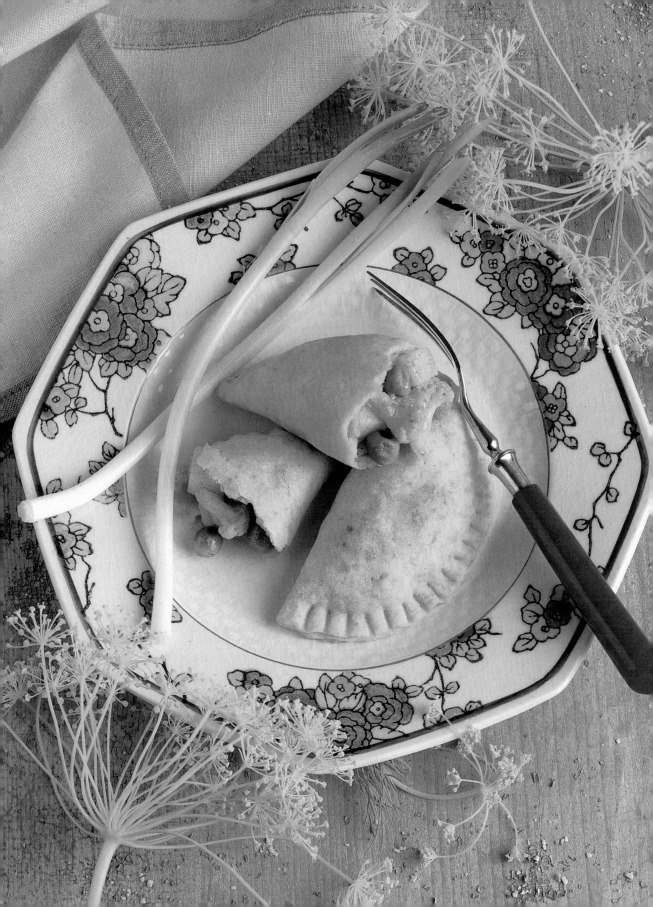

Dolmas

Dolmas can be served chilled or at room temperature.

Makes 4 Servings

1 teaspoon olive oil
$\frac{1}{4}$ cup minced carrot
1 garlic clove, minced
$\frac{1}{4}$ cup thinly sliced scallions
$1\frac{1}{4}$ cups chicken broth
2 ounces regular long-grain rice
3 tablespoons chopped fresh dill
$\frac{1}{4}$ teaspoon grated lemon zest
2 tablespoons fresh lemon juice
12 bottled large grape leaves, drained, soaked and
    rinsed several times
8 large dill sprigs
$\frac{1}{4}$ cup plain nonfat yogurt

1. In medium saucepan heat oil; add carrot and garlic. Cook over low heat, stirring frequently, 4 minutes. Stir in scallions and $\frac{1}{4}$ cup of the broth. Cook, stirring occasionally, until most of the liquid has evaporated, about 5 minutes. Stir in remaining 1 cup chicken broth, the rice, dill, zest and juice. Cook, covered, about 17 minutes, until rice is tender.

2. On clean work surface, arrange 12 grape leaves in a single layer. Spoon equal amounts of the rice mixture onto stem end of each leaf; fold stem end over, then fold sides of leaves over filling to enclose. From stem end, roll leaves, jelly-roll style.

3. In large skillet, arrange dolmas, seam-side down. Place 4 dill sprigs over dolmas.

4. Pour $\frac{1}{2}$ cup water into skillet; bring to a boil. Reduce heat to low; simmer, covered, 30 minutes. Let cool to room temperature.

5. To serve, on each of 4 plates arrange 3 dolmas and 1 tablespoon yogurt; garnish each with a dill sprig.

EACH SERVING (3 dolmas) PROVIDES: $\frac{1}{4}$ Fat, $\frac{1}{2}$ Vegetable, $\frac{1}{2}$ Bread, 15 Optional Calories
PER SERVING: 94 Calories, 4 g Protein, 2 g Fat, 16 g Carbohydrate, 329 mg Sodium, 0 mg Cholesterol, 1 g Dietary Fiber

Polenta and Bean Cakes

Makes 4 Servings

3 ounces uncooked yellow cornmeal
$\frac{3}{4}$ teaspoon salt
4 ounces cooked red beans
2 tablespoons thinly sliced scallions
1 tablespoon chopped fresh cilantro
1 tablespoon tomato paste
2 teaspoons fresh lime juice
$\frac{1}{4}$ teaspoon ground coriander
$\frac{1}{4}$ teaspoon ground cumin
$1\frac{1}{2}$ ounces reduced-fat mozzarella cheese,
    shredded

1. In medium bowl, combine cornmeal and 1 cup water; stir to mix well.

2. In medium saucepan, bring $\frac{2}{3}$ cup water to a boil; stir in cornmeal mixture and $\frac{1}{2}$ teaspoon of the salt. Reduce heat to low; simmer, stirring constantly, until thickened, about 10 minutes. Let stand until room temperature.

3. Meanwhile, in small bowl, with potato masher or back of a spoon, mash beans; stir in scallions, cilantro, tomato paste, juice, coriander, cumin and the remaining $\frac{1}{4}$ teaspoon salt.

4. Preheat oven to 400°F. Spray baking sheet with nonstick cooking spray.

5. Shape cornmeal mixture into 4 equal patties; arrange on prepared baking sheet. Bake 10 minutes. Spoon one-fourth of the bean mixture on each patty; bake 10 minutes. Sprinkle each patty with one-fourth of the cheese; bake 2 minutes longer.

EACH SERVING PROVIDES: $\frac{1}{2}$ Protein, $1\frac{1}{2}$ Breads
PER SERVING: 144 Calories, 7 g Protein, 2 g Fat, 25 g Carbohydrate, 502 mg Sodium, 4 mg Cholesterol, 2 g Dietary Fiber

ORIENTAL RICE CAKES

MAKES 4 SERVINGS

1/4 cup rice-wine vinegar
1 tablespoon + 2 teaspoons granulated sugar
1 teaspoon soy sauce
1 1/2 cups thinly sliced cucumbers
4 ounces uncooked short-grain rice
1/4 teaspoon salt
3 tablespoons minced carrot
3 tablespoons minced red bell pepper
2 tablespoons minced scallions
1 egg white
1 teaspoon peanut oil
1 teaspoon sesame oil

1. In small bowl, combine 2 tablespoons of the vinegar, 2 teaspoons of the sugar and the soy sauce; add cucumbers and toss to mix well. Refrigerate, covered with plastic wrap, at least 1 hour.

2. In medium saucepan, bring 1 1/2 cups water to a boil; stir in rice and salt and return to a boil. Reduce heat to low; cook 20 minutes, until rice is very soft and sticky. Set aside; keep warm.

3. In small saucepan, combine the remaining 2 tablespoons vinegar and the remaining 1 tablespoon sugar. Cook over low heat, stirring occasionally, about 1 minute, until sugar dissolves.

4. Pour vinegar mixture into cooked rice; stir to mix well. Stir in carrot, bell pepper and scallions; let cool to room temperature.

5. Add egg white to rice mixture; stir to mix well. Shape mixture into 8 equal patties, each about 1/2" thick.

6. In large nonstick skillet, heat 1/2 teaspoon of each oil; add 4 of the patties. Cook over medium-high heat about 3 minutes, turning once. Repeat procedure with the remaining 1/2 teaspoon of each oil and 4 patties.

7. To serve, on each of 4 plates spoon one-fourth of the cucumber mixture evenly; top each with 2 patties. Serve immediately.

EACH SERVING (2 cakes + cucumber mixture) PROVIDES: 1/2 Fat, 1 Vegetable, 1 Bread, 25 Optional Calories
PER SERVING: 158 Calories, 3 g Protein, 2 g Fat, 31 g Carbohydrate, 241 mg Sodium, 0 mg Cholesterol, 1 g Dietary Fiber

DEVILED EGGS

MAKES 4 SERVINGS

4 hard-cooked large eggs, cut lengthwise into halves
1 tablespoon finely chopped chutney
2 teaspoons reduced-calorie mayonnaise
1 teaspoon Dijon-style mustard
1/4 teaspoon ground red pepper
1/8 teaspoon salt

1. Remove yolks from egg halves; set whites aside.

2. In small bowl, with fork, mash egg yolks; stir in chutney, mayonnaise, mustard, red pepper and salt, mixing well.

3. Spoon yolk mixture evenly into each reserved egg white.

EACH SERVING (1 egg) PROVIDES: 1/4 Fat, 1 Protein, 10 Optional Calories
PER SERVING: 98 Calories, 6 g Protein, 6 g Fat, 4 g Carbohydrate, 226 mg Sodium, 213 mg Cholesterol, 0 g Dietary Fiber

POTATO-VEGETABLE PANCAKE

MAKES 4 SERVINGS

10 ounces shredded pared Idaho potatoes
3 ounces shredded pared parsnip
$\frac{1}{2}$ cup shredded pared carrot
1 egg
2 tablespoons all-purpose flour
$\frac{3}{4}$ teaspoon salt
$\frac{1}{4}$ teaspoon baking powder
2 teaspoons olive oil

1. In large bowl, combine potatoes, parsnip, carrot, egg, flour, salt and baking powder; stir to mix well.

2. In large nonstick skillet, heat oil until very hot; with spatula spread potato mixture into pan, flattening until even. Cook over medium-high heat 8 minutes, or until crisp, browned and set. Turn pancake; reduce heat to medium and cook 8 minutes, or until crisp, browned and cooked through.

3. To serve, cut pancake into quarters.

EACH SERVING PROVIDES: $\frac{1}{2}$ Fat, $\frac{1}{4}$ Vegetable, $\frac{1}{4}$ Protein, $\frac{3}{4}$ Bread, 15 Optional Calories
PER SERVING: 131 Calories, 4 g Protein, 4 g Fat, 21 g Carbohydrate, 469 mg Sodium, 53 mg Cholesterol, 3 g Dietary Fiber

SCALLION PANCAKES

A light version of an Oriental specialty, this is perfect for a cocktail party, served with a soy sauce–wine vinegar dipping sauce and garnished with minced scallions.

MAKES 4 SERVINGS

$\frac{3}{4}$ cup all-purpose flour
$\frac{3}{4}$ cup skim milk
1 large egg
$\frac{1}{2}$ teaspoon salt
$\frac{1}{4}$ teaspoon ground ginger
$\frac{1}{2}$ cup thinly sliced scallions
1 teaspoon baking powder
2 teaspoons sesame oil

1. In blender, combine flour, milk, egg, 2 tablespoons water, the salt and ginger; purée until smooth. Let stand 30 minutes at room temperature. Add scallions and baking powder; stir to mix well.

2. In large nonstick skillet or on griddle, heat $\frac{1}{2}$ teaspoon of the oil over medium-high heat; pour batter by tablespoons into skillet, making 4 pancakes. Cook 1 minute, or until bubbles appear on surface; turn and cook 20 seconds longer.

3. With spatula, remove pancakes to plate; keep warm. Repeat procedure with the remaining $1\frac{1}{2}$ teaspoons oil and the remaining batter, making 12 more pancakes.

EACH SERVING (4 pancakes) PROVIDES: $\frac{1}{2}$ Fat, $\frac{1}{4}$ Vegetable, $\frac{1}{4}$ Protein, 1 Bread, 15 Optional Calories
PER SERVING: 145 Calories, 6 g Protein, 4 g Fat, 22 g Carbohydrate, 438 mg Sodium, 54 mg Cholesterol, 1 g Dietary Fiber

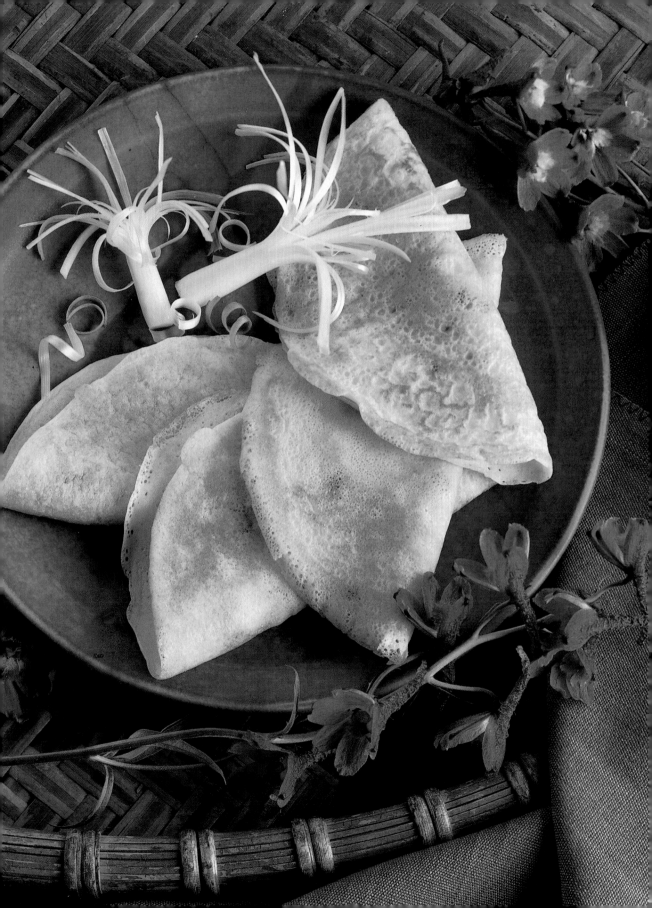

CHICK-PEA AND SPINACH PATTIES

These savory little patties get their flavorings from Middle Eastern cuisine. They're also good at room temperature, so you can take them along for an easy lunch.

MAKES 4 SERVINGS

1 cup packed spinach leaves
12 ounces drained cooked chick-peas
$\frac{1}{4}$ cup + 2 tablespoons plain dried bread crumbs
1 egg
1 tablespoon fresh lemon juice
1 garlic clove, crushed
$\frac{1}{4}$ teaspoon salt
$\frac{1}{4}$ teaspoon ground cumin
1 tablespoon + 1 teaspoon olive oil
$\frac{1}{4}$ cup plain nonfat yogurt
4 lemon wedges to garnish (optional)

1. Thoroughly wash spinach leaves; drain on paper towels.

2. In food processor, combine washed spinach, chick-peas, 3 tablespoons of the bread crumbs, the egg, juice, garlic, salt and cumin; purée until smooth.

3. Shape spinach mixture into 8 equal patties. Gently dip patties in the remaining 3 tablespoons bread crumbs, coating both sides of each.

4. In large nonstick skillet, heat 2 teaspoons of the oil; add 4 of the patties. Cook over medium heat, 1 minute on each side, or until browned and crisp. Repeat procedure with the remaining 2 teaspoons oil and 4 patties.

5. To serve, on each of 4 plates, arrange 2 cooked patties; spoon 1 tablespoon yogurt on each plate. Top with lemon wedge.

EACH SERVING (2 patties) PROVIDES: 1 Fat, $\frac{1}{2}$ Vegetable, $\frac{1}{4}$ Protein, 2 Breads, 10 Optional Calories
PER SERVING: 252 Calories, 12 g Protein, 9 g Fat, 33 g Carbohydrate, 270 mg Sodium, 53 mg Cholesterol, 4 g Dietary Fiber

CHICK-PEA SPREAD

Serve with warm pitas.

MAKES 8 SERVINGS

12 ounces drained cooked chick-peas
$\frac{1}{2}$ cup plain nonfat yogurt
2 tablespoons fresh lemon juice
3 garlic cloves
2 teaspoons olive oil
$\frac{1}{2}$ teaspoon salt
$\frac{1}{2}$ teaspoon ground cumin
$\frac{1}{8}$ teaspoon ground allspice

In food processor or blender, combine chick-peas, yogurt, juice, garlic, olive oil, salt, cumin and allspice with 1 tablespoon water; purée until smooth.

EACH SERVING (2 tablespoons) PROVIDES: $\frac{1}{4}$ Fat, $\frac{3}{4}$ Protein, 10 Optional Calories
PER SERVING: 91 Calories, 5 g Protein, 2 g Fat, 13 g Carbohydrate, 151 mg Sodium, 0 mg Cholesterol, 1 g Dietary Fiber

---

Great Grilling

◆

Looking for a flexible summer appetizer? Get out your grills! Have fun finding the freshest, prettiest vegetables, then making small skewers of mixed vegetables for the grill. Below you'll find some pointers to help you get started.

- *If you're serving a large group, use several small grills, and let friends and family grill their own skewers of vegetables.*
- *Start your fire early enough that cooking can begin as soon as people arrive.*
- *Prepare vegetables in advance, and have them all ready on skewers.*
- *Leftover grilled vegetables? Add them to sandwiches or soups, or mix into pasta or grain salads.*

Guacamole

A little avocado goes a long way, boosted by spinach, buttermilk and the classic guacamole seasonings.

Makes 4 Servings

4 small pitas (1 ounce each), cut into halves
   horizontally
2 cups packed spinach leaves
¼ cup low-fat (1.5%) buttermilk
¼ cup finely chopped red onion
1 tablespoon drained canned chopped green chilies
1 teaspoon fresh lime juice
¼ medium avocado (about 2 ounces), pared and
   sliced
¼ cup chopped plum tomato
¼ cup chopped fresh cilantro

1. Preheat oven to 400°F. Cut each pita half into 4 equal pieces; arrange on baking sheet. Bake 4–5 minutes, or until crisp; set aside.

2. Thoroughly wash spinach leaves. In pot of boiling water, cook spinach 1 minute; drain well and squeeze dry.

3. In food processor, combine spinach, buttermilk, 2 tablespoons of the onion, the chilies and juice; purée until spinach is finely chopped and mixture is well combined (do not over-process).

4. In medium bowl, with potato masher or the back of a spoon, mash avocado. Stir in puréed spinach mixture, tomato, cilantro and remaining onion. Serve with pita chips.

EACH SERVING PROVIDES: ½ Fat, 1¼ Vegetables, 1 Bread,
5 Optional Calories
PER SERVING: 124 Calories, 5 g Protein, 3 g Fat, 20 g Carbohydrate, 212 mg Sodium, 1 mg Cholesterol, 2 g Dietary Fiber

Baba Ghanouj

Makes 4 Servings

1 medium eggplant (about 1 pound)
3 tablespoons chopped fresh cilantro
3 tablespoons plain nonfat yogurt
1 tablespoon + 1 teaspoon fresh lemon juice
1 garlic clove
1 teaspoon paprika
¾ teaspoon ground coriander
¾ teaspoon salt
4 small pitas (1 ounce each)
24 carrot sticks (3 ½" sticks)

1. Preheat oven to 425°F. Line baking sheet with heavy-duty foil; spray with nonstick cooking spray.

2. With knife, pierce eggplant several times; place on prepared baking sheet. Bake 45 minutes, turning once or twice, until soft and skin is charred; let stand until cool enough to handle. Remove and discard skin.

3. In food processor or blender, combine baked eggplant, cilantro, yogurt, juice, garlic, paprika, ground coriander and salt; purée until smooth.

4. To serve, onto each of 4 plates, arrange ⅓ cup baba ghanouj, 1 pita and 6 carrot sticks.

EACH SERVING (⅓ cup Baba Ghanouj, pita and carrot sticks) PROVIDES:
2½ Vegetables, 1 Bread, 5 Optional Calories
PER SERVING: 138 Calories, 5 g Protein, 1 g Fat, 29 g Carbohydrate, 595 mg Sodium, 0 mg Cholesterol, 4 g Dietary Fiber

MOROCCAN RED BEAN DIP

The fruit and warm spices typical of Moroccan cuisine give this dip a marvelous, mysterious flavor. Serve it with crisp vegetable slices or toasted pita wedges.

MAKES 4 SERVINGS

1 teaspoon olive oil
$\frac{1}{4}$ cup chopped red onion
1 garlic clove, finely chopped
$\frac{1}{4}$ cup chopped tomato
1 tablespoon golden raisins
3 dried apricot halves, chopped
1 tablespoon orange juice
8 ounces drained cooked kidney beans
$\frac{1}{4}$ teaspoon ground cumin
$\frac{1}{8}$ teaspoon cinnamon
$\frac{1}{8}$ teaspoon ground cloves
$\frac{1}{8}$ teaspoon curry powder
$\frac{1}{8}$ teaspoon chili powder
$\frac{1}{8}$ teaspoon salt

1. In medium nonstick skillet, heat oil; add onion and garlic. Sauté over medium-high heat, stirring frequently, 2–3 minutes, until just softened. Reduce heat to low; cook covered, 2 minutes. Add tomato, raisins, apricots and juice; stir to combine. Cook, covered, 2 minutes.

2. Add beans, cumin, cinnamon, cloves, curry powder, chili powder and salt; stir to mix well. Remove from heat; let cool slightly. In food processor or blender, purée mixture until smooth. Refrigerate, covered, until ready to serve.

EACH SERVING PROVIDES: $\frac{1}{4}$ Fat, $\frac{1}{4}$ Fruit, $\frac{1}{4}$ Vegetable, 1 Bread, 2 Optional Calories
PER SERVING: 106 Calories, 5 g Protein, 2 g Fat, 19 g Carbohydrate, 74 mg Sodium, 0 mg Cholesterol, 3 g Dietary Fiber

SPICED RED BEAN DIP

MAKES 4 SERVINGS

1 teaspoon olive oil
$\frac{1}{3}$ cup finely chopped onion
8 ounces drained cooked red beans
2 teaspoons fresh lime juice
$\frac{1}{2}$ teaspoon dried oregano leaves
$\frac{1}{4}$ teaspoon salt
$\frac{1}{4}$ teaspoon hot red pepper sauce, or to taste
$\frac{1}{2}$ ounce coarsely chopped pecans
2 tablespoons finely chopped parsley

1. In small nonstick skillet, heat $\frac{1}{4}$ cup water and the oil; add onion. Cook over low heat, stirring occasionally, 5–7 minutes, or until soft.

2. In food processor, combine beans, $\frac{1}{4}$ cup water, juice, oregano, salt and red pepper sauce; purée until smooth. Add cooked onion, pecans and parsley; pulse just until combined.

EACH SERVING ($\frac{1}{4}$ cup) PROVIDES: $\frac{3}{4}$ Fat, 1 Bread
PER SERVING: 113 Calories, 5 g Protein, 4 g Fat, 15 g Carbohydrate, 145 mg Sodium, 0 mg Cholesterol, 3 g Dietary Fiber

HERBED YOGURT CHEESE

Your cheese of choice could well be this one you make yourself. Easy to prepare, it works equally well in savory or sweet variations. Try it with your favorite herb combination, spreadable fruit or a combination of nuts and seeds.

MAKES 4 SERVINGS

3 cups plain nonfat yogurt
8 unpeeled garlic cloves
$\frac{1}{2}$ teaspoon fresh lemon juice
1 tablespoon thinly sliced scallion
2 teaspoons chopped fresh oregano, or $\frac{3}{4}$ teaspoon dried leaves
$\frac{1}{4}$ teaspoon salt
2 cups thinly sliced kirby or European cucumber
4 scallions, made into brushes to garnish (optional)

1. To prepare yogurt cheese, spoon yogurt into a coffee filter or cheesecloth-lined sieve; place over bowl. Refrigerate, covered with plastic wrap, 24 hours. Discard liquid.

2. Preheat oven to 400°F. Cut a 12" sheet of foil.

3. Wrap garlic in foil; arrange on baking sheet. Bake 30 minutes, or until soft. Let stand until cool enough to handle; unwrap. Squeeze garlic from skins. In mini food processor, purée garlic with juice until smooth.

4. In medium bowl, combine yogurt cheese, puréed garlic, sliced scallion, oregano and salt; mix until well blended.

5. To serve, line each of 4 plates with $\frac{1}{4}$ cup of the cucumber slices. Line a $\frac{1}{3}$-cup dry measuring cup with plastic wrap; spoon yogurt cheese into cup. Unmold onto center of 1 cucumber-lined plate. Repeat procedure, mounding $\frac{1}{3}$ cup of the yogurt cheese onto the 3 remaining plates. Garnish each with a scallion brush.

EACH SERVING PROVIDES: 1 Milk, 1 Vegetable
PER SERVING: 90 Calories, 8 g Protein, 1 g Fat, 12 g Carbohydrate, 212 mg Sodium, 0 mg Cholesterol, 1 g Dietary Fiber

ROASTED RED PEPPER DIP

Keep a container of this in your refrigerator for "free" snacking; it complements any cut-up vegetables and is a fabulous baked potato topper.

MAKES 4 SERVINGS

2 large red bell peppers
2 teaspoons tomato paste
2 teaspoons balsamic vinegar
1 garlic clove
$\frac{1}{8}$ teaspoon ground red pepper

1. Preheat broiler. Line baking sheet with heavy-duty foil.

2. Arrange peppers on prepared baking sheet; broil 3" from source of heat, turning frequently, until charred on all sides. Let stand about 15 minutes, until cool enough to handle.

3. Fit strainer over small bowl. Peel peppers over strainer, removing and discarding stem ends and seeds and allowing juices to drip into bowl.

4. In food processor, combine roasted peppers and juice, tomato paste, vinegar, garlic, and ground red pepper; purée until almost smooth.

EACH SERVING ($\frac{1}{4}$ cup) PROVIDES: 2 Vegetables
PER SERVING: 16 Calories, 1 g Protein, 0 g Fat, 4 g Carbohydrate, 23 mg Sodium, 0 mg Cholesterol, 1 g Dietary Fiber

CAPONATA

Commercial caponata is loaded with fat, so try this tasty version instead. Caponata can be served chilled or at room temperature.

MAKES 4 SERVINGS

2 cups pared cubed eggplant (¾" cubes)
1½ teaspoons coarse kosher salt
2 teaspoons olive oil
½ cup chopped onion
3 garlic cloves, minced
½ cup diced celery
1 cup canned chopped tomatoes (with liquid)
2 tablespoons golden raisins
1 tablespoon chopped fresh mint
1 tablespoon drained capers, rinsed
1 teaspoon chopped fresh thyme leaves
8 ounces Belgian endive, separated into leaves

1. In colander, toss eggplant with kosher salt; let set over bowl 1 hour. Rinse well under cold running water; drain and dry thoroughly with paper towels.

2. In large nonstick skillet, heat oil; add onion and garlic. Cook over medium-high heat, stirring frequently, about 2 minutes. Add ¼ cup water and cook, stirring, until vegetables are soft, about 5 minutes.

3. Add celery and 2 tablespoons water; cook, covered, 5 minutes. Add prepared eggplant and ⅓ cup water; cook, covered, 5 minutes. Stir in tomatoes, raisins, mint, capers and thyme; cook, covered, 10 minutes. Uncover; cook 4 minutes longer.

4. To serve, on each of 4 plates, arrange one-fourth of the endive leaves; top each with one-fourth of the caponata.

EACH SERVING PROVIDES: ½ Fat, ¼ Fruit, 2½ Vegetables
PER SERVING: 79 Calories, 2 g Protein, 3 g Fat, 14 g Carbohydrate, 356 mg Sodium, 0 mg Cholesterol, 3 g Dietary Fiber

MANGO AND BLACK BEAN SALSA

MAKES 4 SERVINGS

½ cup diced red onion
1½ small mangoes, pared, pitted and diced
½ cup diced red bell pepper
½ cup fresh or thawed frozen whole-kernel corn
2 ounces drained cooked black beans
2 tablespoons fresh lime juice
¼ teaspoon salt
8 Boston lettuce leaves

1. In small bowl, cover onion with 1 cup ice water; soak 30 minutes. Drain; dry well.

2. In medium bowl, combine onion, mangoes, bell pepper, corn, black beans, juice and salt; stir to mix well.

3. To serve, line 4 plates with 2 lettuce leaves each; top each with one-fourth of the mango mixture.

EACH SERVING PROVIDES: ¾ Fruit, ¾ Vegetable, ½ Bread
PER SERVING: 90 Calories, 3 g Protein, 1 g Fat, 21 g Carbohydrate, 140 mg Sodium, 0 mg Cholesterol, 2 g Dietary Fiber

Just Plain Muffins (page 74)

CHAPTER FOUR

BREADS

BASIC WHITE BREAD

Baking your own bread is enormously satisfying—plus you can vary it to suit your mood! Try the Parmesan variation for a loaf with extra flavor, the raisin bread to make morning toast a treat.

MAKES 16 SERVINGS

1 envelope active dry yeast
$\frac{1}{2}$ cup lukewarm (105°–115°F) skim milk
2 teaspoons granulated sugar
$\frac{1}{4}$ cup lukewarm (105°–115°F) water
2 cups all-purpose flour (reserve 1 tablespoon)*
1 teaspoon salt
1 teaspoon skim milk

1. In small bowl, combine yeast with lukewarm milk, sugar and lukewarm water; let stand 10 minutes, until dissolved.

2. In large bowl or food processor, combine flour and salt; add yeast mixture. Mix well, or process 1 minute.

3. If mixing by hand, sprinkle work surface with 1 tablespoon reserved flour; turn dough out onto prepared work surface and knead until dough is smooth and no longer sticky, about 10 minutes.

4. Spray large bowl with nonstick cooking spray; place dough in bowl. Cover loosely with plastic wrap or a damp towel and let rise in a warm, draft-free place until dough doubles in volume, about 40–50 minutes.

5. Punch down dough; sprinkle work surface with 1 tablespoon reserved flour. Turn dough out onto prepared work surface. Pat into an 8 × 12" rectangle. Fold into thirds lengthwise, pinching seams to seal, and form into an 8" loaf. Spray an 8 × 4" loaf pan with nonstick cooking spray. Place dough in pan, seam-side down. Cover with plastic wrap or a damp towel and let rise in a warm, draft-free place until dough doubles in volume, about 35–40 minutes.

6. Brush bread with 1 teaspoon skim milk and place on center oven rack. Set oven to 425°F and bake 20 minutes. Lower heat to 375°F and bake about 25–30 minutes more, until bread is golden brown and loaf sounds hollow when tapped. Turn out onto a rack and cool thoroughly before slicing.

* If mixing by hand (step 3), reserve an additional 1 tablespoon flour.

EACH SERVING (1-ounce slice) PROVIDES: $\frac{1}{2}$ Bread, 20 Optional Calories
PER SERVING: 64 Calories, 2 g Protein, 0 g Fat, 13 g Carbohydrate, 142 mg Sodium, 0 mg Cholesterol, 1 g Dietary Fiber

CHEESE BREAD

Add $\frac{3}{4}$ ounce (2 tablespoons + 1 teaspoon) grated Parmesan cheese, 3 ounces grated extra sharp cheddar cheese and a pinch each of ground red pepper and nutmeg with the flour.

EACH SERVING PROVIDES: $\frac{1}{4}$ Protein, $\frac{1}{2}$ Bread, 20 Optional Calories
PER SERVING: 91 Calories, 4 g Protein, 2 g Fat, 13 g Carbohydrate, 200 mg Sodium, 7 mg Cholesterol, 1 g Dietary Fiber

RAISIN BREAD

Add 1 teaspoon cinnamon to flour, and knead in $\frac{1}{2}$ cup raisins just before shaping loaf.

EACH SERVING PROVIDES: $\frac{1}{4}$ Fruit, $\frac{1}{2}$ Bread, 20 Optional Calories
PER SERVING: 78 Calories, 2 g Protein, 0 g Fat, 17 g Carbohydrate, 143 mg Sodium, 0 mg Cholesterol, 1 g Dietary Fiber

---

Yeast Bread Tips

◆

Choose a warm, draft-free spot to place rising dough; a gas oven lit only by a pilot light is ideal. When using plastic wrap to cover dough as it rises, spray wrap with nonstick cooking spray. Cover dough, sprayed side down to avoid sticking.

To test whether dough has risen sufficiently, poke two fingers into the dough. If it pops back right away, the dough is ready.

When dough has doubled in bulk, which should take about an hour, make a fist and punch it down to work out air and return dough to its original, unleavened size. Now it's ready for the second rising.

WHOLE-WHEAT BREAD

MAKES 12 SERVINGS

1 tablespoon + 1 teaspoon honey
1 cup lukewarm (105°–115°F) water
1 envelope dry active yeast
2½ cups whole-wheat flour (reserve 1 tablespoon)*
1 teaspoon salt

1. In small bowl combine honey with lukewarm water and sprinkle evenly with yeast. Let stand 10 minutes, until dissolved.

2. In large bowl or food processor, combine flour and salt; add yeast mixture. Mix well, or process until the dough forms a ball.

3. If mixing by hand, sprinkle work surface with 1 tablespoon reserved flour; turn dough out onto prepared work surface, and knead until dough is smooth and no longer sticky, about 10 minutes.

4. Spray large bowl with nonstick cooking spray and place dough in bowl. Cover loosely with plastic wrap or a damp towel and let rise until dough doubles in volume, about 1 hour.

5. Punch down dough; sprinkle work surface with 1 tablespoon reserved flour. Turn dough out onto prepared work surface. Pat into an 8 × 12" rectangle. Fold into thirds lengthwise; pinch seams to seal, and form into an 8" loaf. Spray an 8 × 4" loaf pan with nonstick cooking spray. Place dough in pan, seam-side down. Cover loosely with plastic wrap or a damp towel and let rise in a warm, draft-free place until dough doubles in volume, about 1 hour.

6. Preheat oven to 350°F. Bake on center oven rack for 1 hour, or until loaf sounds hollow when tapped. Turn out onto a rack and cool thoroughly before slicing. Makes one loaf.

*If mixing by hand (step 3), reserve an additional 1 tablespoon flour.

EACH SERVING PROVIDES: 1 Bread, 15 Optional Calories
PER SERVING: 95 Calories, 4 g Protein, 2 g Fat, 20 g Carbohydrate, 185 mg Sodium, 0 mg Cholesterol, 2 g Dietary Fiber

WHOLE-WHEAT SANDWICH BREAD

Whole wheat provides extra nutrition in this easy bread, perfect for the whole family's sandwiches.

MAKES 16 SERVINGS

1 envelope dry active yeast
1 cup lukewarm (105°–115°F) water
1 cup whole-wheat flour
½ teaspoon salt
1 tablespoon canola or safflower oil
2 cups all-purpose flour or bread flour

1. In large bowl, sprinkle yeast evenly over lukewarm water; let stand 5 minutes, until dissolved.

2. In medium bowl, mix whole-wheat flour and salt; stir into the yeast mixture. Stir in oil and 1¾ cups of the all-purpose flour; when dough forms, sprinkle work surface with remaining ¼ cup flour; turn dough out onto prepared work surface and knead until dough becomes elastic.

3. Spray large bowl with nonstick cooking spray and place dough in bowl; cover loosely with plastic wrap or a damp towel and let rise in a warm, draft-free place until dough doubles in volume, about 1 hour.

4. Spray an 8 × 4" loaf pan with nonstick cooking spray; punch down dough and shape into loaf; place in pan. Cover loosely with plastic wrap or a damp towel and let rise in a warm, draft-free place until loaf has risen about 2½–3" above the pan, about 1 hour.

5. After dough has risen for 25 minutes, preheat oven to 375°F.

6. Bake for 35–40 minutes; turn out onto a rack. To keep the crust soft, drape with a clean towel and cool thoroughly before slicing.

EACH SERVING PROVIDES: 1 Bread, 10 Optional Calories
PER SERVING: 92 Calories, 3 g Protein, 1 g Fat, 18 g Carbohydrate, 70 mg Sodium, 0 mg Cholesterol, 1 g Dietary Fiber

RYE BREAD

MAKES 10 SERVINGS

½ cup lukewarm (105°–115°F) skim milk
2 teaspoons dark brown sugar
¼ cup lukewarm (105°–115°F) water
1 envelope active dry yeast
1 cup minus 1 tablespoon whole-wheat flour
  (reserve 1 tablespoon)*
1 cup minus 1 tablespoon all-purpose flour
1 tablespoon + 1 teaspoon caraway seeds
2 teaspoons salt
1 egg white beaten with 2 teaspoons water
  (optional)

1. In small bowl, combine the lukewarm milk, lukewarm water and sugar; sprinkle evenly with yeast. Let stand 10 minutes, until dissolved.

2. In large bowl or food processor combine whole-wheat flour, all-purpose flour, seeds and salt. Add yeast mixture and mix well, or process until the dough forms a ball.

3. If mixing by hand, sprinkle work surface with 1 tablespoon reserved flour; turn dough out onto prepared work surface, and knead for 10 minutes, until smooth and no longer sticky. Spray large bowl with nonstick cooking spray; place dough in bowl. Cover loosely with plastic wrap or a damp towel and let rise in a warm, draft-free place until dough doubles in volume, about 1½–2 hours.

4. Punch down dough; sprinkle work surface with 1 tablespoon reserved flour. Turn dough out onto prepared work surface. Shape into a plump oval loaf, 8" long. Spray baking sheet with nonstick cooking spray; place loaf on sheet. Cover loosely with plastic wrap or a damp towel and let rise in warm, draft-free place until dough doubles in volume, about 1 hour.

5. Preheat oven to 375°F. Slash loaf diagonally with sharp knife or single-edge razor blade; brush with water and bake on center oven rack for 50–55 minutes, or until loaf sounds hollow when tapped. If desired, brush the loaf with the egg-white mixture five minutes before it is done and return it to the oven to glaze. Cool thoroughly on a rack before slicing.

* If mixing by hand (step 3), reserve an additional 1 tablespoon flour.

EACH SERVING PROVIDES: 1 Bread, 15 Optional Calories
PER SERVING: 97 Calories, 4 g Protein, 1 g Fat, 19 g Carbohydrate, 454 mg Sodium, 0 mg Cholesterol, 2 g Dietary Fiber

◆

SOURDOUGH WHITE BREAD

Sourdough bread is based on using a "starter" instead of plain yeast. You'll want to begin this piquant bread at least two days before you'd like to bake it.

MAKES 12 SERVINGS

Starter:
1 envelope active dry yeast
¾ cup lukewarm (105°–115°F) water
¾ cup all-purpose flour
Bread:
1½ cups all-purpose flour (reserve 1 tablespoon +
  1 teaspoon)*
2 teaspoons salt

1. To prepare starter, in a glass bowl, combine yeast with lukewarm water and ¾ cup flour. Cover and let stand 2 days at room temperature. Mixture should be bubbly and have a grapefruit-like odor.

2. To prepare bread, in large bowl or food processor, combine flour and salt. Add starter, and mix well, or process 1 minute. If mixing by hand, sprinkle work surface with 1 tablespoon reserved flour; turn dough out onto prepared work surface and knead until no longer sticky, about 10 minutes.

3. Spray a large bowl with nonstick cooking spray and place dough in bowl. Cover loosely with plastic wrap or a damp towel and let rise in a warm, draft-free place until dough doubles in volume, about 1 hour.

4. Punch down dough; sprinkle work surface with 1 tablespoon reserved flour. Turn dough out onto prepared work surface. Form into a round, 6" loaf. Spray a baking sheet with nonstick cooking spray and place the dough on it. Cover loosely with plastic wrap or a damp towel and let rise in a warm, draft-free place until dough doubles in volume, about 1 hour.

5. Place a pan of boiling water on lowest oven rack. Dust loaf with remaining 1 teaspoon reserved flour, and slash dough twice vertically and twice horizontally with a sharp knife or single-edge razor blade. Set oven to 400°F and bake 20 minutes. Lower heat to 350°F and continue baking for 20–30 minutes, or until bread is well browned, and sounds hollow when tapped. Turn out onto a rack and cool thoroughly before slicing.

* If mixing by hand (step 2), reserve an additional 1 tablespoon flour.

EACH SERVING PROVIDES: 1 Bread
PER SERVING: 86 Calories, 3 g Protein, 0 g Fat, 17 g Carbohydrate, 368 mg Sodium, 0 mg Cholesterol, 1 g Dietary Fiber

WHOLE-WHEAT SOURDOUGH DATE BREAD

MAKES 14 SERVINGS

Starter:
1 teaspoon active dry yeast
$\frac{1}{4}$ cup + 2 tablespoons lukewarm (105°–115°F) water
$\frac{1}{4}$ cup all-purpose flour or bread flour
$\frac{1}{4}$ cup whole-wheat flour
Bread:
$\frac{1}{2}$ teaspoon salt
2 tablespoons whole-wheat flour
2 cups all-purpose flour or bread flour (reserve 2 tablespoons)
$5\frac{1}{4}$ ounces dried dates, cut into $\frac{1}{4}$-inch slices

1. To prepare the starter, in a large bowl, sprinkle yeast over lukewarm water; when the yeast appears moistened, add $\frac{1}{4}$ cup all-purpose flour and $\frac{1}{4}$ cup whole-wheat flour and stir briskly. Scrape sides of bowl so all the dough is together in one sticky mass; cover loosely with plastic wrap or a damp towel and set aside at room temperature for 2–3 days.

2. With a sturdy spoon, beat $\frac{1}{2}$ cup cold water into the starter; combine the 2 tablespoons whole-wheat flour with the salt and stir into the starter; add all except reserved all-purpose flour and stir into the starter to form a single mass of dough.

3. Sprinkle work surface with 1 tablespoon reserved flour; turn dough out onto prepared work surface and knead until very resilient and bouncy, about 15 minutes.

4. Spray a large bowl with nonstick cooking spray; place dough in bowl. Cover loosely with plastic wrap or a damp towel and let rise in a warm, draft-free place until dough doubles in volume.

5. Spray an 8 × 4" loaf pan with nonstick cooking spray and set aside.

6. Punch down dough; sprinkle work surface with 1 tablespoon reserved flour. Turn dough out onto prepared work surface. Sprinkle with dates; then knead slowly until the dates are evenly distributed.

7. Return to bowl and let rest for 10 minutes. Meanwhile, preheat oven to 375°F.

8. Shape dough into a loaf and place in prepared loaf pan; cover loosely with plastic wrap or a damp towel and let rise in a warm, draft-free place until dough doubles in volume. Bake on center rack of oven for 40 minutes. Turn out onto rack and cool thoroughly before slicing.

EACH SERVING PROVIDES: $\frac{1}{2}$ Fruit, 1 Bread
PER SERVING: 115 Calories, 3 g Protein, 0 g Fat, 26 g Carbohydrate, 79 mg Sodium, 0 mg Cholesterol, 2 g Dietary Fiber

SOURDOUGH PUMPERNICKEL

MAKES 12 SERVINGS

Starter:
1 envelope active dry yeast
1 cup lukewarm (105°–115°F) water
1 cup whole-wheat flour
Bread:
1¼ cups rye flour
½ cup whole-wheat flour (reserve 2 tablespoons)
1 tablespoon + 1 teaspoon unsweetened cocoa
2 teaspoons salt
2 tablespoons + 2 teaspoons molasses
2 teaspoons instant coffee dissolved in 2 teaspoons hot water
½ cup raisins
2 teaspoons caraway seeds
1 teaspoon cornmeal

1. To prepare starter, in a glass bowl, combine yeast with lukewarm water and the flour. Beat well; cover and let stand 2 days at room temperature. Mixture should be bubbly, and have a grapefruit-like odor.

2. In large bowl or food processor, combine rye flour, whole-wheat flour, cocoa and salt. Add molasses and coffee to starter; then combine with flour mixture, stirring well, or process 1 minute. If mixing by hand, sprinkle work surface with 1 tablespoon reserved flour; turn dough out onto prepared work surface and knead 10 minutes. Dough will be slightly sticky. (If using processor or dough hook, finish kneading by hand on prepared board for a few minutes to make sure it is well blended.)

3. Spray a large bowl with nonstick cooking spray and place dough in bowl. Cover loosely with plastic wrap or a damp towel and let rise in warm, draft-free place until dough doubles in volume, about 1 hour.

4. Punch down dough; sprinkle work surface with 1 tablespoon reserved flour. Turn dough out onto prepared work surface. Knead in raisins and caraway seeds, and form into an oval 8" loaf. Spray a baking sheet with nonstick cooking spray. Sprinkle bottom of dough with cornmeal and place it on baking sheet. Cover loosely with plastic wrap or a damp towel and let rise in a warm, draft-free place until dough doubles in volume, about 1 hour.

5. Place baking sheet on center rack of oven and set oven to 350°F. Bake for 50–60 minutes or until bread is well browned and sounds hollow when tapped. Turn out onto rack and cool thoroughly before slicing.

EACH SERVING PROVIDES: ½ Fruit, 1 Bread, 45 Optional Calories
PER SERVING: 125 Calories, 4 g Protein, 1 g Fat, 28 g Carbohydrate, 371 mg Sodium, 0 mg Cholesterol, 4 g Dietary Fiber

◆

CHALLAH

This traditional Jewish bread makes a lovely braided loaf and can even serve as a centerpiece! Leftover challah makes exceptional French toast.

MAKES 10 SERVINGS

1 envelope active dry yeast
½ cup lukewarm (105°–115°F) water
2 cups minus 2 tablespoons all-purpose flour (reserve 1 tablespoon)*
2 teaspoons granulated sugar
¾ teaspoon salt
1 large egg, beaten
2 teaspoons corn oil
1 egg white, beaten with 1 teaspoon water
½ teaspoon poppy seeds

1. In small bowl, sprinkle yeast over lukewarm water; add 1 tablespoon of the flour; let stand 10 minutes.

2. In large bowl or food processor, combine the remaining flour, the sugar and salt. Add egg and oil to the yeast mixture, and stir into the flour mixture. (If using processor, process 1 minute.)

3. If mixing by hand, sprinkle work surface with 1 tablespoon reserved flour; turn dough out onto prepared work surface and knead for 10 minutes.

4. Spray large bowl with nonstick cooking spray; place dough in bowl. Cover loosely with plastic wrap or a damp towel and let rise in a warm, draft-free place until dough doubles in volume, about 1 hour.

5. Punch down dough; sprinkle work surface with 1 tablespoon reserved flour. Turn dough out onto prepared work surface. Divide into 3 equal pieces. Roll each piece between your palms into an 18"-long rope. Pinch the 3 ropes together at one end and braid loosely to allow room for rising. Spray a baking sheet with nonstick cooking spray; gently transfer the braided loaf onto it. Cover loosely with plastic wrap or a damp towel and let rise in a warm, draft-free place until dough doubles in volume, about 1 hour.

6. Preheat oven to 350°F. Brush loaf with half of egg white mixture and bake 20 minutes. Brush with remainder of egg-white mixture, sprinkle with poppy seeds, and bake about 10–15 minutes more, or until loaf sounds hollow when tapped on bottom. Turn out onto rack and cool thoroughly before slicing.

* If mixing by hand (step 3), reserve an additional 1 tablespoon flour.

EACH SERVING PROVIDES: 1 Bread, 20 Optional Calories
PER SERVING: 110 Calories, 4 g Protein, 2 g Fat, 19 g Carbohydrate, 177 mg Sodium, 21 mg Cholesterol, 1 g Dietary Fiber

◆

ITALIAN BREAD

MAKES 12 SERVINGS

1 envelope active dry yeast
¾ cup lukewarm (105°–115°F) water
2 cups + 1 teaspoon all-purpose flour*
¼ cup whole-wheat flour
1½ teaspoons salt
1 teaspoon cornmeal

1. In small bowl, sprinkle yeast evenly over ¼ cup of the lukewarm water.

2. In large bowl or in food processor, combine all except 1 teaspoon of the all-purpose flour, the whole-wheat flour and salt.

3. Add the remaining ½ cup lukewarm water and the yeast mixture to flour mixture, and mix well, or process 1 minute.

4. If mixing by hand, sprinkle work surface with 1 tablespoon reserved flour; turn dough out onto prepared work surface and knead for 10 minutes.

5. Spray a large bowl with nonstick cooking spray. Place the dough in the bowl and cover loosely with plastic wrap or a damp towel and let rise in a warm, draft-free place until dough doubles in volume, about 40–50 minutes.

6. Punch down dough, and turn out onto work surface. Spray baking sheet with nonstick cooking spray; sprinkle cornmeal in a 12"-long strip down the center. Form the dough into a 12 × 6" rectangle. Fold into thirds lengthwise and pinch seam to seal; turn over and form into a tapered oval loaf 12" long. Place on prepared sheet. Cover loosely with plastic wrap or a damp towel and let rise in warm, draft-free place until dough doubles in volume, about 30 minutes.

7. Dust loaf with the 1 teaspoon reserved flour and slash top with a sharp knife or single-edge razor blade. Place in upper third of cold oven, and set oven to 400°F. Bake for 20 minutes. Lower heat to 350°F, and bake 25–30 minutes more, or until loaf sounds hollow when tapped. Cool on rack.

* If mixing by hand (step 4), reserve 1 tablespoon flour.

EACH SERVING PROVIDES: 1 Bread, 2 Optional Calories
PER SERVING: 89 Calories, 3 g Protein, 1 g Fat, 18 g Carbohydrate, 275 mg Sodium, 0 mg Cholesterol, 1 g Dietary Fiber

FOCACCIA

Focaccia is an Italian bread of great versatility. You may want to experiment with your own toppings, such as fresh herbs.

MAKES 12 SERVINGS

1 envelope active dry yeast
1 cup minus 1 tablespoon lukewarm (105°–115°F) water
2 cups + 2 tablespoons all-purpose flour (reserve 1 tablespoon)*
2 tablespoons whole-wheat flour
1 teaspoon salt
Topping (recipes follow)

1. In small bowl, sprinkle yeast evenly over lukewarm water; let stand 10 minutes.

2. In large bowl or in food processor, combine all-purpose flour, whole-wheat flour and salt. Add yeast mixture and mix well or process 1 minute. If mixing by hand, sprinkle work surface with 1 tablespoon reserved flour; turn dough out onto prepared work surface, and knead 5 minutes. Dough will be sticky. Spray large bowl with non-stick cooking spray; place dough in bowl. Cover loosely with plastic wrap or a damp towel and let rise until dough doubles in volume, about 1 hour.

3. Spray a baking sheet with nonstick cooking spray. Punch down dough. Flour hands with 1 tablespoon reserved flour, and form dough into a ball. Place it on prepared sheet, and press out into a 10" circle. Cover loosely with plastic wrap or a damp towel and let rise in a warm, draft-free place until dough doubles in volume, about 30 minutes.

4. Meanwhile, prepare topping. When dough has risen, preheat oven to 425°F for 15 minutes. Without piercing the dough, make dimples all over it with fingertips. Cover with topping (see right), and bake on center rack of oven, 15–20 minutes, or until crust is nicely browned. Serve hot or at room temperature.

*If mixing by hand (step 2), reserve an additional 1 tablespoon flour.

EACH SERVING (without topping) PROVIDES: 1 Bread

POTATO-TOMATO TOPPING

$\frac{1}{4}$ cup boiling water
4 sun-dried tomato halves (not packed in oil), minced
1 medium onion, thinly sliced
3 garlic cloves, minced
2 teaspoons olive oil
4 ounces cooked new potatoes, thinly sliced
$1\frac{1}{2}$ teaspoons chopped fresh basil
$1\frac{1}{2}$ teaspoons chopped fresh parsley
$\frac{1}{8}$ teaspoon pepper
1 tablespoon + $1\frac{1}{2}$ teaspoons Parmesan cheese

1. In small bowl, pour boiling water over the sun-dried tomatoes; let soak 10 minutes; drain well.

2. Add the onion, garlic and olive oil to the tomatoes, and toss to coat. Add potatoes, basil, parsley and pepper; toss gently.

3. Distribute evenly over focaccia crust, and sprinkle evenly with Parmesan cheese. Bake as directed.

EACH SERVING (topping only) PROVIDES: $\frac{1}{4}$ Vegetable, 15 Optional Calories
PER SERVING: 116 Calories, 4 g Protein, 2 g Fat, 22 g Carbohydrate, 208 mg Sodium, 1 mg Cholesterol, 1 g Dietary Fiber

FETA CHEESE TOPPING

3 shallots, thinly sliced
3 garlic cloves, minced
2 teaspoons olive oil
$1\frac{1}{2}$ ounces drained feta cheese, crumbled
6 large black olives, chopped
1 tablespoon chopped fresh parsley
$\frac{1}{2}$ teaspoon oregano
$\frac{1}{8}$ teaspoon pepper

1. In small bowl, toss shallots and garlic with olive oil. Add cheese, olives, parsley, oregano and pepper; mix well.

2. Distribute evenly over focaccia crust, and bake as directed.

EACH SERVING (topping only) PROVIDES: 20 Optional Calories
PER SERVING: 110 Calories, 3 g Protein, 2 g Fat, 19 g Carbohydrate, 245 mg Sodium, 3 mg Cholesterol, 1 g Dietary Fiber

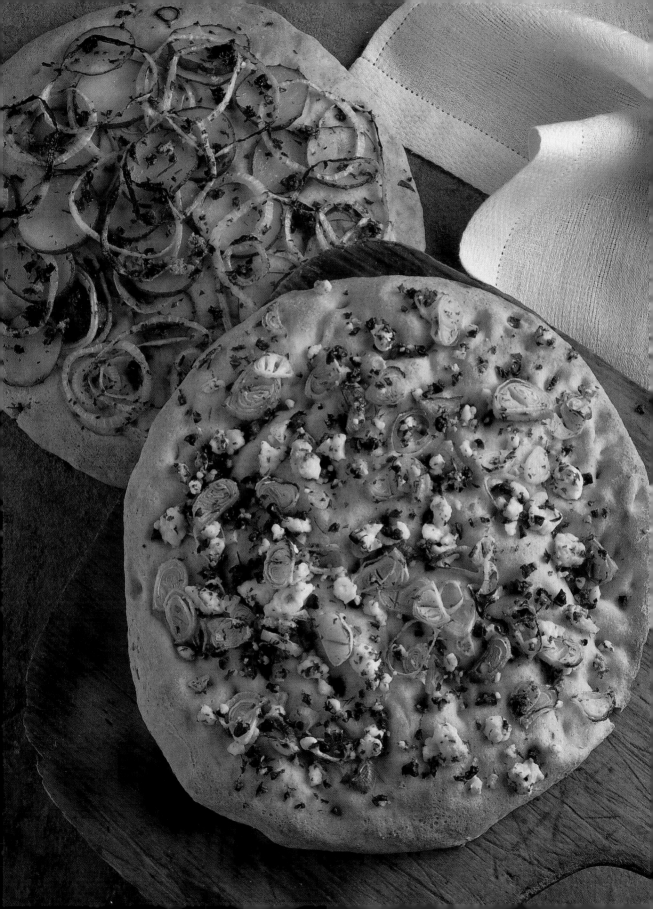

MICROWAVE-BAKED ENGLISH MUFFIN BREAD

Your microwave gives you hearty bread in short order! And, just like regular English muffins, this bread is best toasted before serving.

MAKES 11 SERVINGS

2 cups + 1 tablespoon all-purpose flour
1 package dry active yeast
2 teaspoons granulated sugar
$\frac{1}{2}$ teaspoon salt
1 cup lukewarm (105–115ºF) skim milk
$\frac{1}{4}$ teaspoon baking soda

1. In large bowl, mix together flour, yeast, sugar and salt.

2. Pour milk onto dry ingredients, and with a sturdy spoon, stir together to form a very thick batter. Beat vigorously for 15–20 seconds (the batter will become very stretchy as you beat). Cover loosely with plastic wrap or a damp towel and let rise in a warm, draft-free place until dough doubles in volume, about 45 minutes.

3. Spray an 8 × 4" glass loaf pan with nonstick cooking spray.

4. Blend baking soda and 1 tablespoon water together and beat it into the bread batter until it becomes stretchy once again.

5. Scrape batter into prepared loaf pan and cover loosely with plastic wrap or a damp towel. Let rise in a warm, draft-free place until it fills the pan about two-thirds to three-quarters full, about 40 minutes.

6. Microwave on high (100%), uncovered, for 4 minutes, or until no wet spots remain on the top of the loaf.

7. Cool in the pan for 10 minutes, then gently but firmly pull back on the sides of the loaf to release from the pan, unmold and cool completely on a rack. Toast before serving.

EACH SERVING PROVIDES: 1 Bread, 10 Optional Calories
PER SERVING: 99 Calories, 3 g Protein, 0 g Fat, 20 g Carbohydrate, 140 mg Sodium, 0 mg Cholesterol, 1 g Dietary Fiber

BRAN BREAD

MAKES 12 SERVINGS

1 envelope active dry yeast
$1\frac{1}{3}$ cups lukewarm (105°–115°F) water
2 cups all-purpose flour*
$\frac{1}{2}$ cup plus 2 tablespoons whole-wheat flour
$3\frac{1}{2}$ ounces wheat bran
2 teaspoons salt

1. In small bowl, sprinkle yeast evenly over lukewarm water; let stand 10 minutes or until dissolved. In large bowl or food processor, combine all-purpose flour, whole-wheat flour, bran and salt. Add yeast mixture and mix well, or process 1 minute. If mixing by hand, sprinkle work surface with 1 tablespoon reserved flour; turn dough out onto prepared work surface and knead until dough is no longer sticky, about 10 minutes.

2. Spray large bowl with nonstick cooking spray and place dough in bowl. Cover loosely with plastic wrap or a damp towel and let rise in a warm draft-free place until dough doubles in volume, about 1 hour.

3. Punch down dough. Cover loosely with plastic wrap or a damp towel and let rise in warm, draft-free place for 30 minutes.

4. Spray an 8 × 4" loaf pan with nonstick cooking spray. Form the dough into a rectangle about 12 × 8". Fold the dough into thirds to form an 8 × 4" loaf, pinching seam to seal; place in pan, seam-side down. Cover loosely with plastic wrap or a damp towel and let rise until dough comes to 1" above rim of pan, about 1 hour.

5. Preheat oven to 375°F. Brush dough with water and bake on center rack about 45–50 minutes, or until golden brown and loaf sounds hollow when tapped. Turn out onto a rack and cool thoroughly, preferably overnight, before slicing.

* If mixing by hand (step 1), reserve 1 tablespoon flour.

EACH SERVING PROVIDES: $1\frac{1}{2}$ Breads, 2 Optional Calories
PER SERVING: 118 Calories, 5 g Protein, 1 g Fat, 26 g Carbohydrate, 368 mg Sodium, 0 mg Cholesterol, 5 g Dietary Fiber

TOASTED OATMEAL BREAD

MAKES 12 SERVINGS

$1\frac{1}{2}$ ounces rolled oats
1 envelope active dry yeast
2 tablespoons lukewarm (105°–115°F) water
$\frac{1}{2}$ cup lukewarm (105°–115°F) skim milk
1 tablespoon + 1 teaspoon honey
1 teaspoon salt
$1\frac{1}{4}$ cups + 2 tablespoons all-purpose flour (reserve 1 tablespoon)*
$\frac{1}{2}$ cup whole-wheat flour

1. In a pie tin, toast oats at 325°F for 15–20 minutes, stirring once or twice to toast evenly. Set aside.

2. Sprinkle yeast evenly over lukewarm water; let stand 10 minutes, until dissolved.

3. Combine lukewarm milk, honey and salt with yeast mixture.

4. In a large bowl or food processor, combine all-purpose flour and whole-wheat flour; add yeast mixture. Mix until well blended, or process until dough forms a ball, about 1 minute. If mixing by hand, sprinkle work surface with 1 tablespoon reserved flour; turn dough out onto prepared work surface and knead 10 minutes.

5. Spray large bowl with nonstick cooking spray; place dough in bowl. Cover loosely with plastic wrap or a damp towel and let rise in a warm, draft-free place until dough doubles in volume, about 1 hour.

6. Punch down dough; sprinkle work surface with 1 tablespoon reserved flour. Turn dough out onto prepared work surface. Pat out dough about $\frac{1}{2}$" thick, and knead in the reserved toasted oats until well incorporated. Pat into a 12 × 18" rectangle; fold into thirds lengthwise, pinching seam to seal. Spray an 8 × 4" loaf pan with nonstick cooking spray, and place dough in pan, seam-side down. Cover loosely with plastic wrap or a damp towel and let rise in a warm, draft-free place until dough doubles in volume, about $1\frac{1}{2}$ hours.

7. Place in center of cold oven and set to 350°F. Bake for 50–60 minutes, or until loaf sounds hollow when tapped. Turn onto rack and cool thoroughly before slicing.

* If mixing by hand (step 4), reserve an additional 1 tablespoon flour.

EACH SERVING PROVIDES: 1 Bread, 10 Optional Calories
PER SERVING: 96 Calories, 3 g Protein, 1 g Fat, 20 g Carbohydrate, 190 mg Sodium, 0 mg Cholesterol, 2 g Dietary Fiber

ANADAMA BREAD

MAKES 14 SERVINGS

$\frac{1}{4}$ cup cornmeal
1 cup boiling water
1 envelope active dry yeast
$\frac{1}{4}$ cup lukewarm (105°–115°F) water
2 tablespoons + 2 teaspoons molasses
1 teaspoon salt
2 cups all-purpose flour
$\frac{1}{4}$ cup whole-wheat flour

1. In large bowl or food processor, stir cornmeal and boiling water together until smooth. Let stand 30 minutes.

2. In small bowl, sprinkle yeast evenly over lukewarm water; let stand 10 minutes. Add molasses, salt and yeast mixture to the cornmeal mixture. Stir or process briefly. Add all-purpose flour and whole-wheat flour; mix well, or process, until well blended. Dough will be sticky. Spray an 8 × 4" loaf pan with nonstick cooking spray. Place dough in pan; cover with plastic wrap or a damp towel and let rise in a warm, draft-free place until dough doubles in volume, about 1 hour.

3. Preheat oven to 350°F. Bake bread on center rack about 45–50 minutes, or until golden brown and loaf sounds hollow when tapped. Turn out onto a when tapped rack and cool thoroughly before slicing.

EACH SERVING PROVIDES: 1 Bread, 10 Optional Calories
PER SERVING: 94 Calories, 3 g Protein, 0 g Fat, 20 g Carbohydrate, 159 mg Sodium, 0 mg Cholesterol, 1 g Dietary Fiber

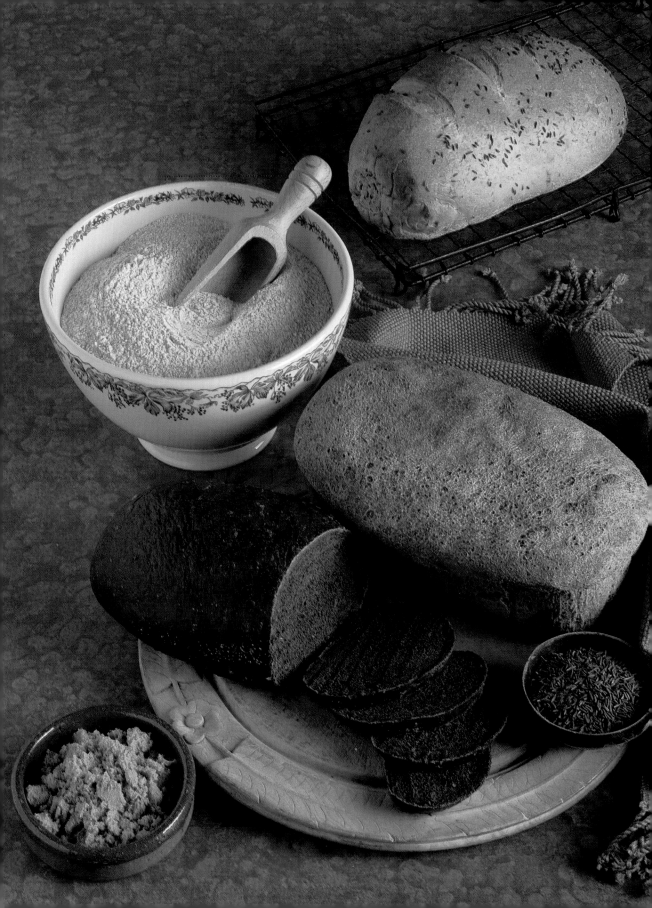

FIVE-GRAIN BEER BREAD

MAKES 20 SERVINGS

1 envelope active dry yeast
3 tablespoons lukewarm (105°–115°F) water
10 fluid ounces dark beer, room temperature
1¼ cups whole-wheat flour (reserve 1 tablespoon)
1 cup all-purpose flour
½ cup rye flour
½ cup oat flour
¼ cup buckwheat flour
¼ cup cornmeal
1½ teaspoons salt

1. In large bowl, sprinkle yeast evenly over lukewarm water. Let stand 10 minutes until dissolved.

2. Add beer; stir in whole-wheat flour and all-purpose flour to form a thick batter. Beat well, with mixer or by hand, for 3 minutes. With a rubber spatula, scrape down the sides of bowl. Cover loosely with plastic wrap or a damp towel and let rise in a warm, draft-free place until dough doubles in volume, about 1 hour.

3. In small bowl, combine rye flour, oat flour, buckwheat flour, cornmeal and salt. Stir flour mixture into the beer mixture.

4. Sprinkle work surface with 1 tablespoon reserved flour; turn dough out onto prepared work surface and knead for 5 minutes. Dough will be sticky. Spray large bowl with nonstick cooking spray; place dough in bowl. Cover loosely with plastic wrap or a damp towel and let rise in a warm, draft-free place until dough doubles in volume, about 1 hour.

5. Spray an 8 × 4" loaf pan with nonstick cooking spray. Place dough in pan; cover loosely with plastic wrap or a damp towel and let rise until dough doubles in volume, about 1 hour.

6. Preheat oven to 375°F. Bake on center oven rack 40–50 minutes, until loaf sounds hollow when tapped. Turn out onto rack and cool thoroughly before slicing.

*Five-Grain Beer Bread, Rye Bread(page 58),
Sourdough Pumpernickel (page 60)*

EACH SERVING PROVIDES: 1 Bread, 10 Optional Calories
PER SERVING: 87 Calories, 3 g Protein, 0 g Fat, 17 g Carbohydrate, 166 mg Sodium, 0 mg Cholesterol, 1 g Dietary Fiber

CORN BREAD

Corn bread is a quick addition to a meal and would be especially nice with Vegetarian Bean Chili (page 290).

MAKES 12 SERVINGS

1¼ cups yellow cornmeal
¾ cup all-purpose flour
1 tablespoon + 1 teaspoon granulated sugar
2½ teaspoons baking powder
½ teaspoon salt
1 egg
1 cup + 2 tablespoons low-fat (1.5%) buttermilk

1. Preheat oven to 400°F. Spray a 9" square pan or a 12-muffin tin with nonstick cooking spray.

2. In large bowl, combine cornmeal, flour, sugar, baking powder and salt. In small bowl, beat egg with buttermilk.

3. Add buttermilk mixture to flour mixture and mix just until blended. Do not overblend.

4. Spoon into prepared pan and bake 20–25 minutes or until golden brown and toothpick comes out clean. Cool 10 minutes on a rack; turn out and serve warm.

EACH SERVING PROVIDES: 1 Bread, 35 Optional Calories
PER SERVING: 105 Calories, 3 g Protein, 1 g Fat, 20 g Carbohydrate, 223 mg Sodium, 19 mg Cholesterol, 1 g Dietary Fiber

CHEESE CORN BREAD

Omit sugar, and add 1½ ounces grated extra sharp cheddar cheese, 1½ ounces grated Parmesan cheese, 1 cup cooked or frozen corn kernels and 1–2 teaspoons minced jalapeño chilies.

EACH SERVING PROVIDES: ¼ Protein, 1¼ Breads, 25 Optional Calories
PER SERVING: 145 Calories, 6 g Protein, 4 g Fat, 22 g Carbohydrate, 313 mg Sodium, 26 mg Cholesterol, 1 g Dietary Fiber

TOMATO-HERB ROLLS

MAKES 12 SERVINGS

12 sun-dried tomato halves (not packed in oil)
1 envelope active dry yeast
1 ¼ cups lukewarm (105°–115°F) water
3 ½ cups all-purpose flour (reserve 1 tablespoon)*
1½ teaspoons salt
2 teaspoons minced fresh rosemary (or 1 teaspoon dried leaves)
2 teaspoons fresh sage (or ½ teaspoon dried leaves)
½ teaspoon dried oregano leaves
¼ teaspoon freshly ground black pepper
1 egg white beaten with 2 teaspoons water

1. Cut tomatoes into slivers, and place in small bowl. Cover with boiling water and soak 5 minutes. Drain well.

2. In small bowl, sprinkle yeast evenly over lukewarm water. Let stand 10 minutes until dissolved.

3. In large bowl or food processor, combine the flour and salt. Add the yeast mixture, and mix well, or process until the dough forms a ball.

4. If mixing by hand, sprinkle work surface with 1 tablespoon reserved flour; turn dough out onto prepared work surface and knead for 10 minutes, until smooth and no longer sticky. Spray large bowl with nonstick cooking spray; place dough in bowl. Cover loosely with plastic wrap or a damp towel and let rise in a warm, draft-free place until dough doubles in volume, about 1 hour.

5. Punch down dough; sprinkle work surface with 1 tablespoon reserved flour. Turn dough out onto prepared work surface and knead in the tomatoes, herbs and pepper, until they are evenly distributed. Divide dough into 12 equal pieces, forming each piece into an oval with tapered ends.

6. Spray a baking sheet with nonstick cooking spray and place rolls 3 inches apart on sheet. Cover loosely with plastic wrap or a damp towel and let rise in a warm, draft-free place until dough doubles in volume, about 1 hour.

7. Preheat oven to 400°F. Bake on center oven rack 20 minutes; brush with egg-white mixture and continue baking until rolls are golden brown and sound hollow when tapped. Turn out onto rack and cool rolls thoroughly before serving.

* If mixing by hand (step 4), reserve an additional 1 tablespoon flour.

EACH SERVING PROVIDES: ½ Vegetable, 1½ Breads, 5 Optional Calories
PER SERVING: 147 Calories, 5 g Protein, 1 g Fat, 30 g Carbohydrate, 284 mg Sodium, 0 mg Cholesterol, 2 g Dietary Fiber

TOMATO-HERB LOAF

This dough may be made into a single loaf. After kneading in the tomatoes, herbs and pepper, pat dough out into a 16 × 12" rectangle. Fold lengthwise into thirds; pinch seam to seal. Turn it over and mold into a 16"-long loaf with tapered ends. Transfer to sprayed baking sheet, and proceed as directed above.

◆

PITA

MAKES 16 SERVINGS

6 cups all-purpose flour or bread flour (reserve 2 tablespoons)
1 package dry active yeast
1 teaspoon salt
2 cups very warm water

1. In large bowl, mix together flour, yeast and salt; add water and stir with a wooden spoon to form a dough. Sprinkle work surface with 2 tablespoons reserved flour; turn dough out onto prepared work surface, and knead until dough is flexible and resilient, about 8 minutes.

2. Spray large bowl with nonstick cooking spray; place dough in bowl. Cover loosely with plastic wrap or a damp towel and let rise in a warm, draft-free place for 2 hours.

3. Preheat oven to 400°F. Divide the dough into 16 equal pieces; roll each into a 4" circle; bake until well puffed and colored, 15–20 minutes.

EACH SERVING PROVIDES: 2 Breads
PER SERVING: 172 Calories, 5 g Protein, 1 g Fat, 36 g Carbohydrate, 139 mg Sodium, 0 mg Cholesterol, 1 g Dietary Fiber

WHOLE-WHEAT PIZZA DOUGH

You can create endless pizza variations with this delicious dough. Try the tomato-basil topping, below. It's the luscious topping on our front cover! You can also add mushrooms and olives, feta cheese and scallions, sliced cooked turkey, cooked shrimp or any combination of your favorites.

MAKES 8 SERVINGS

Sponge:
2 teaspoons active dry yeast
$\frac{1}{4}$ cup lukewarm (105°–115°) water
$\frac{1}{4}$ cup all-purpose flour
Pizza Dough:
$\frac{1}{2}$ cup skim milk
$1\frac{1}{3}$ cups all-purpose flour (reserve 1 tablespoon)
$\frac{1}{2}$ cup whole-wheat flour
$\frac{1}{4}$ teaspoon salt

1. To prepare the sponge, in large bowl, sprinkle yeast evenly over lukewarm water; when yeast appears wet, add $\frac{1}{4}$ cup all-purpose flour and stir hard to make a sponge; cover loosely and set aside at room temperature for 40 minutes.

2. Stir milk into the sponge. In medium bowl combine all-purpose flour, whole-wheat flour and the salt. Mix well; add flour mixture to the sponge and stir to mix.

3. Sprinkle work surface with 1 tablespoon reserved flour; turn dough out onto prepared work surface and knead until it becomes elastic and resilient, about 10–12 minutes.

4. Spray a large bowl with nonstick cooking spray. Place dough in bowl; cover loosely with plastic wrap or a damp towel and let rise in a warm, draft-free place until dough doubles in volume, about 45–60 minutes.

5. Punch down dough and roll into a circle about 14" in diameter; place on 14" pizza pan or large baking sheet.

6. Arrange the toppings of your choice on crust and bake at 500°F for 10 minutes.

EACH SERVING PROVIDES: $1\frac{1}{4}$ Breads, 20 Optional Calories
PER SERVING: 124 Calories, 4 g Protein, 1 g Fat, 25 g Carbohydrate, 77 mg Sodium, 0 mg Cholesterol, 2 g Dietary Fiber

TOMATO-BASIL TOPPING

MAKES 8 SERVINGS

2 cups sliced ripe red medium tomatoes
2 cups sliced red and yellow cherry tomatoes
2–3 tablespoons fresh basil leaves
Whole-Wheat Pizza Dough (left)
2 tablespoons olive oil
$1\frac{1}{2}$ ounces coarsely grated Parmesan cheese

1. Arrange tomatoes and whole or shredded basil leaves on prepared (unbaked) pizza dough.

2. Drizzle evenly with olive oil and sprinkle evenly with cheese. Bake as directed.

EACH SERVING (topping only) PROVIDES: $\frac{3}{4}$ Fat, 1 Vegetable, $\frac{1}{4}$ Protein
PER SERVING: 69 Calories, 3 g Protein, 5 g Fat, 4 g Carbohydrate, 105 mg Sodium, 4 mg Cholesterol, 1 g Dietary Fiber

CALZONE

Calzone, originally from Naples, are pizza turnovers. Traditionally stuffed with heavy cheeses, our lightened spinach-and-cheese version keeps all the great flavor of the original.

MAKES 6 SERVINGS

Dough:
1¼ teaspoons (about ½ envelope) active dry yeast
¾ cup lukewarm (105°–115°F) water
1¾ cups + 3 tablespoons all-purpose flour*
¼ teaspoon salt

Filling:
¼ cup minced shallots
5 garlic cloves, minced
2 teaspoons olive oil
¾ cup thawed frozen chopped spinach, squeezed dry
½ cup part-skim ricotta cheese
2¼ ounces feta cheese, crumbled
1 egg, lightly beaten
3 tablespoons chopped fresh mint
1 teaspoon dried oregano leaves
¾ teaspoon salt
¼ teaspoon pepper

1. In measuring cup, dissolve yeast in ¼ cup of the lukewarm water and let stand 10 minutes. In bowl of electric mixer, combine all except 2 tablespoons of the flour with salt. Beat in yeast mixture and remaining ½ cup lukewarm water until well combined. If using a dough hook, knead lightly until dough is smooth and elastic. If mixing by hand, sprinkle work surface with 1 tablespoon reserved flour; turn dough out onto prepared work surface and knead by hand.

2. Spray medium bowl with nonstick cooking spray; place dough in bowl. Cover loosely with plastic wrap or a damp towel and let rise in a warm, draft-free place until dough doubles in volume, about 1 hour.

3. Meanwhile, in small nonstick skillet, sauté shallots and garlic in oil until soft, about 7 minutes. Add spinach; cook 2 minutes. Transfer to medium bowl. Stir in ricotta, feta cheese, egg, mint, oregano, salt and pepper.

4. Preheat oven to 400°F. Spray baking sheet with nonstick cooking spray; set aside.

5. Sprinkle work surface with remaining 2 tablespoons flour; turn dough out onto prepared work surface. Form dough into a cylinder and divide into 6 equal parts; then roll each part into a 6"-diameter circle. For each calzone, put about 2 heaping tablespoons of filling on one side of circle, wet rim all around the edge and seal with a wet thumb. Bake 20–25 minutes or until golden brown and crisped.

* If mixing by hand (step 1), reserve 1 additional tablespoon flour.

EACH SERVING (1 calzone) PROVIDES: ¼ Fat, ¼ Vegetable, 1½ Proteins, 1½ Breads, 25 Optional Calories
PER SERVING: 250 Calories, 10 g Protein, 7 g Fat, 36 g Carbohydrate, 542 mg Sodium, 51 mg Cholesterol, 2 g Dietary Fiber

---

In a Pinch

◆

Sometimes you can't avoid using a substitute when baking. If you're ever caught short-handed, try these easy baking substitutes:

Instead of:	*Use:*
1 teaspoon baking powder	*¼ teaspoon baking soda and ½ teaspoon cream of tartar, combined*
1 package active dry yeast	*1 cake compressed yeast*
1 teaspoon finely shredded lemon peel	*½ teaspoon lemon extract*
1 cup skim milk	*⅓ cup instant nonfat dry milk powder + water to make 1 cup*

SCONES

A British teatime treat, scones are perfect for breakfast, for parties or any time you'd like a sweet bread. They are also good served with spreadable fruit.

MAKES 12 SERVINGS

1 cup + 2 tablespoons all-purpose flour (reserve 1 tablespoon)
$\frac{1}{4}$ cup + 2 tablespoons dried currants
1 teaspoon granulated sugar
1 teaspoon baking powder
$\frac{1}{4}$ teaspoon baking soda
$\frac{1}{4}$ teaspoon salt
$\frac{1}{2}$ cup low-fat (1.5%) buttermilk
1 egg
1 teaspoon margarine, melted
$\frac{1}{4}$ teaspoon butter flavoring

1. Preheat oven to 425°F. Spray a baking sheet with nonstick cooking spray.

2. In large bowl, combine flour, currants, sugar, baking powder, baking soda, and salt. In small bowl, combine buttermilk, egg, margarine and butter flavoring.

3. Add buttermilk mixture to flour mixture, and stir just until flour disappears; do not overblend. Sprinkle work surface with 1 tablespoon reserved flour; turn dough out onto prepared work surface and pat out $\frac{1}{4}$" thick. Cut into 12 rounds with a 2" cutter, or into 12 triangles with a sharp knife, and place on baking sheet an inch apart. Place in upper third of oven and turn oven down to 400°F. Bake for 12–15 minutes or until golden brown and crusty. Serve hot.

EACH SERVING (1 scone) PROVIDES: $\frac{1}{4}$ Fruit, $\frac{1}{2}$ Bread, 15 Optional Calories
PER SERVING: 72 Calories, 2 g Protein, 1 g Fat, 13 g Carbohydrate, 131 mg Sodium, 18 mg Cholesterol, 1 g Dietary Fiber

NAAN

An Indian bread, naan is excellent to serve when you'd like to tone down spicy dishes.

MAKES 8 SERVINGS

2 cups all-purpose flour (reserve 1 tablespoon)*
1$\frac{1}{2}$ teaspoons baking powder
1 teaspoon granulated sugar
$\frac{1}{4}$ teaspoon salt
$\frac{1}{8}$ teaspoon baking soda
$\frac{1}{2}$ cup skim milk
1 large egg

1. In large bowl, combine flour, baking powder, sugar, salt and baking soda, to blend thoroughly. In small bowl, beat together the milk and egg, and add them to the flour mixture, stirring constantly, until very well blended. (If using a food processor, combine flour with the other dry ingredients, and add the milk mixture in a slow stream, while processing for 1 minute.)

2. If mixing by hand, sprinkle work surface with 1 tablespoon reserved flour; turn dough out onto prepared work surface and knead for 10 minutes. Spray a bowl with nonstick cooking spray; place dough in bowl. Cover loosely with plastic wrap or a damp towel and let rise in a warm, draft-free place for 3 hours.

3. Place a large baking sheet on the center oven rack, and preheat to 450°F. Sprinkle work surface with 1 tablespoon reserved flour; turn dough out onto prepared work surface. Divide dough into 8 equal pieces and flatten each piece into a teardrop-shaped leaf, $\frac{3}{8}$" thick.

4. Arrange the naan on the preheated sheet, and bake 10–12 minutes, or until firm. Slide briefly under a broiler to brown the tops lightly. Serve hot or at room temperature.

*If mixing by hand (step 2), reserve an additional 1 tablespoon flour.

EACH SERVING (1 naan) PROVIDES: 1$\frac{1}{4}$ Breads, 25 Optional Calories
PER SERVING: 131 Calories, 5 g Protein, 1 g Fat, 25 g Carbohydrate, 195 mg Sodium, 27 mg Cholesterol, 1 g Dietary Fiber

NAAN WITH CUMIN SEEDS

Toast 2 teaspoons whole cumin seed in a 325°F oven for 10 minutes, stirring occasionally, and add to the flour in step #1.

◆

WHOLE-WHEAT NAAN

MAKES 18 SERVINGS

3 cups finely chopped onions
$\frac{1}{2}$ teaspoon ground cumin
$\frac{1}{8}$ teaspoon black pepper
2 teaspoons stick margarine
1 cup lukewarm (105º–115ºF) skim milk
$1\frac{1}{2}$ teaspoons salt
3 cups all-purpose flour
1 cup + 2 tablespoons whole-wheat flour (reserve 1 tablespoon)

1. In large skillet, sauté onions, cumin and black pepper in 1 teaspoon of the margarine over medium-low heat until very soft; set aside.

2. In large bowl, combine lukewarm milk, onion mixture, salt, the remaining 1 teaspoon margarine, the all-purpose flour and the whole-wheat flour. Stir with a sturdy wooden spoon until a mass of dough forms. Sprinkle work surface with 1 tablespoon reserved flour; turn dough out onto prepared work surface and knead until dough is slightly firm and no longer sticky, about 2–3 minutes.

3. Form into 18" cylinder and cut off 1" pieces. Roll each into a ball. Cover loosely with plastic wrap or a damp towel and let rise for 5 minutes.

4. Preheat oven to 425°F. Roll each piece of dough into a 3" round about $\frac{1}{4}$" thick. Bake 25 minutes until puffed and lightly browned.

EACH SERVING PROVIDES: $\frac{1}{4}$ Vegetable, 1 Bread, 30 Optional Calories
PER SERVING: 120 Calories, 4 g Protein, 1 g Fat, 24 g Carbohydrate, 197 mg Sodium, 0 mg Cholesterol, 2 g Dietary Fiber

BIALYS

MAKES 8 SERVINGS

1 envelope active dry yeast
1 teaspoon granulated sugar
1 cup lukewarm (105°–115°F) water
2 cups all-purpose flour*
$\frac{1}{2}$ cup whole-wheat flour
2 teaspoons salt
$\frac{1}{2}$ cup minced onion
2 teaspoons poppy seeds
1 teaspoon vegetable oil

1. In small bowl, sprinkle yeast and sugar over 1 cup lukewarm water; let stand 10 minutes or until yeast is dissolved.

2. In large bowl or in food processor, combine all-purpose flour, whole-wheat flour and salt. Stir in yeast mixture; mix thoroughly by hand or process 1 minute. If mixing by hand, sprinkle work surface with 1 tablespoon reserved flour; turn dough out onto prepared work surface and knead for 10 minutes. Spray large bowl with nonstick cooking spray; place dough in bowl. Cover loosely with plastic wrap or a damp towel and let rise in a warm, draft-free place until dough doubles in volume, about 30–45 minutes.

3. Punch dough down and turn out onto work surface. Divide dough into 8 equal pieces.

4. Spray baking sheet with nonstick cooking spray. Form each piece of dough into a ball and flatten into a 4" disk. Place on prepared baking sheet; cover with plastic wrap or a damp towel and let rise in a warm, draft-free place until dough doubles in volume, about 30 minutes.

5. In small bowl, combine onion, poppy seeds and oil. With your thumb, press out a $1\frac{1}{2}$" well in the center of each piece of dough. Fill each well with 1 tablespoon of the onion mixture. Cover loosely with plastic wrap or a damp towel and let rise until dough doubles in volume, about 30 minutes.

6. Preheat oven to 425°F. Bake bialys on upper oven rack 12–15 minutes. Do not overbake; bialys should be chewy, not crisp. Cool on rack; serve at once or freeze.

*If mixing by hand (step 2), reserve an additional 1 tablespoon flour.

EACH SERVING (1 bialy) PROVIDES: ¼ Vegetable, 1½ Breads, 25 Optional Calories
PER SERVING: 158 Calories, 5 g Protein, 2 g Fat, 31 g Carbohydrate, 552 mg Sodium, 0 mg Cholesterol, 2 g Dietary Fiber

♦

STICKY BUNS

MAKES 8 SERVINGS

1 envelope active dry yeast
2 tablespoons lukewarm (105°–115°F) water
2 ¼ cups all-purpose flour*
2 tablespoons + 2 teaspoons granulated sugar
1½ teaspoons cinnamon
½ teaspoon salt
½ cup lukewarm (105°–115°F) skim milk
1 large egg
2 teaspoons stick margarine, melted
½ teaspoon butter flavoring
½ cup dark raisins
2 teaspoons skim milk
¼ cup confectioners sugar
½ teaspoon vanilla extract

1. In small bowl, sprinkle yeast evenly over lukewarm water. Let stand 10 minutes, until yeast is dissolved.

2. In large bowl or food processor, whisk together flour, granulated sugar, cinnamon and salt.

3. In small bowl, combine the lukewarm milk, egg, margarine and butter flavoring. Stir into yeast mixture and add to dry ingredients.

4. Process 1 minute or, if mixing by hand, sprinkle work surface with 1 tablespoon reserved flour; turn dough out onto prepared work surface and knead for 10 minutes. Spray bowl with nonstick cooking spray; place dough in bowl. Cover loosely with plastic wrap or a damp towel and let rise in a warm, draft-free place until dough doubles in volume, about 30–45 minutes.

5. Punch down dough and turn out onto prepared work surface. Knead in raisins and divide dough into 8 equal pieces.

6. Spray an 8" cake pan with nonstick cooking spray. Roll each piece of dough into an 8" cylinder and form each into a coil. Place coiled dough into prepared pan; cover loosely with plastic wrap or a damp towel and let rise until dough doubles in volume, about 35–40 minutes.

7. Preheat oven to 375°F. Brush tops of buns evenly with the 2 teaspoons skim milk. Bake on center oven rack 20–25 minutes.

8. While buns are baking, in small bowl, combine confectioners sugar, 1½ teaspoons warm water and vanilla extract. Spread evenly over buns as soon as they are removed from oven. Serve warm.

*If mixing by hand (step 4), reserve 1 tablespoon flour.

EACH SERVING (1 bun) PROVIDES: ¼ Fat, ½ Fruit, 1½ Breads, 50 Optional Calories
PER SERVING: 215 Calories, 6 g Protein, 2 g Fat, 44 g Carbohydrate, 167 mg Sodium, 27 mg Cholesterol, 2 g Dietary Fiber

---

Bake a Better Muffin

♦

- *Spray muffin tins with nonstick cooking spray; fill tins two-thirds full with batter; add a few tablespoons water to the empty spaces to keep empty cups from burning.*
- *For easier removal, allow muffins to "rest" in tins a few moments after baking.*
- *To reheat muffins, wrap loosely in foil, then heat in a 450°F oven about 5 minutes.*

JUST PLAIN MUFFINS

MAKES 12 SERVINGS

1 cup skim milk
1 egg
1 tablespoon + 1 teaspoon stick margarine, melted
$\frac{1}{2}$ teaspoon butter flavoring
1 $\frac{3}{4}$ cups all-purpose flour
1 tablespoon + 1 teaspoon granulated sugar
2 teaspoons baking powder
$\frac{1}{2}$ teaspoon salt

1. Preheat oven to 400°F. Spray a 12-muffin (2") tin with nonstick cooking spray.

2. In small bowl, combine milk, egg, margarine and butter flavoring. In larger bowl, combine the flour, sugar, baking powder and salt.

3. Add milk mixture to flour mixture, and stir just until flour disappears; do not overblend. Spoon into muffin tin and bake 20–25 minutes, or until toothpick comes out clean and muffins are golden brown. Cool on rack for 5 minutes; remove from pan and serve hot.

EACH SERVING (1 muffin) PROVIDES: $\frac{1}{4}$ Fat, $\frac{3}{4}$ Bread, 25 Optional Calories
PER SERVING: 99 Calories, 3 g Protein, 2 g Fat, 17 g Carbohydrate, 204 mg Sodium, 18 mg Cholesterol, 0 g Dietary Fiber

BERRY MUFFINS

Add $\frac{3}{4}$ cup fresh blueberries or raspberries to flour mixture. Increase Optional Calories to 30.

PER SERVING: 104 Calories, 3 g Protein, 2 g Fat, 18 g Carbohydrate, 204 mg Sodium, 18 mg Cholesterol, 1 g Dietary Fiber

SWEET MUFFINS

Use same amount of dark brown sugar or maple sugar instead of granulated.

PER SERVING: 99 Calories, 3 g Protein, 2 g Fat, 17 g Carbohydrate, 204 mg Sodium, 18 mg Cholesterol, 0 g Dietary Fiber

ORANGE MUFFINS

Substitute $\frac{1}{2}$ cup skim milk, $\frac{1}{2}$ cup fresh orange juice (milk will curdle) and 2 teaspoons orange zest for skim milk in basic recipe.

PER SERVING: 100 Calories, 3 g Protein, 2 g Fat, 17 g Carbohydrate, 198 mg Sodium, 18 mg Cholesterol, 1 g Dietary Fiber

LEMON MUFFINS

Substitute $\frac{3}{4}$ cup + 2 tablespoons skim milk, 2 tablespoons lemon juice (milk will curdle) and 2 teaspoons lemon zest for skim milk in basic recipe. Reduce Optional Calories to 20.

PER SERVING: 99 Calories, 3 g Protein, 2 g Fat, 17 g Carbohydrate, 203 mg Sodium, 18 mg Cholesterol, 0 g Dietary Fiber

PINEAPPLE MUFFINS

Add $\frac{1}{2}$ cup well-drained crushed pineapple to milk mixture. Increase Optional Calories to 30.

PER SERVING: 105 Calories, 3 g Protein, 2 g Fat, 18 g Carbohydrate, 204 mg Sodium, 18 mg Cholesterol, 2 g Dietary Fiber

CHOCOLATE MUFFINS

Use 2 tablespoons unsweetened cocoa powder and 1$\frac{1}{2}$ cups flour, and increase sugar to 2 tablespoons + 2 teaspoons. Add 1 teaspoon vanilla extract to liquid. Dust with 1 teaspoon confectioners sugar when slightly cooled.

EACH SERVING (1 muffin) PROVIDES: $\frac{1}{4}$ Fat, $\frac{1}{2}$ Bread, 35 Optional Calories
PER SERVING: 99 Calories, 3 g Protein, 2 g Fat, 17 g Carbohydrate, 204 mg Sodium, 18 mg Cholesterol, 2 g Dietary Fiber

◆

YOGURT BISCUITS

These biscuits make a good base for fruit shortcake or topping for chicken pot pie. They freeze very well.

MAKES 16 SERVINGS

2 cups minus 1 tablespoon all-purpose flour
    (reserve 1 tablespoon)
1 cup plain nonfat yogurt
1 teaspoon granulated sugar
2 teaspoons baking powder
$\frac{1}{2}$ teaspoon baking soda
$\frac{1}{2}$ teaspoon salt

1. In small bowl, combine 1 cup of the flour with the yogurt, blending until very smooth. Sprinkle with sugar; cover loosely with plastic wrap or a damp towel and let stand in a warm, draft-free place at least 4 hours, or overnight.

2. Preheat oven to 425°F. In separate bowl, combine remaining flour, the baking powder, baking soda and salt. Add to yogurt mixture, mixing until blended. Sprinkle work surface with 1 tablespoon reserved flour; turn dough out onto prepared work surface and pat into an 8 × 6" rectangle. Cut into 16 even pieces. Spray baking sheet with nonstick cooking spray; place biscuits on sheet, 1 inch apart. Bake 10 minutes; lower heat to 400°F and bake 10 minutes more, or until medium brown. Serve hot.

EACH SERVING (1 biscuit) PROVIDES: $\frac{1}{2}$ Bread, 20 Optional Calories
PER SERVING: 63 Calories, 2 g Protein, 0 g Fat, 13 g Carbohydrate, 178 mg Sodium, 0 mg Cholesterol, 0 g Dietary Fiber

PUMPKIN APPLE BREAD

MAKES 10 SERVINGS

2 cups all-purpose flour
$\frac{1}{4}$ cup + 1 teaspoon granulated sugar
1 teaspoon baking powder
$\frac{1}{2}$ teaspoon baking soda
$\frac{1}{2}$ teaspoon salt
$\frac{1}{2}$ teaspoon cinnamon
1 large egg
1 cup low-fat (1.5%) buttermilk
1 medium (6-ounce) apple, peeled, cored and grated
$\frac{1}{2}$ cup cooked puréed pumpkin or canned pumpkin purée
1 teaspoon confectioners sugar

1. Preheat oven to 350°F. Spray a 9 × 5" loaf pan with nonstick cooking spray.

2. In large bowl, combine flour, granulated sugar, baking powder, baking soda, salt and cinnamon.

3. In small bowl, beat egg; add buttermilk, apple and pumpkin.

4. Add egg mixture to flour mixture, and mix just until blended. Do not overblend.

5. Spoon into prepared pan and bake about 1–1$\frac{1}{4}$ hours, or until a toothpick inserted near center comes out clean. Cool for 10 minutes; turn out onto a rack and cool thoroughly. Dust with confectioners sugar and serve.

EACH SERVING PROVIDES: 1 Bread, 50 Optional Calories
PER SERVING: 155 Calories, 4 g Protein, 2 g Fat, 30 g Carbohydrate, 262 mg Sodium, 23 mg Cholesterol, 2 g Dietary Fiber

BANANA BREAD

MAKES 12 SERVINGS

1$\frac{3}{4}$ cups all-purpose flour
2 tablespoons + 2 teaspoons firmly packed light brown sugar
2$\frac{1}{4}$ teaspoons baking powder
$\frac{1}{2}$ teaspoon salt
$\frac{1}{2}$ teaspoon cinnamon
8 dried dates, chopped
6 dried apricot halves, chopped
1 egg
1 very ripe medium banana, mashed
$\frac{1}{4}$ cup skim milk

1. Preheat oven to 350°F. Spray an 8 × 4" loaf pan with nonstick cooking spray.

2. In medium bowl, combine flour, sugar, baking powder, salt and cinnamon. Add dates and apricots.

3. In small bowl, beat egg; add the mashed banana and milk.

4. Add the banana mixture to the flour mixture, and mix just until blended. Do not overblend.

5. Pour into prepared pan and bake about 1 hour, or until a toothpick inserted near center comes out clean. Cool thoroughly on rack.

EACH SERVING PROVIDES: $\frac{1}{2}$ Fruit, $\frac{3}{4}$ Bread, 25 Optional Calories
PER SERVING: 119 Calories, 3 g Protein, 1 g Fat, 26 g Carbohydrate, 193 mg Sodium, 18 mg Cholesterol, 1 g Dietary Fiber

Leni's Honey Loaf

*While very nice as a sweet bread, slices can also be
served as an easy dessert.*

Makes 12 Servings

$\frac{1}{4}$ cup + 2 tablespoons raisins
1 cup whole-wheat flour
$\frac{1}{2}$ cup all-purpose flour
2 teaspoons orange zest
$1\frac{1}{4}$ teaspoons baking powder
$\frac{1}{2}$ teaspoon salt
$\frac{1}{2}$ teaspoon baking soda
$\frac{3}{4}$ cup skim milk
$\frac{1}{4}$ cup honey
$\frac{1}{2}$ teaspoon walnut extract
1 ounce chopped walnuts

1. Preheat oven to 275°F. Spray an 8 × 4"
loaf pan with nonstick cooking spray.

2. Steam raisins in a covered strainer over
boiling water until soft and plumped, about 5
minutes. Set aside.

3. Combine whole-wheat flour, all-purpose
flour, zest, baking powder, salt and baking soda.
Add milk, honey and walnut extract, and beat by
hand or with a mixer just until smooth. Do not
overbeat. Fold in raisins and nuts.

4. Spoon into prepared pan and bake on center rack for 45–60 minutes until tester comes out
clean. Cool thoroughly on a rack before slicing.

EACH SERVING PROVIDES: $\frac{1}{4}$ Fruit, $\frac{1}{2}$ Bread, 50 Optional Calories
PER SERVING: 110 Calories, 3 g Protein, 2 g Fat, 22 g Carbo-
hydrate, 204 mg Sodium, 0 mg Cholesterol, 2 g Dietary Fiber

Zucchini Bread

Makes 7 Servings

1 egg
2 tablespoons + 2 teaspoons granulated sugar
$1\frac{1}{4}$ cups plus 1 tablespoon all-purpose flour
2 teaspoons baking powder
$\frac{1}{2}$ teaspoon salt
$\frac{1}{4}$ teaspoon nutmeg
$\frac{1}{2}$ cup low-fat (1.5%) buttermilk
2 teaspoons stick margarine, melted
1 teaspoon grated lemon zest
$\frac{1}{2}$ teaspoon butter flavoring
1 cup (4 ounces) zucchini, grated and squeezed dry

1. Preheat oven to 425°F. Spray an 8 × 4"
loaf pan with nonstick cooking spray.

2. In a large bowl, beat egg until pale yellow,
gradually adding sugar.

3. Sift flour, baking powder, salt and nutmeg
onto a sheet of waxed paper.

4. In small bowl, whisk together buttermilk,
margarine, zest and butter flavoring.

5. Alternately beat half the flour mixture and
half the buttermilk mixture into the egg mixture.
Fold in the zucchini, and spoon into the prepared
pan. Batter will be thick.

6. Bake in upper third of oven for 10 minutes. Reduce oven temperature to 400°F and bake
50–60 minutes longer, or until a cake tester
inserted near the center comes out clean. Cool on
a rack for 10 minutes; turn out and cool thoroughly before slicing.

EACH SERVING (1 ounce) PROVIDES: $\frac{1}{4}$ Fat, $\frac{1}{4}$ Vegetable, 1 Bread, 35
Optional Calories
PER SERVING: 136 Calories, 4 g Protein, 2 g Fat, 24 g Carbo-
hydrate, 337 mg Sodium, 31 mg Cholesterol, 1 g Dietary Fiber

SWEET BROWN BREAD

MAKES 12 SERVINGS

1¼ cups + 1 tablespoon whole-wheat flour
1 teaspoon baking powder
1 teaspoon grated orange or lemon zest
½ teaspoon baking soda
½ teaspoon cinnamon
⅛ teaspoon salt
½ cup low-fat (1.5%) buttermilk
1 egg
2 tablespoons + 2 teaspoons molasses
2 tablespoons + 2 teaspoons firmly packed dark brown sugar

1. Preheat oven to 375°F. Spray an 8 × 4" loaf pan with nonstick cooking spray.

2. In medium bowl, combine flour, baking powder, zest, baking soda, cinnamon and salt. In another bowl, combine buttermilk, egg, molasses and sugar.

3. Add molasses mixture to flour mixture, mixing quickly to blend. Do not overblend.

4. Pour into prepared pan and bake about 35–40 minutes, or until a toothpick inserted near the center comes out clean. Cool thoroughly on a rack before slicing.

EACH SERVING PROVIDES: ½ Bread, 35 Optional Calories
PER SERVING: 81 Calories, 3 g Protein, 2 g Fat, 16 g Carbohydrate, 135 mg Sodium, 18 mg Cholesterol, 2 g Dietary Fiber

IRISH SODA BREAD

MAKES 10 SERVINGS

1 cup low-fat (1.5%) buttermilk
2 tablespoons + 2 teaspoons honey
1½ cups + 1 tablespoon all-purpose flour (reserve 1 tablespoon)
½ cup whole-wheat flour
½ cup dried currants
2 teaspoons caraway seeds
2 teaspoons lemon zest
1 teaspoon baking soda
½ teaspoon salt
1 teaspoon granulated sugar

1. Preheat oven to 350°F. Spray baking sheet with nonstick cooking spray.

2. In small bowl, combine buttermilk and honey. In a larger bowl, combine all-purpose flour, whole-wheat flour, currants, caraway seeds, zest, baking soda and salt.

3. Add milk mixture to flour mixture, and stir just until flour disappears; do not overblend. Sprinkle work surface with 1 tablespoon reserved flour; turn dough out onto prepared work surface, flour hands and knead lightly seven times. Form into a 7" round loaf, and place on prepared baking sheet. Slash a cross on the top with a sharp knife or single-edge razor blade; sprinkle with the sugar and bake in upper third of oven about 40–45 minutes, or until nicely browned, and a toothpick inserted near center comes out clean. Cool on rack; serve at room temperature.

EACH SERVING PROVIDES: ¼ Fruit, 1 Bread, 50 Optional Calories
PER SERVING: 146 Calories, 4 g Protein, 1 g Fat, 31 g Carbohydrate, 263 mg Sodium, 2 mg Cholesterol, 2 g Dietary Fiber

CORNCAKES

MAKES 10 SERVINGS

¼ cup cornmeal
¼ cup boiling water
¼ cup all-purpose flour
1½ teaspoons baking powder
1 teaspoon granulated sugar
¼ teaspoon salt
½ cup cooked corn kernels, well drained
1 egg
¼ cup skim milk
2 teaspoons stick margarine, melted
½ teaspoon butter flavoring

1. In large bowl, stir boiling water into the cornmeal and let stand 30 minutes. In small bowl, combine flour, baking powder, granulated sugar and salt. Stir in the corn kernels. In another small bowl, combine egg, milk, margarine and butter flavoring.

2. Add egg mixture to soaked cornmeal; mix well. Add flour mixture, and beat just until well blended. Do not overbeat.

3. Heat a nonstick skillet over medium heat until a drop of water sizzles in it. Drop batter by 1½ tablespoonfuls onto skillet, and cook until bubbles form all over the top of batter. Turn; cook the other side until golden brown. You can do several at a time in a large skillet or griddle. Serve hot.

EACH SERVING (3 cakes) PROVIDES: ¼ Bread, 35 Optional Calories
PER SERVING: 52 Calories, 2 g Protein, 1 g Fat, 8 g Carbohydrate, 147 mg Sodium, 21 mg Cholesterol, 1 g Dietary Fiber

SOUR CREAM BLUEBERRY-LEMON PANCAKES

Using a nonstick skillet and nonstick cooking spray reduces the fat in these luscious pancakes dramatically! Blueberry and lemon add a fresh and unexpected taste to everyday pancakes.

MAKES 5 SERVINGS

1 cup minus 1 tablespoon all-purpose flour
1 tablespoon granulated sugar
1 teaspoon baking powder
¼ teaspoon salt
1 cup skim milk
¼ cup nonfat sour cream
¼ cup + 1 tablespoon egg substitute
1 teaspoon vanilla extract
1 tablespoon + 2 teaspoons margarine, melted
½ cup blueberries
Finely chopped zest of 1 lemon

1. In large bowl, combine flour, sugar, baking powder and salt; mix well.

2. In medium bowl, beat together milk, sour cream, egg substitute and vanilla.

3. Pour milk mixture over dry ingredients, and with a sturdy spoon, mix until batter is just smooth; stir in margarine. Gently fold in blueberries and lemon zest.

4. Spray nonstick skillet with nonstick cooking spray and set over medium heat; when hot, ladle a scant ½ cup of the batter into the pan to make a 6" pancake; when the top of the pancake is full of holes, flip the pancake and cook very briefly on the second side, just long enough to brown the second side. Slip onto plate and keep warm. Repeat with remaining batter.

EACH SERVING (1 pancake) PROVIDES: 1 Fat, ¼ Protein, 1 Bread, 45 Optional Calories
PER SERVING: 182 Calories, 7 g Protein, 5 g Fat, 27 g Carbohydrate, 312 mg Sodium, 1 mg Cholesterol, 1 g Dietary Fiber

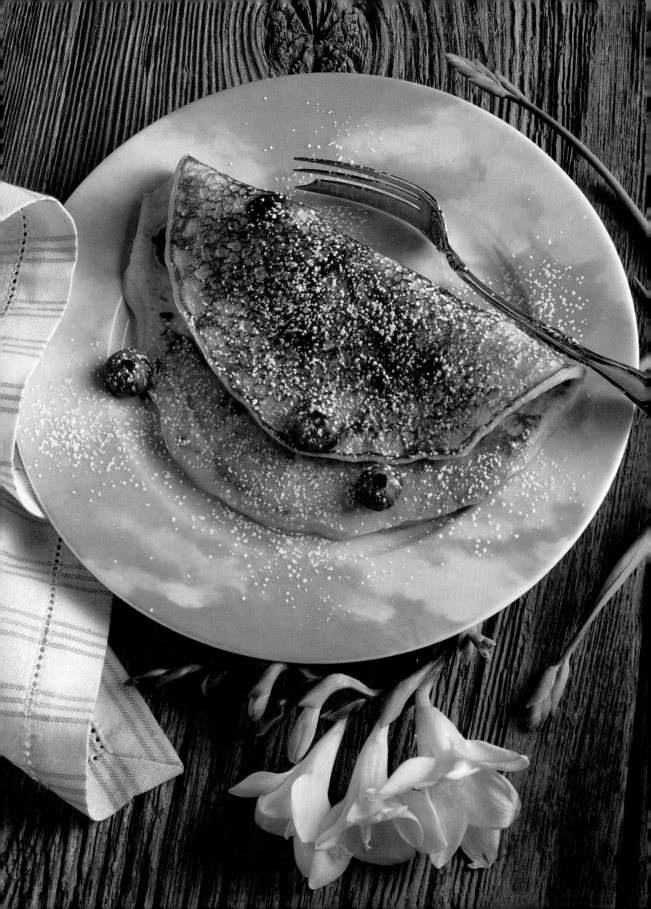

BAKED GERMAN PANCAKE

MAKES 4 SERVINGS

1 large egg, separated
½ cup skim milk
2½ teaspoons grated lemon zest
2 teaspoons granulated sugar
½ cup all-purpose flour
½ teaspoon baking powder
½ teaspoon salt
2 teaspoons stick margarine, melted
½ teaspoon butter flavoring
3 egg whites
2 tablespoons lemon juice
2 teaspoons confectioners sugar

1. Preheat oven to 450°F. Spray an 8" oven-proof skillet or cake pan with nonstick cooking spray.

2. In large bowl, beat egg yolk with milk, lemon zest and sugar. Sift flour, baking powder and salt together, and gradually whisk into yolk mixture. Add margarine and butter flavoring, and beat until smooth.

3. In another bowl, beat the four egg whites until stiff but not dry; fold into yolk mixture. Pour into prepared skillet and bake 10 minutes. Reduce heat to 350°F and bake 7–10 minutes more, or until toothpick inserted near center comes out clean. Sprinkle with lemon juice and confectioners sugar, and serve immediately.

EACH SERVING PROVIDES: ½ Fat, ½ Protein, ½ Bread, 40 Optional Calories
PER SERVING: 134 Calories, 7 g Protein, 4 g Fat, 18 g Carbohydrate, 431 mg Sodium, 54 mg Cholesterol, 0 g Dietary Fiber

Cold Carrot Soup with Indian Spices (page 96),
Vichyssoise (page 97), Chilled Spinach Soup (page 96)

CHAPTER FIVE

SOUPS

PISTOU

Pistou is a hearty French vegetable soup that uses a variation of pesto to create a rich flavor.

MAKES 4 SERVINGS

1 cup diagonally sliced carrots
5 ounces cubed pared yellow or white potato
  ($\frac{1}{2}$" cubes)
1 cup sliced, thoroughly washed leeks (white part
  only)
$\frac{3}{4}$ teaspoon salt
$\frac{1}{4}$ teaspoon pepper
1 cup sliced zucchini
1 cup trimmed green beans, cut into 1" pieces
3 ounces uncooked rotelle (spiral pasta)
4 ounces rinsed drained canned lima beans or red
  kidney beans
$\frac{3}{4}$ ounce grated Parmesan cheese
1 tablespoon tomato paste
2 tablespoons minced fresh basil
1 garlic clove, minced
1 tablespoon + 1 teaspoon olive oil

1. In large saucepan, combine carrots, potato, leeks, salt, pepper and 6 cups water. Bring to a boil; reduce heat. Simmer, covered, 30 minutes, stirring occasionally.

2. Add zucchini, green beans and pasta; stir to combine. Simmer, stirring occasionally, 10 minutes. Stir in lima beans.

3. In small bowl, whisk together Parmesan cheese, tomato paste, basil and garlic. Whisk in oil in a slow, steady stream. Stir $\frac{1}{2}$ cup of the hot broth into the basil mixture, then gradually stir into soup.

EACH SERVING (1$\frac{3}{4}$ cups) PROVIDES: 1 Fat, 2 Vegetables, $\frac{3}{4}$ Protein, 1$\frac{1}{4}$ Breads
PER SERVING: 251 Calories, 10 g Protein, 7 g Fat, 39 g Carbohydrate, 748 mg Sodium, 4 mg Cholesterol, 5 g Dietary Fiber

BLACK BEAN SOUP

You'll notice this soup thickens as it stands. When you reheat any leftover soup, thin it with a little water.

MAKES 4 SERVINGS

6 ounces dried turtle beans
2 teaspoons olive oil
1 cup + 2 tablespoons chopped onions
2 tablespoons chopped jalapeño peppers (about 2
  peppers, seeded)
1 garlic clove, minced
2 cups low-sodium chicken broth
1 teaspoon ground cumin
1 teaspoon ground coriander
2 tablespoons dry sherry
1 teaspoon lime juice
$\frac{1}{2}$ teaspoon salt
2 tablespoons chopped fresh cilantro

1. Rinse beans. Place in 3-quart saucepan; add water to cover and bring to a boil. Remove from heat; cover. Let stand 1 hour; drain.

2. In same saucepan, heat oil. Add 1 cup of the onions, the jalapeño peppers and garlic; sauté until soft, about 5 minutes. Stir in beans, broth, 1 cup water, cumin and coriander. Bring to a boil; reduce heat. Simmer, covered, 45 minutes, or until beans are tender. Remove from heat; stir in sherry, lime juice and salt. Let cool slightly.

3. In food processor or blender, purée soup until smooth. Pour back into saucepan and heat to serving temperature. Top each serving with equal amounts of the remaining 2 tablespoons chopped onion and the cilantro.

EACH SERVING ($\frac{3}{4}$ cup) PROVIDES: $\frac{1}{2}$ Fat, $\frac{1}{2}$ Vegetable, 2 Proteins, 15 Optional Calories
PER SERVING: 213 Calories, 11 g Protein, 4 g Fat, 33 g Carbohydrate, 308 mg Sodium, 0 mg Cholesterol, 6 g Dietary Fiber

NAVY BEAN AND ESCAROLE SOUP

MAKES 4 SERVINGS

6 ounces dried navy beans
1 teaspoon olive oil
$\frac{1}{2}$ cup chopped onion
$\frac{1}{2}$ cup slivered fresh fennel
$1\frac{1}{2}$ teaspoons finely chopped garlic clove
$\frac{1}{2}$ teaspoon dried thyme leaves
1 bay leaf
$1\frac{1}{2}$ cups packed escarole, cut into 1" pieces
$\frac{1}{2}$ cup diagonally sliced carrot
1 teaspoon salt
$\frac{1}{8}$ teaspoon pepper
2 tablespoons chopped fresh parsley
1 teaspoon grated lemon zest
1 garlic clove, minced
1 tablespoon fresh lemon juice

1. Rinse beans. Place in 3-quart saucepan; cover with 2 inches water and bring to a boil. Cook, partially covered, 1 hour, or until tender; drain.

2. In same saucepan, heat oil; add onion, fennel and finely chopped garlic. Sauté until soft, about 5 minutes. Add beans, 4 cups water, thyme and bay leaf. Bring to a boil; reduce heat. Simmer, partially covered, 30 minutes.

3. Add escarole, carrot, salt and pepper. Cook, uncovered, 15 minutes or until carrots are tender and escarole has wilted.

4. In small bowl, combine parsley, lemon zest and garlic; stir in juice. Stir into soup. Remove bay leaf.

EACH SERVING (1 cup) PROVIDES: $\frac{1}{4}$ Fat, $1\frac{1}{2}$ Vegetables, 2 Proteins
PER SERVING: 179 Calories, 11 g Protein, 2 g Fat, 32 g Carbohydrate, 582 mg Sodium, 0 mg Cholesterol, 6 g Dietary Fiber

MINESTRONE

While delicious when freshly made, this soup tastes even better when refrigerated and served the next day!

MAKES 8 SERVINGS

3 cups low-sodium chicken broth
2 cups shredded green cabbage
1 cup chopped onions
1 cup diagonally sliced carrots
1 cup diagonally sliced celery
1 cup julienned pared purple turnip
1 cup canned whole tomatoes
5 ounces pared julienned potato
2 teaspoons Italian seasoning
1 teaspoon salt
$\frac{1}{4}$ teaspoon pepper
1 cup trimmed green beans, cut into 1" pieces
1 cup halved lengthwise and sliced zucchini
6 ounces rinsed drained canned Roman or red kidney beans
1 cup cooked thin spaghetti, broken into halves
$1\frac{1}{2}$ ounces grated Romano or Parmesan cheese

1. In large saucepan, combine broth, 3 cups water, the cabbage, onions, carrots, celery, turnip, tomatoes, potato, Italian seasoning, salt and pepper. Bring to a boil; cover. Simmer 20 minutes.

2. Stir in green beans and zucchini; cover and cook 15 minutes longer. Stir in beans and spaghetti; heat to serving temperature. Sprinkle each serving with an equal amount of Romano cheese.

EACH SERVING ($1\frac{1}{2}$ cups) PROVIDES: $2\frac{1}{4}$ Vegetables, $\frac{1}{4}$ Protein, $\frac{3}{4}$ Bread, 10 Optional Calories
PER SERVING: 134 Calories, 7 g Protein, 3 g Fat, 22 g Carbohydrate, 491 mg Sodium, 6 mg Cholesterol, 4 g Dietary Fiber

ORIENTAL MUSHROOM-TOFU SOUP

Toasted sesame oil and brown rice udon can be found in health food or Asian food stores.

MAKES 4 SERVINGS

1 cup (1 ounce) dried Oriental mushrooms
2 cups boiling water
1½ cups low-sodium chicken broth
1 cup julienned snow peas, strings removed
½ cup sliced scallions
2 teaspoons toasted sesame oil or sesame oil
8 ounces firm tofu, cut into ¼"-thick slices, then into 1" cubes
3 ounces brown rice udon, broken into halves and cooked
⅛ teaspoon salt
⅛ teaspoon white pepper
1½ teaspoons white-wine vinegar

1. In small bowl, soak mushrooms in boiling water 10 minutes. Strain liquid into a 3-quart saucepan. Add broth and bring to a boil.

2. Meanwhile, trim tough stems from mushrooms; cut into strips.

3. To boiling broth, add mushrooms, snow peas, scallions and oil; heat 1 minute. Add tofu, brown rice udon, salt and white pepper; heat to serving temperature. Stir in vinegar and serve.

EACH SERVING (1¼ cups) PROVIDES: ½ Fat, 1¼ Vegetables, 1 Protein, 1 Bread, 10 Optional Calories
PER SERVING: 232 Calories, 14 g Protein, 8 g Fat, 27 g Carbohydrate, 105 mg Sodium, 0 mg Cholesterol, 2 g Dietary Fiber

HERBED SPLIT PEA SOUP

Turkey ham gives you the great flavor of ham, without a lot of fat, in this slimmed-down version of classic split pea soup.

MAKES 4 SERVINGS

6 ounces dried green or yellow split peas
2 teaspoons olive oil
½ cup chopped onion
½ cup chopped carrot
1 garlic clove, minced
2 ounces slivered no-sugar-added turkey ham
1 teaspoon dried marjoram
¾ teaspoon salt
⅛ teaspoon pepper

1. Sort and rinse peas. Place in 3-quart saucepan; cover with 2 inches water and bring to a boil. Remove from heat; cover. Let stand 1 hour; drain.

2. In same saucepan, heat oil; add onion, carrot and garlic. Sauté until soft, about 5 minutes. Add peas and 4 cups water. Bring to a boil; reduce heat. Simmer, covered, 1 hour, or until peas are tender, stirring once.

3. Add turkey ham, marjoram, salt and pepper; heat to serving temperature. Soup thickens upon standing. When reheating, add additional water to thin.

EACH SERVING (1 cup) PROVIDES: ½ Fat, ½ Vegetable, 2½ Proteins
PER SERVING: 198 Calories, 14 g Protein, 4 g Fat, 29 g Carbohydrate, 565 mg Sodium, 9 mg Cholesterol, 3 g Dietary Fiber

Lentil and Swiss Chard Soup

Makes 4 Servings

2 teaspoons olive oil
$\frac{1}{2}$ cup chopped onion
1 garlic clove, minced
2 cups low-sodium beef broth
6 ounces dried lentils
1 cup shredded Swiss chard, packed
1 tablespoon chopped fresh cilantro
$\frac{1}{4}$ teaspoon ground cumin
$\frac{1}{4}$ teaspoon salt
$\frac{1}{8}$ teaspoon pepper
2 teaspoons fresh lemon juice
Cilantro sprigs to garnish (optional)

1. In 3-quart nonstick saucepan, heat oil; add onion and garlic. Sauté until soft, about 5 minutes. Add broth, 2 cups water and lentils. Bring to a boil; reduce heat. Simmer, covered, 45 minutes.

2. Add Swiss chard, cilantro, cumin, salt and pepper; cook 5 minutes or until chard has wilted. Stir in juice. Garnish with cilantro sprig.

EACH SERVING (1 cup) PROVIDES: $\frac{1}{2}$ Fat, $\frac{3}{4}$ Vegetable, 2 Proteins, 10 Optional Calories
PER SERVING: 182 Calories, 13 g Protein, 3 g Fat, 28 g Carbohydrate, 167 mg Sodium, 0 mg Cholesterol, 5 g Dietary Fiber

Beef Barley Soup

This soup thickens after standing, so when reheating, add a bit of water to thin it.

Makes 4 Servings

10 ounces boneless round steak, cut into eighteen 1" cubes
3 ounces barley
$1\frac{1}{2}$ ounces dried lima beans
$\frac{3}{4}$ cup chopped onions
$\frac{3}{4}$ cup chopped carrots
$\frac{1}{2}$ cup sliced celery
1 teaspoon salt
$\frac{1}{4}$ teaspoon fennel seeds (optional)
$\frac{1}{8}$ teaspoon pepper
1 cup sliced mushrooms

1. In large saucepan, combine meat, barley, lima beans and 5 cups water. Bring to a boil; skim off foam. Add onions, carrots, celery, salt, fennel seed if using, and pepper. Bring back to a boil; reduce heat. Simmer, covered, $1\frac{1}{2}$ hours.

2. Add mushrooms. Cook, covered, 15 minutes longer, or until meat is tender.

EACH SERVING ($1\frac{1}{2}$ cups) PROVIDES: $1\frac{1}{2}$ Vegetables, 2 Proteins, $1\frac{1}{2}$ Breads
PER SERVING: 236 Calories, 22 g Protein, 4 g Fat, 28 g Carbohydrate, 617 mg Sodium, 41 mg Cholesterol, 7 g Dietary Fiber

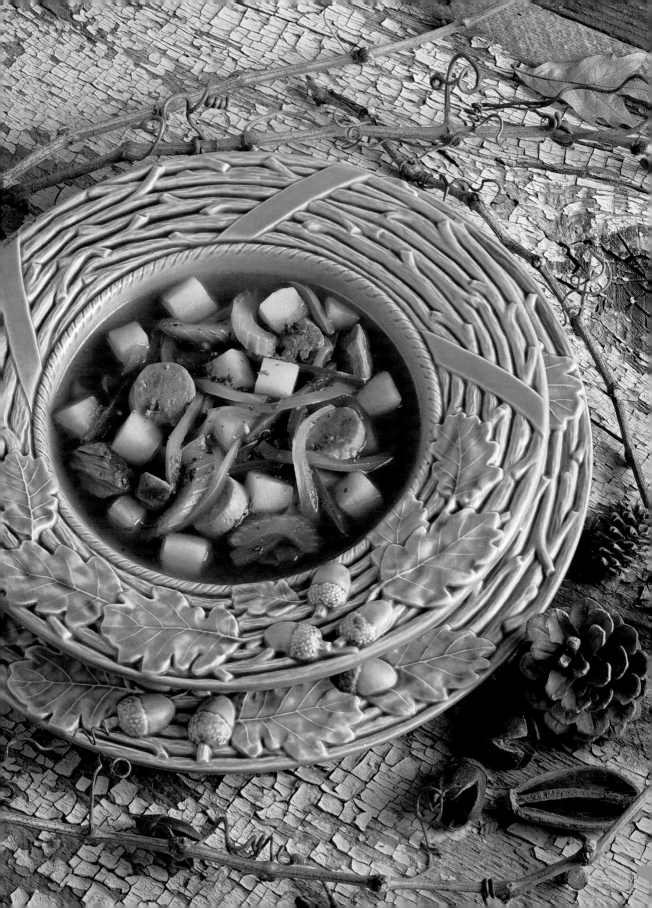

VEAL AND SAUSAGE PEPPERPOT

Veal is substituted for the tripe usually called for in the traditional pepperpot.

MAKES 4 SERVINGS

1 tablespoon + 1 teaspoon olive oil
1 pound, 2 ounces meaty veal shanks
4 ounces 90% fat-free hot Italian turkey sausage
3 cups low-sodium beef broth
1 cup sliced onions
3 parsley sprigs
1 teaspoon Italian seasoning
$\frac{1}{2}$ teaspoon black peppercorns
1 bay leaf
1 cup slivered red onion
$\frac{1}{2}$ cup diagonally sliced celery
1 cup slivered red bell pepper
1 cup slivered green bell pepper
10 ounces cubed pared potatoes ($\frac{1}{2}$" cubes)
1 teaspoon salt
$\frac{1}{2}$ teaspoon pepper
2 tablespoons chopped fresh parsley

1. In large saucepan, heat 1 tablespoon of the oil. Slowly brown veal shanks and sausage. Remove sausage; cool; slice and refrigerate.

2. To same saucepan, add broth, 3 cups hot water, sliced onions, parsley sprigs, Italian seasoning, peppercorns and bay leaf. Bring to a boil; reduce heat. Simmer, partially covered, 1 hour, or until veal is tender.

3. Remove shanks from stock; cool. Strain stock through colander lined with a double thickness of cheesecloth into a very large bowl; measure 5 cups. Reserve any remaining stock for future use. Skim off surface fat (or refrigerate overnight, cooling meat and stock separately). Remove meat from bones; meat should weigh 9 ounces. Cut into cubes.

4. In large nonstick skillet, heat the remaining 1 teaspoon oil. Add red onion and celery; sauté until soft, about 3–5 minutes. Add bell pepper; sauté until soft, about 5–10 minutes.

5. Meanwhile, bring the 5 cups of stock to a boil in large saucepan. Add potatoes, salt and pepper; cook 10 minutes. Add sautéed vegetables, cooked veal and sausage; cook 10 minutes longer. Sprinkle each serving with parsley.

EACH SERVING (1$\frac{1}{2}$ cups) PROVIDES: $\frac{1}{4}$ Fat, 2$\frac{1}{4}$ Vegetables, 3 Proteins, $\frac{1}{2}$ Bread, 45 Optional Calories
PER SERVING: 264 Calories, 21 g Protein, 9 g Fat, 26 g Carbohydrate, 817 mg Sodium, 64 mg Cholesterol, 4 g Dietary Fiber

◆

CORN CHOWDER

MAKES 4 SERVINGS

2 slices turkey bacon, cut into $\frac{1}{2}$" pieces
$\frac{1}{2}$ cup chopped onion
$\frac{1}{2}$ cup chopped yellow bell pepper
2$\frac{1}{2}$ cups low-sodium chicken broth
10 ounces cubed pared potatoes ($\frac{1}{2}$" cubes)
2 cups whole corn kernels
$\frac{1}{4}$ cup light cream

1. In 3-quart saucepan, cook bacon in 2 tablespoons water. Remove with slotted spoon to paper towel; discard liquid.

2. Add onion and bell pepper and 2 teaspoons water to saucepan; sauté until soft, about 5 minutes. Add broth and potatoes. Bring to a boil; lower heat. Simmer, partially covered, 10 minutes, or until potatoes are tender. Add corn; simmer 5 minutes longer. Remove from heat; cool slightly.

3. Place 2 cups soup into food processor or blender; purée until smooth. Pour back into saucepan. Stir in cream and heat to serving temperature. Top each serving evenly with bacon pieces.

EACH SERVING (1 cup) PROVIDES: $\frac{1}{2}$ Vegetable, 1$\frac{1}{2}$ Breads, 60 Optional Calories
PER SERVING: 198 Calories, 76 g Protein, 6 g Fat, 32 g Carbohydrate, 149 mg Sodium, 15 mg Cholesterol, 4 g Dietary Fiber

GUMBO

Gumbo gives you the best of all worlds, showcasing shrimp, chicken and kielbasa in a savory broth. For speed, you'll find that frozen, sliced okra works well in this recipe.

MAKES 4 SERVINGS

1 tablespoon + 1 teaspoon reduced-calorie tub margarine
1 cup coarsely chopped green bell pepper
$\frac{1}{2}$ cup chopped celery
$\frac{1}{2}$ cup sliced scallions
1 garlic clove, minced
2 cups canned no-salt-added tomatoes with juice
2 cups low-sodium chicken broth
1 cup trimmed sliced ($\frac{1}{2}$" slices) fresh or frozen okra, thawed
$\frac{1}{2}$ teaspoon dried thyme leaves
1 bay leaf
$\frac{1}{8}$ to $\frac{1}{4}$ teaspoon ground red pepper
3 ounces uncooked regular long-grain rice
12 medium-size peeled deveined shrimp
4 ounces boneless chicken breast, cut into $\frac{1}{2}$" pieces
2 ounces cooked kielbasa, cut into 8 slices

1. In large nonstick saucepan, melt margarine. Add bell pepper, celery, scallions and garlic; sauté until soft, about 5 minutes. Add tomatoes, broth, okra, thyme, bay leaf and red pepper. Bring to a boil; lower heat. Simmer, covered, 15 minutes.

2. Stir in rice and simmer, covered, 15 minutes longer. Add shrimp, chicken and kielbasa; simmer, covered, 5 minutes longer or until shrimp is opaque, chicken is not pink and rice is tender. Remove bay leaf.

EACH SERVING (1$\frac{1}{2}$ cups) PROVIDES: $\frac{1}{2}$ Fat, 2$\frac{1}{2}$ Vegetables, 2 Proteins, $\frac{3}{4}$ Bread, 10 Optional Calories
PER SERVING: 279 Calories, 22 g Protein, 8 g Fat, 29 g Carbohydrate, 332 mg Sodium, 91 mg Cholesterol, 3 g Dietary Fiber

BOUILLABAISSE

MAKES 4 SERVINGS

2 teaspoons olive oil
$\frac{1}{2}$ cup chopped shallots
1 garlic clove, minced
2 cups no-salt-added canned tomatoes
$\frac{1}{2}$ cup clam juice
4 fluid ounces ($\frac{1}{2}$ cup) dry white wine
1 tablespoon chopped fresh parsley
1 tablespoon tomato paste
$\frac{1}{2}$ teaspoon dried thyme leaves
1 bay leaf
$\frac{1}{8}$ teaspoon crushed saffron (dissolved in 1 tablespoon hot water)
$\frac{1}{8}$ teaspoon fennel seed, crushed
10 ounces boneless firm white fish (tilefish, red snapper or monkfish), cut in $\frac{1}{2}$" chunks
Four 3-ounce fresh or thawed frozen lobster tails, halved
12 medium littleneck clams, scrubbed
2 cups cooked regular long-grain rice

1. In large nonstick saucepan, heat oil; add shallots and garlic. Sauté until soft, about 3 minutes. Add tomatoes, 1$\frac{1}{2}$ cups water, clam juice, wine, parsley, tomato paste, thyme, bay leaf, saffron and fennel seed; stir to combine. Bring to a boil; reduce heat. Simmer, covered, 30 minutes.

2. Add fish, lobster and clams; return to a boil; reduce heat. Simmer, covered, 6–8 minutes, until clams open and fish and lobster are cooked through. Remove bay leaf.

3. To serve, spoon rice into 4 shallow soup bowls; ladle bouillabaise evenly over rice.

EACH SERVING (1$\frac{3}{4}$ cups) PROVIDES: $\frac{1}{2}$ Fat, 1$\frac{1}{4}$ Vegetables, 3 Proteins, 1 Bread, 25 Optional Calories
PER SERVING: 348 Calories, 29 g Protein, 5 g Fat, 40 g Carbohydrate, 334 mg Sodium, 40 mg Cholesterol, 2 g Dietary Fiber

FISH CHOWDER

This versatile chowder lets you take advantage of the freshest fish available at the market.

MAKES 4 SERVINGS

1 tablespoon + 1 teaspoon reduced-calorie tub margarine
$\frac{1}{2}$ cup chopped onion
$\frac{1}{2}$ cup chopped carrot
1 garlic clove, minced
4 cups low-sodium chicken broth
5 ounces diced pared potato
13 ounces boneless firm white fish (orange roughy, red snapper, tilefish or sea bass), cut into $\frac{1}{2}$" chunks
3 tablespoons chopped fresh parsley
1 tablespoon snipped fresh dill
$\frac{1}{8}$ teaspoon white pepper
1 cup skim milk

1. In 3-quart nonstick saucepan, melt margarine. Add onion, carrot and garlic; sauté until soft, about 5 minutes. Add broth and potato. Bring to a boil; lower heat. Simmer, covered, 15 minutes or until potato is tender.

2. Add fish, parsley, dill and white pepper. Simmer, covered, 5 minutes or until fish flakes easily when tested with a fork. Stir in milk. Heat to serving temperature.

EACH SERVING (1¼ cups) PROVIDES: ½ Fat, ½ Vegetable, 1¼ Proteins, ¼ Bread, 30 Optional Calories
PER SERVING: 218 Calories, 18 g Protein, 10 g Fat, 13 g Carbohydrate, 173 mg Sodium, 19 mg Cholesterol, 1 g Dietary Fiber

CREAMY CLAM CHOWDER

MAKES 4 SERVINGS

10 ounces diced pared potatoes ($\frac{1}{2}$" dice)
$\frac{1}{2}$ cup chopped celery
$\frac{1}{2}$ cup chopped onion
1 tablespoon + 1 teaspoon reduced-calorie tub margarine
1 tablespoon all-purpose flour
1 cup skimmed milk
1 cup evaporated skimmed milk
8 ounces drained canned clams, $\frac{1}{2}$ cup juice reserved
$\frac{1}{2}$ teaspoon dried thyme leaves
$\frac{1}{8}$ teaspoon white pepper
2 strips crisp cooked bacon, crumbled (optional)*

1. In 3-quart saucepan, combine potatoes, 1 cup water, celery, onion and margarine. Bring to a boil; reduce heat. Simmer, covered, 13–15 minutes, or until potatoes are tender.

2. Place flour in a medium bowl. Stir in milk and evaporated skimmed milk. Add to potatoes in saucepan. Add clams with reserved $\frac{1}{2}$ cup juice, thyme and white pepper. Cook and stir over medium heat until chowder has thickened slightly, about 10 minutes. Do not boil. Sprinkle each serving evenly with crumbled bacon, if desired.

*If using bacon, increase Optional Calories to 25.

EACH SERVING (1¼ cups) PROVIDES: ¾ Milk, ½ Fat, ½ Vegetable, 1 Protein, ½ Bread, 10 Optional Calories
PER SERVING: 246 Calories, 24 g Protein, 3 g Fat, 30 g Carbohydrate, 288 mg Sodium, 42 mg Cholesterol, 2 g Dietary Fiber

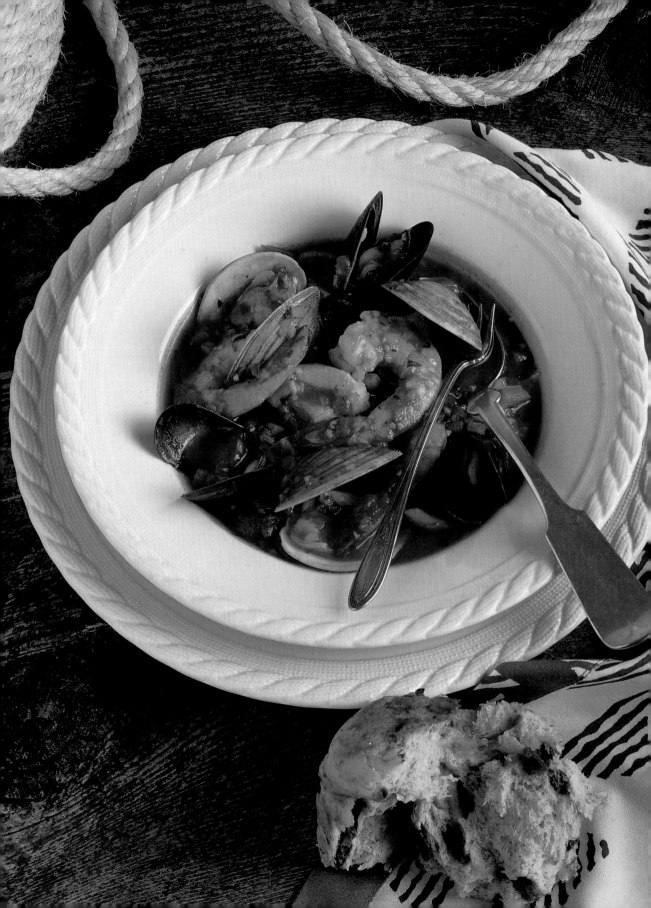

CIOPPINO

MAKES 4 SERVINGS

2 teaspoons olive oil
½ cup finely chopped onion
½ cup diced green bell pepper
1½ teaspoons finely chopped garlic
2 cups canned tomatoes
8 fluid ounces (1 cup) dry white wine
¼ cup tomato paste
¼ cup chopped fresh flat-leaf (Italian) parsley
¼ teaspoon pepper
¼ teaspoon dried basil
¼ teaspoon dried oregano
1 bay leaf
10 ounces boneless firm white fish (hake, tilefish, monkfish), cut in 1½" chunks
12 medium littleneck clams, scrubbed
12 medium mussels, scrubbed and debearded
8 medium shelled and deveined shrimp

1. In large nonstick saucepan, heat oil. Add onion, bell pepper and garlic; sauté until soft, about 5 minutes. Stir in tomatoes, wine, ½ cup water, tomato paste, parsley, pepper, basil, oregano and bay leaf. Bring to a boil; reduce heat. Simmer, covered, 30 minutes.

2. Add fish; simmer, uncovered, 3 to 5 minutes. Add clams and mussels; simmer, covered, 3 to 5 minutes. Add shrimp; simmer, covered, 3 to 5 minutes, until clams and mussels are open and shrimp are opaque. Remove bay leaf.

EACH SERVING (1¾ cups) PROVIDES: ½ Fat, 2 Vegetables, 2½ Proteins, 50 Optional Calories
PER SERVING: 257 Calories, 27 g Protein, 6 g Fat, 14 g Carbohydrate, 507 mg Sodium, 61 mg Cholesterol, 1 g Dietary Fiber

MULLIGATAWNY SOUP

An east Indian curry soup.

MAKES 4 SERVINGS

1 tablespoon + 1 teaspoon reduced-calorie tub margarine
½ cup chopped onion
½ cup chopped carrot
½ cup chopped celery
½ cup chopped green bell pepper
1 small tart green apple, pared, cored and diced
¼ cup all-purpose flour
2 teaspoons curry powder
⅛ teaspoon mace
1 whole clove
2 cups low-sodium chicken broth
1 cup chopped seeded peeled tomatoes
1 teaspoon lemon juice
6 ounces cooked diced chicken
¼ teaspoon salt

In 3-quart nonstick saucepan, melt margarine. Add onion, carrot, celery, bell pepper and apple; sauté until vegetables are soft, about 5 minutes. Add flour, curry, mace and clove; cook and stir 1 minute. Gradually stir in chicken broth. Add tomatoes and lemon juice. Bring to a boil, stirring occasionally; lower heat. Simmer, covered, 30 minutes, stirring occasionally. Add chicken and salt; simmer 5 minutes longer.

EACH SERVING (1 cup) PROVIDES: ½ Fat, ¼ Fruit, 1½ Vegetables, 1½ Proteins, ¼ Bread, 20 Optional Calories
PER SERVING: 199 Calories, 15 g Protein, 6 g Fat, 18 g Carbohydrate, 259 mg Sodium, 38 mg Cholesterol, 3 g Dietary Fiber

CHICKEN SOUP WITH HERBED MATZO BALLS

MAKES 4 SERVINGS

1 large egg, separated
1 large egg white
Pinch cream of tartar
1 tablespoon seltzer
$\frac{1}{8}$ teaspoon salt
$\frac{1}{4}$ cup + 2 tablespoons matzo meal
1 tablespoon minced scallions
1 tablespoon snipped fresh dill
4 cups low-sodium chicken broth
$\frac{1}{4}$ cup julienned carrot
$\frac{1}{4}$ cup julienned parsnip
Dill sprigs to garnish (optional)

1. With electric mixer at high speed, beat both egg whites with cream of tartar until stiff, but not dry, peaks form; set aside.

2. In small bowl, beat egg yolk with seltzer and salt until thick and doubled in volume. Fold in egg whites. Combine matzo meal with scallions and dill; fold into egg mixture. Refrigerate at least 30 minutes.

3. In large saucepan, bring 2 quarts water to boiling (add pinch of salt, if desired). Shape matzo mixture into 8 equal-size balls. Drop into boiling water. Simmer, covered, 20–30 minutes.

4. Meanwhile, in 3-quart saucepan, bring chicken broth, carrot and parsnip to a boil; reduce heat. Simmer, covered, 5 minutes, or until vegetables are tender. Lift matzo balls from water with slotted spoon to soup; heat to serving temperature. Ladle soup and equal amounts of vegetables into 4 soup bowls, with 2 matzo balls each. Garnish with dill sprig.

EACH SERVING (1 cup soup + vegetables, 2 matzo balls) PROVIDES: $\frac{1}{4}$ Vegetable, $\frac{1}{4}$ Protein, $\frac{1}{2}$ Bread, 25 Optional Calories
PER SERVING: 112 Calories, 6 g Protein, 3 g Fat, 14 g Carbohydrate, 156 mg Sodium, 53 mg Cholesterol, 1 g Dietary Fiber

---

Soup Economics

◆

Soup is an economical dish, as it comfortably incorporates leftovers and uses its tasty broth to extend the meal. Try making soups such as Minestrone (page 83) and Mulligatawny (page 91) when you have leftover vegetables. You can also get the maximum use from chicken and beef bones by making your own stocks—see pages 349 and 350. Homemade broth freezes well and can be easily stored for soup whenever you please. And fans of croutons can make their own from leftover bread—see page 357.

TORTELLINI IN CHICKEN BROTH

In Italy this soup is called tortellini en brodo.

MAKES 4 SERVINGS

2 cups low-sodium chicken broth
2 cups cooked cheese tortellini
1 cup slivered watercress leaves, thick stems removed
2 tablespoons sliced scallions
Few drops hot red pepper sauce (optional)
$\frac{3}{4}$ ounce grated Romano or Parmesan cheese
Freshly ground black pepper

In 3-quart saucepan, heat broth and $\frac{2}{3}$ cup water. Add cooked tortellini, watercress and scallions. Cook over medium heat 2 minutes or until tortellini is hot and watercress has wilted. Add red pepper sauce, if using. Serve sprinkled with cheese and black pepper to taste.

EACH SERVING (1 cup) PROVIDES: $\frac{1}{2}$ Vegetable, 1 Protein, $\frac{1}{2}$ Bread, 25 Optional Calories
PER SERVING: 212 Calories, 13 g Protein, 5 g Fat, 29 g Carbohydrate, 356 mg Sodium, 38 mg Cholesterol, 0 g Dietary Fiber

POTATO–SWEET POTATO SOUP

MAKES 4 SERVINGS

2 teaspoons reduced-calorie tub margarine
$\frac{1}{2}$ cup chopped shallots or onion
10 ounces diced pared white or all-purpose potatoes ($\frac{1}{2}$" dice)
8 ounces diced pared sweet potatoes ($\frac{1}{2}$" dice)
$1\frac{1}{2}$ cups low-sodium chicken broth
$\frac{1}{4}$ teaspoon salt
$\frac{1}{8}$ teaspoon white pepper
$\frac{1}{4}$ teaspoon mace
1 cup evaporated skimmed milk
1 tablespoon chopped fresh parsley to garnish (optional)

1. In 3-quart saucepan, melt margarine. Add shallots and sauté until soft, about 3 minutes. Add white potatoes and sweet potatoes, broth, salt, white pepper and mace. Bring to a boil; lower heat. Simmer, covered, 6–8 minutes, or until potatoes are tender. Remove from heat; cool slightly.

2. In food processor or blender, purée 1 cup of the potatoes with some stock until smooth. Pour back into saucepan. Stir in evaporated milk. Heat to serving temperature. Sprinkle each serving with parsley.

EACH SERVING (1 cup) PROVIDES: $\frac{1}{2}$ Milk, $\frac{1}{4}$ Fat, $\frac{1}{4}$ Vegetable, 1 Bread, 10 Optional Calories
PER SERVING: 200 Calories, 9 g Protein, 2 g Fat, 38 g Carbohydrate, 261 mg Sodium, 3 mg Cholesterol, 3 g Dietary Fiber

PUMPKIN SOUP WITH CINNAMON TOAST TRIANGLES

If you like, you can substitute frozen butternut squash* for the pumpkin. This soup is also delicious served cold.

MAKES 4 SERVINGS

1 cup canned pumpkin purée
2 cups frozen yellow turnips, cooked
1 cup low-sodium chicken broth
$\frac{1}{4}$ teaspoon salt
$\frac{1}{4}$ teaspoon ground ginger
$\frac{1}{4}$ teaspoon cinnamon
$\frac{1}{8}$ teaspoon ground nutmeg
Dash white pepper
1 cup evaporated skimmed milk
1 tablespoon + 1 teaspoon reduced-calorie tub margarine
$\frac{3}{4}$ teaspoon granulated sugar
2 slices 9-grain or whole-wheat bread
Parsley sprigs to garnish (optional)

1. In 3-quart saucepan, combine pumpkin, turnips, broth, $\frac{1}{4}$ cup water, salt, ginger, $\frac{1}{8}$ teaspoon of the cinnamon, the nutmeg and white pepper. Blend in evaporated milk. Heat slowly to serving temperature, stirring occasionally.

2. Meanwhile, in small bowl, combine margarine, sugar and the remaining $\frac{1}{8}$ teaspoon cinnamon. Spread equally over bread slices. Toast in toaster oven or under broiler until golden. Cut each slice into 4 triangles. Ladle soup into bowls; serve 2 bread triangles with each bowl and garnish with parsley sprig.

*If using squash, add $\frac{1}{4}$ Bread Selection per serving and reduce Vegetable Selection to 1.

EACH SERVING (1$\frac{1}{4}$ cups soup + 2 toast triangles) PROVIDES: $\frac{1}{2}$ Milk, $\frac{1}{2}$ Fat, $1\frac{1}{2}$ Vegetables, $\frac{1}{2}$ Bread, 10 Optional Calories
PER SERVING: 134 Calories, 7 g Protein, 3 g Fat, 20 g Carbohydrate, 331 mg Sodium, 3 mg Cholesterol, 2 g Dietary Fiber

ONION SOUP GRATINÉE

This recipe can easily be doubled when you'd like to serve four. To make short work of slivering the onion, first cut it into quarters, then sliver each quarter.

MAKES 2 SERVINGS

1 tablespoon reduced-calorie tub margarine
1½ cups slivered Spanish onion
½ cup thoroughly washed sliced leeks (white part only)
1 cup low-sodium beef broth
⅛ teaspoon pepper
2 slices (1 ounce each) semolina bread, toasted
1 tablespoon + 1 teaspoon grated Parmesan cheese
1½ ounces shredded reduced-fat Swiss cheese

1. In 2-quart nonstick saucepan, melt margarine. Add onion and leeks; sauté over medium heat, stirring occasionally, until onion is golden, about 15 minutes.

2. Add broth, 1 cup water and pepper. Bring to a boil; lower heat. Simmer, covered, 15 minutes.

3. Preheat broiler. Set 2 flameproof bowls on baking sheet. Ladle half the soup into each bowl; top each portion with 1 slice bread. Sprinkle each with half the Parmesan cheese and then half the Swiss cheese. Broil until cheese is melted, about 2 minutes.

EACH SERVING (1 cup) PROVIDES: ¾ Fat, 2 Vegetables, 1 Protein, 1 Bread, 30 Optional Calories
PER SERVING: 284 Calories, 15 g Protein, 9 g Fat, 30 g Carbohydrate, 321 mg Sodium, 18 mg Cholesterol, 4 g Dietary Fiber

CREAM OF BROCCOFLOWER SOUP

Broccoflower is a new vegetable that is a combination of broccoli and cauliflower. If it is unavailable, simply substitute broccoli or a mixture of broccoli and cauliflower.

MAKES 4 SERVINGS

1½ cups low-sodium chicken broth or Vegetable Stock (page 349)
2 cups coarsely chopped broccoflower
½ cup chopped scallions
2 tablespoons reduced-calorie stick margarine
2 tablespoons all-purpose flour
½ teaspoon dried marjoram leaves
¼ teaspoon salt
⅛ teaspoon white pepper
1 cup evaporated skimmed milk
Broccoflower florets to garnish (optional)

1. In 3-quart saucepan, combine broth, broccoflower and scallions. Bring to a boil; reduce heat. Simmer, covered, 10 minutes, or until broccoflower is tender. Remove from heat; cool slightly. Place soup in food processor or blender; purée until smooth.

2. In saucepan, melt margarine. Blend in flour, marjoram, salt and white pepper. Gradually stir in evaporated milk until mixture is smooth. Cook and stir over medium heat until mixture thickens and bubbles. Stir in puréed soup. Heat to serving temperature. Garnish with broccoflower florets.

EACH SERVING (¾ cup) PROVIDES: ½ Milk, 1 Fat, 1¼ Vegetables, 25 Optional Calories
PER SERVING: 116 Calories, 7 g Protein, 4 g Fat, 14 g Carbohydrate, 306 mg Sodium, 3 mg Cholesterol, 2 g Dietary Fiber

TOMATO-ORANGE SOUP

This soup is lovely served hot or cold. If you are serving it hot, you may like to add ¹/₂ cup cooked brown or white rice to each serving for extra body. If you do, add one Bread Selection per serving .

MAKES 4 SERVINGS

1 tablespoon reduced-calorie tub margarine
¹/₄ cup chopped shallots or onion
1 tablespoon all-purpose flour
1 cup low-sodium chicken broth
1 cup canned no-salt-added crushed tomatoes
¹/₂ teaspoon granulated sugar
¹/₄ teaspoon salt
¹/₂ cup orange juice
¹/₄ teaspoon ground allspice
¹/₄ cup plain low-fat yogurt
Orange triangles to garnish (optional)

In 3-quart nonreactive saucepan, melt margarine. Add shallots; sauté until soft, about 5 minutes. Stir in flour. Gradually stir in broth, then add tomatoes, sugar and salt. Bring to a boil, stirring frequently; lower heat. Simmer, covered, 15 minutes. Stir in juice and allspice; heat to serving temperature. Top each serving with 1 tablespoon of yogurt. Garnish with orange triangle, if desired.

EACH SERVING (³/₄ cup) PROVIDES: ¹/₄ Fat, ¹/₄ Fruit, ¹/₂ Vegetable, 25 Optional Calories
PER SERVING: 72 Calories, 3 g Protein, 2 g Fat, 11 g Carbohydrate, 192 mg Sodium, 2 mg Cholesterol, 1 g Dietary Fiber

HERBED CUCUMBER AND YOGURT SOUP

In Greece, this refreshing cold soup is called Tzatiki.

MAKES 4 SERVINGS

3 cups plain low-fat yogurt
1¹/₂ cups chopped seeded pared cucumber
1 tablespoon snipped fresh dill
1 tablespoon minced fresh mint
1 tablespoon snipped fresh chives
1 garlic clove, minced
1 teaspoon lemon juice (optional)
¹/₄ teaspoon salt
¹/₈ teaspoon white pepper
Mint, dill or chive to garnish (optional)

In large bowl, combine yogurt, cucumber, 1 cup water, dill, mint, chives, garlic, juice, salt and white pepper; blend thoroughly. Cover and refrigerate until well chilled. Garnish with mint, dill or chive.

EACH SERVING (1¹/₄ cups) PROVIDES: 1 Milk, ³/₄ Vegetable
PER SERVING: 117 Calories, 9 g Protein, 3 g Fat, 14 g Carbohydrate, 258 mg Sodium, 10 mg Cholesterol, 0 g Dietary Fiber

---

Power Lunches

◆

Soup is a wonderful lunch, whether it's a warm soup on a chilly day or a cold soup when it's warm and sultry. And soup is easy to take to work or school, even if you don't have access to a refrigerator or a microwave oven. Just pour it into a vacuum container, and you can enjoy a hot or cold soup whenever you please. After using your vacuum container, wash thoroughly and rinse with boiling water. Before filling with hot soup, rinse again with hot water. You may also want to buy a lunch box, which helps to keep food well insulated and in which you can also tote along other lunchtime treats!

CHILLED SPINACH SOUP

MAKES 4 SERVINGS

1 tablespoon reduced-calorie tub margarine
$\frac{1}{2}$ cup chopped onion or scallions
1 package (10 ounces) frozen chopped spinach,
    partially thawed
2 cups low-sodium chicken broth
$\frac{1}{4}$ teaspoon salt
$\frac{1}{8}$ teaspoon pepper
$\frac{1}{8}$ teaspoon ground nutmeg
$\frac{1}{2}$ cup evaporated skimmed milk
2 teaspoons minced fresh mint
1 teaspoon grated lemon zest
Lemon slices and mint sprigs to garnish (optional)

1. In 3-quart nonstick saucepan, melt margarine. Add onion and sauté until soft, about 5 minutes. Add spinach, broth, salt, pepper and nutmeg. Bring to a boil; lower heat. Simmer, covered, 10 minutes, or until spinach is tender. Remove from heat; cool slightly.

2. Pour mixture into food processor or blender container; purée until smooth. Pour into medium bowl. Stir in milk, minced mint and lemon zest. Cover and refrigerate until well chilled. Garnish each serving with a lemon slice and mint sprig, if desired.

EACH SERVING (1 cup) PROVIDES: $\frac{1}{4}$ Milk, $\frac{1}{4}$ Fat, 1$\frac{1}{4}$ Vegetables, 15 Optional Calories
PER SERVING: 78 Calories, 6 g Protein, 2 g Fat, 9 g Carbohydrate, 286 mg Sodium, 1 mg Cholesterol, 2 g Dietary Fiber

COLD CARROT SOUP WITH INDIAN SPICES

MAKES 4 SERVINGS

2 teaspoons olive oil
$\frac{1}{2}$ cup chopped onion
2 teaspoons curry powder
$\frac{1}{4}$ teaspoon ground coriander
$\frac{1}{4}$ teaspoon ground cardamom
4 cups chopped pared carrots (1" chunks)
3 cups low-sodium chicken broth
$\frac{1}{4}$ cup plain low-fat yogurt
Carrot curls and mint sprigs to garnish (optional)

1. In 3-quart nonstick saucepan, heat oil. Add onion and sauté until soft, about 5 minutes.

2. Add curry powder, coriander and cardamom; cook and stir 1 minute. Add carrots and broth. Bring to a boil; reduce heat. Simmer, covered, 20 minutes, or until carrots are tender. Strain broth into a large bowl.

3. In food processor or blender, purée carrots with part of the broth until smooth. Stir purée into broth. Cover and refrigerate until well chilled. Top each serving with 1 tablespoon yogurt; garnish with carrot curl and mint sprig, if desired.

EACH SERVING ($\frac{3}{4}$ cup) PROVIDES: $\frac{1}{2}$ Fat, 2$\frac{1}{4}$ Vegetables, 25 Optional Calories
PER SERVING: 110 Calories, 4 g Protein, 4 g Fat, 16 g Carbohydrate, 90 mg Sodium, 1 mg Cholesterol, 4 g Dietary Fiber

---

Cold Soups

◆

We are used to thinking of soups as warm and cozy, but they are also delightful hot-weather fare. Cold soups are a boon to cooks, as they can be prepared ahead of time and then whisked out of the refrigerator when needed. Try Herbed Cucumber and Yogurt Soup (page 95), Chilled Spinach Soup (above) or Summer Squash Soup (page 97) as refreshing starters. Hearty Vichyssoise (page 97), Borscht (page 98) or Gazpacho with 9-Grain Croutons (page 100) makes a wonderful meal. And, for a different dessert, try the luscious Cherry-Berry Soup (page 98).

SUMMER SQUASH SOUP

MAKES 4 SERVINGS

2 teaspoons olive oil
$\frac{1}{2}$ cup chopped scallions
$\frac{1}{2}$ cup chopped celery
1 garlic clove, minced
$1\frac{3}{4}$ cups coarsely shredded zucchini
$1\frac{3}{4}$ cups coarsely shredded yellow squash
$1\frac{1}{2}$ cups low-sodium chicken broth
$\frac{1}{4}$ teaspoon salt
$\frac{1}{4}$ teaspoon white pepper
$\frac{1}{4}$ cup chopped fresh basil
$\frac{1}{4}$ cup nonfat sour cream
Julienned zucchini or yellow squash and basil
    sprigs to garnish (optional)

1. In 3-quart nonstick saucepan, heat oil. Add scallions, celery and garlic; sauté until soft, about 5 minutes. Add zucchini, yellow squash, broth, salt and white pepper. Bring to a boil; lower heat. Simmer, uncovered, 15 minutes. Remove from heat; cool slightly.

2. In food processor or blender, purée soup with basil until smooth. Pour into a large bowl. Cover and refrigerate until well chilled. When ready to serve, swirl in sour cream. Garnish with julienned zucchini and basil sprig, if desired.

EACH SERVING ($\frac{3}{4}$ cup) PROVIDES: $\frac{1}{2}$ Fat, $2\frac{1}{4}$ Vegetables, 20 Optional Calories
PER SERVING: 71 Calories, 4 g Protein, 3 g Fat, 8 g Carbohydrate, 183 mg Sodium, 0 mg Cholesterol, 1 g Dietary Fiber

VICHYSSOISE

An elegant French soup that is wonderful in warm weather; it's also an elegant first course.

MAKES 4 SERVINGS

1 tablespoon + 1 teaspoon reduced-calorie tub
    margarine
$\frac{1}{2}$ cup sliced thoroughly washed leeks (white part
    only)
10 ounces cubed pared yellow or white potatoes
    ($\frac{1}{4}$" cubes)
2 cups low-sodium chicken broth
1 cup evaporated skimmed milk
$\frac{1}{4}$ teaspoon salt
$\frac{1}{4}$ teaspoon white pepper
$\frac{1}{4}$ teaspoon ground nutmeg
$\frac{1}{4}$ cup light cream
Chive sprigs to garnish (optional)

1. In 3-quart nonstick saucepan, melt margarine. Add leeks and sauté until soft, about 2 minutes. Add potatoes, broth, milk, salt, pepper and nutmeg. Bring to a boil over high heat; reduce heat. Simmer, uncovered, 3 minutes or until potatoes are fork-tender. Remove from heat; cool slightly.

2. In food processor or blender, purée soup until smooth. Pour into a large bowl. Stir in cream. Cover and refrigerate until well chilled. Garnish with chive sprigs, if desired.

EACH SERVING (1 cup) PROVIDES: $\frac{1}{2}$ Milk, $\frac{1}{2}$ Fat, $\frac{1}{4}$ Vegetable, $\frac{1}{2}$ Bread, 40 Optional Calories
PER SERVING: 176 Calories, 8 g Protein, 6 g Fat, 23 g Carbohydrate, 285 mg Sodium, 12 mg Cholesterol, 1 g Dietary Fiber

BORSCHT

MAKES 4 SERVINGS

2 cups low-sodium chicken broth
2 cups shredded fresh beets
½ cup sliced scallions
½ teaspoon firmly packed light brown sugar
½ cup shredded red cabbage
2 tablespoons snipped fresh dill
1 teaspoon grated lemon zest
2 tablespoons fresh lemon juice
¼ teaspoon salt
⅛ teaspoon white pepper
¼ cup light sour cream
Fresh dill sprigs to garnish

1. In 3-quart nonreactive saucepan, combine broth, beets, scallions, brown sugar and 1½ cups water. Bring to a boil; lower heat. Simmer, covered, 15 minutes. Add cabbage and dill. Cook, covered, 5 minutes longer or until beets and cabbage are soft. Remove from heat.

2. Stir in lemon zest and juice, salt and pepper. Pour into medium bowl. Cover and refrigerate until well chilled. Top each serving with 1 tablespoon sour cream and a dill sprig.

EACH SERVING (1 cup) PROVIDES: 1½ Vegetables, 30 Optional Calories
PER SERVING: 82 Calories, 4 g Protein, 3 g Fat, 12 g Carbohydrate, 215 mg Sodium, 5 mg Cholesterol, 1 g Dietary Fiber

CHERRY-BERRY SOUP

MAKES 4 SERVINGS

2 cups canned tart red pitted cherries packed in juice
1½ cups sliced strawberries
2 tablespoons granulated sugar
1 tablespoon cornstarch
2 teaspoons grated orange zest
¼ teaspoon cinnamon
½ cup orange juice
2 fluid ounces (¼ cup) sweet red wine
¼ cup vanilla-flavored nonfat yogurt (sweetened with aspartame)
Mint sprigs to garnish (optional)

1. Drain juice from cherries into food processor or blender. Remove eight perfect cherries; set aside in refrigerator. Add remaining cherries to food processor or blender. Add strawberries, sugar, cornstarch, orange zest and cinnamon; purée until smooth.

2. Pour puréed fruit into a 3-quart nonreactive saucepan. Stir in orange juice and wine. Bring to a boil over medium-low heat, stirring constantly, until mixture thickens slightly; boil 1 minute.

3. Pour mixture into a sieve set over a medium bowl; press out pulp using the back of wooden spoon. Cover and refrigerate until well chilled.

4. When ready to serve, ladle soup evenly into 4 chilled soup bowls. Top each serving with 1 tablespoon of the yogurt, 2 reserved cherries and a mint sprig, if desired.

EACH SERVING (¾ cup) PROVIDES: 1¾ Fruits, 60 Optional Calories
PER SERVING: 125 Calories, 2 g Protein, 0 g Fat, 28 g Carbohydrate, 19 mg Sodium, 0 mg Cholesterol, 2 g Dietary Fiber

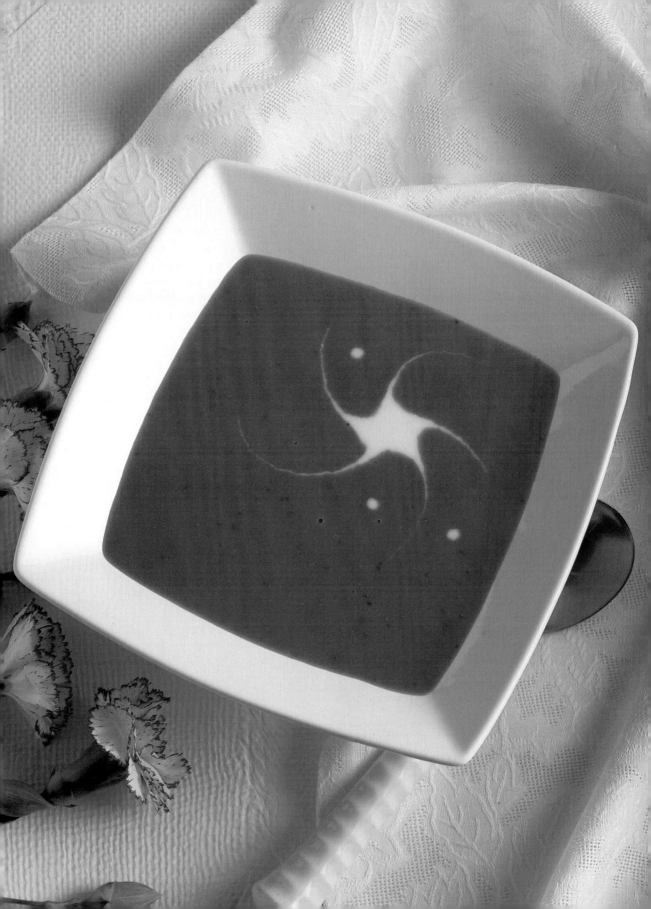

GAZPACHO WITH 9-GRAIN CROUTONS

This is virtually a floating salad! The croutons add crunch and texture to this refreshing soup.

MAKES 4 SERVINGS

1½ cups sliced peeled plum tomatoes
½ cup chopped unpared cucumber
½ cup sliced scallions
2 tablespoons tarragon wine vinegar
1 large garlic clove
2 cups spicy mixed vegetable juice or low-sodium mixed vegetable juice
1 teaspoon dried tarragon
¼ teaspoon hot red pepper sauce*
Salt to taste
1 tablespoon reduced-calorie tub margarine
2 teaspoons olive oil
1 garlic clove, minced
2 slices 9-grain or whole-wheat bread, cut in 1" cubes

1. In food processor or blender, place tomatoes, cucumber, scallions, vinegar and whole garlic clove; process, in pulses, until vegetables are chunky. Pour into a large bowl. Stir in vegetable juice, tarragon and pepper sauce, if using. Salt to taste. Cover and refrigerate until well chilled.

2. Just before serving, in medium skillet, melt margarine with oil; add the minced garlic. Add bread cubes; toss to coat. Cook and stir just until bread begins to brown, about 2–3 minutes. Top each serving equally with croutons.

*Omit liquid red pepper sauce if using spicy vegetable juice.

EACH SERVING (1 cup) PROVIDES: ¾ Fat, 2¼ Vegetables, ½ Bread, 5 Optional Calories
PER SERVING: 113 Calories, 3 g Protein, 4 g Fat, 17 g Carbohydrate, 491 mg Sodium, 0 mg Cholesterol, 2 g Dietary Fiber

SWEET AND SOUR CABBAGE SOUP

This soup tastes even better the next day.

MAKES 4 SERVINGS

2 teaspoons canola or vegetable oil
1 cup chopped onions
6 cups shredded green cabbage
4 cups low-sodium beef broth
1 cup canned crushed tomatoes in tomato purée
¼ cup dark raisins
2 tablespoons firmly packed light brown sugar
2 tablespoons fresh lemon juice
1 teaspoon salt
¼ teaspoon caraway seeds
Pinch black pepper

In large nonstick saucepan, heat oil; add onions. Sauté over medium-low heat until golden, about 5 minutes, stirring frequently. Add cabbage, broth, 2 cups water, tomatoes, raisins, brown sugar, juice, salt, caraway seeds and pepper. Bring to a boil; reduce heat. Simmer, covered, 1 hour, stirring occasionally.

EACH SERVING (1½ cups) PROVIDES: ½ Fat, ½ Fruit, 4 Vegetables, 45 Optional Calories
PER SERVING: 143 Calories, 4 g Protein, 3 g Fat, 29 g Carbohydrate, 670 mg Sodium, 0 mg Cholesterol, 4 g Dietary Fiber

Marinated Three-Bean Salad (page 130),
German Potato Salad (page 130)

CHAPTER SIX

VEGETABLES AND SALADS

HERB-STUFFED ARTICHOKES

MAKES 4 SERVINGS

4 medium artichokes (12 ounces each)
$\frac{1}{2}$ lemon
$\frac{3}{4}$ cup plain dried bread crumbs
1 cup chopped tomato
2 tablespoons chopped fresh parsley
2 tablespoons chopped fresh basil
2 tablespoons chopped fresh tarragon
2 tablespoons lemon juice
$\frac{1}{2}$ teaspoon chopped fresh rosemary
1 teaspoon grated lemon zest
$\frac{1}{2}$ teaspoon salt
$\frac{1}{4}$ teaspoon freshly ground black pepper

1. With large stainless steel knife, cut off stem of each artichoke flush with base so that artichokes will stand upright; remove and discard center leaves and choke. With scissors, trim 1" from the top of each artichoke; rub cut ends with lemon.

2. In large saucepan with 2 quarts of water, arrange prepared artichokes and lemon half; bring to a boil. Reduce heat to low; simmer 15–20 minutes, until tender. Meanwhile, preheat oven to 350°F.

3. On baking sheet, sprinkle bread crumbs; toast in oven 15–20 minutes, or until lightly browned, and transfer to bowl; add tomato, parsley, basil, tarragon, lemon juice, rosemary, lemon zest, salt and pepper; toss to mix well.

4. Fill center of each artichoke with one-fourth of the bread crumb mixture; arrange stuffed artichokes on baking sheet. Bake 25–30 minutes, until heated through.

EACH SERVING PROVIDES: 1$\frac{1}{2}$ Vegetables, 1 Bread
PER SERVING: 160 Calories, 8 g Protein, 2 g Fat, 33 g Carbo-hydrate, 583 mg Sodium, 0 mg Cholesterol, 9 g Dietary Fiber

BRAISED BELGIAN ENDIVE WITH LEMON

MAKES 4 SERVINGS

4 medium Belgian endive (about 4 ounces each), trimmed, with discolored leaves removed
$\frac{1}{2}$ cup chicken broth
1 tablespoon fresh lemon juice
2 teaspoons chopped fresh parsley
$\frac{1}{4}$ teaspoon grated lemon zest
$\frac{1}{4}$ teaspoon salt
$\frac{1}{4}$ teaspoon freshly ground black pepper

1. Preheat oven to 350°F. In a 13 × 9" baking pan, arrange endive; add broth and lemon juice. Cover with foil; bake 25 minutes, until fork-tender.

2. Remove foil; bake 5 minutes longer. To serve, sprinkle with parsley, lemon zest, salt and pepper.

EACH SERVING PROVIDES: 1 Vegetable, 3 Optional Calories
PER SERVING: 20 Calories, 1 g Protein, 0 g Fat, 4 g Carbohydrate, 266 mg Sodium, 0 mg Cholesterol, 2 g Dietary Fiber

---

Great Greens

◆

The key to exciting salads is variety, and there is a whole world of salad greens beyond iceberg lettuce. Try mixing and matching different combinations of the greens listed below, then top with your favorite dressing. See pages 136–137 for fresh dressing recipes.

Bibb lettuce	*Romaine*	*Chicory*
Boston lettuce	*Cabbage*	*Beet greens*
Spinach	*Escarole*	*Chard*
Arugula	*Watercress*	*Collard greens*
Radicchio	*Mustard*	*Belgian endive*
Nasturtium		

Oven-Roasted Beets and Garlic

Makes 4 Servings

4 large beets (2½" diameter), trimmed, pared and
  quartered (about 2 cups)
6 garlic cloves, quartered
2½ teaspoons chopped fresh thyme
2 teaspoons olive oil
¼ cup + 1 tablespoon orange juice

1. Preheat oven to 375°F. In medium bowl,
combine beets, garlic, oil and 1½ teaspoons of the
thyme. Transfer to a 9 × 13" baking pan.

2. In same bowl, combine juice and 2 tablespoons water; pour over beet mixture. Roast, covered with foil, 50 minutes, until tender. Remove
foil; roast 10 minutes longer. To serve, sprinkle
with the remaining teaspoon of thyme.

EACH SERVING PROVIDES: ½ Fat, 1 Vegetable, 10 Optional Calories
PER SERVING: 65 Calories, 1 g Protein, 2 g Fat, 10 g Carbohydrate, 43 mg Sodium, 0 mg Cholesterol, 2 g Dietary Fiber

◆

Broccoli-Garlic Sauté

Makes 4 Servings

2 teaspoons olive oil
4 cups chopped broccoli, steamed until tender-
  crisp
3 garlic cloves, minced
¼ teaspoon dried oregano leaves, crushed
¼ cup julienned roasted red bell pepper

1. In large nonstick skillet, heat oil; add broccoli, garlic and oregano. Sauté over medium-high
heat, stirring, 3 minutes, until garlic is golden.

2. Add bell pepper to skillet; cook, stirring
frequently, 2 minutes.

EACH SERVING PROVIDES: ½ Fat, 2 Vegetables
PER SERVING: 51 Calories, 3 g Protein, 3 g Fat, 6 g Carbohydrate,
24 mg Sodium, 0 mg Cholesterol, 3 g Dietary Fiber

Brussels Sprouts Sauté

Makes 4 Servings

2 teaspoons olive oil
¼ cup chopped red onion
2 ounces julienned boiled ham
2 cups Brussels sprouts, steamed until tender-crisp
  and quartered
⅓ cup orange sections
1 tablespoon cider vinegar
1 teaspoon caraway seeds

1. In large nonstick skillet, heat oil; add
onion. Cook over medium-high heat, stirring frequently, 3–4 minutes, until translucent. Add ham;
cook, stirring frequently, 2 minutes.

2. Add Brussels sprouts, orange sections,
vinegar and caraway seeds to skillet; sauté, stirring
frequently, 1 minute, until heated through.

EACH SERVING PROVIDES: ½ Fat, 1 Vegetable, ½ Protein, 15
Optional Calories
PER SERVING: 73 Calories, 5 g Protein, 3 g Fat, 7 g Carbohydrate,
183 mg Sodium, 8 mg Cholesterol, 3 g Dietary Fiber

STIR-FRIED ASPARAGUS AND CARROTS

MAKES 4 SERVINGS

$\frac{1}{3}$ cup low-sodium chicken broth
2 teaspoons reduced-sodium soy sauce
1 teaspoon cornstarch
$\frac{1}{2}$ teaspoon granulated sugar
1 teaspoon vegetable oil
24 asparagus spears, cut into $\frac{1}{2}$" diagonal pieces
$\frac{1}{2}$ cup thinly sliced carrot

1. In small bowl, combine broth, soy sauce, cornstarch and sugar; stir until cornstarch and sugar are dissolved.

2. In large nonstick skillet, heat oil over high heat; add asparagus. Cook 2 minutes, stirring constantly, until bright green. Add broth mixture and carrot; cook 3 minutes, stirring constantly, until asparagus is tender and sauce is thickened.

EACH SERVING PROVIDES: $\frac{1}{4}$ Fat, $1\frac{1}{4}$ Vegetables, 5 Optional Calories
PER SERVING: 43 Calories, 3 g Protein, 1 g Fat, 6 g Carbohydrate, 111 mg Sodium, 0 mg Cholesterol, 1 g Dietary Fiber

◆

DILLED CARROTS

MAKES 4 SERVINGS

4 cups sliced carrots ($\frac{1}{4}$" slices)
2 bay leaves
1 cinnamon stick
$\frac{1}{2}$ teaspoon salt
$\frac{1}{4}$ cup fresh lemon juice
2 tablespoons chopped fresh dill
1 tablespoon + 1 teaspoon olive oil
1 teaspoon granulated sugar
$\frac{1}{8}$ teaspoon ground red pepper

1. In large skillet, combine carrots, bay leaves, cinnamon stick and salt; add water to cover and bring to a boil. Reduce heat to low; simmer 10 minutes, or until tender. Drain well; set aside.

2. In medium bowl, whisk together juice, dill, oil, sugar and red pepper. Add cooked carrots; toss to coat. Refrigerate, covered, 1 hour. Serve at room temperature.

EACH SERVING PROVIDES: 1 Fat, 2 Vegetables, 5 Optional Calories
PER SERVING: 98 Calories, 1 g Protein, 5 g Fat, 14 g Carbohydrate, 313 mg Sodium, 0 mg Cholesterol, 4 g Dietary Fiber

◆

HONEY-GLAZED CARROTS

MAKES 4 SERVINGS

4 pared medium carrots, cut into 3" sticks
2 tablespoons fresh lemon juice
2 tablespoons honey
2 teaspoons unsalted stick margarine
2 teaspoons grated lemon zest
Pinch ground coriander
1 tablespoon chopped fresh cilantro
$\frac{1}{8}$ teaspoon freshly ground black pepper

1. In large nonstick skillet, combine carrots, juice, 2 tablespoons water, the honey, margarine, lemon zest and coriander; bring to a boil. Reduce heat to low; simmer, covered, 5 minutes, just until tender.

2. Uncover and increase heat to medium; cook, stirring occasionally, 3 minutes, until most of the liquid has evaporated and carrots are glazed. To serve, sprinkle with cilantro and pepper.

EACH SERVING PROVIDES: $\frac{1}{2}$ Fat, 2 Vegetables, 30 Optional Calories
PER SERVING: 95 Calories, 1 g Protein, 2 g Fat, 20 g Carbohydrate, 58 mg Sodium, 0 mg Cholesterol, 3 g Dietary Fiber

BRAISED RED CABBAGE WITH GINGER

MAKES 4 SERVINGS

2 teaspoons olive oil
$\frac{1}{2}$ cup thinly sliced onion
2 tablespoons chopped fresh ginger root
4 cups thinly sliced red cabbage
$\frac{2}{3}$ cup chicken broth

1. In medium saucepan, heat oil; add onion and ginger. Cook over medium heat, stirring frequently, 1 minute; stir in cabbage and broth.

2. Reduce heat to low; simmer, covered, stirring occasionally, 20 minutes, until cabbage is tender.

EACH SERVING PROVIDES: $\frac{1}{2}$ Fat, $2\frac{1}{4}$ Vegetables, 5 Optional Calories
PER SERVING: 53 Calories, 2 g Protein, 3 g Fat, 7 g Carbohydrate, 174 mg Sodium, 0 mg Cholesterol, 2 g Dietary Fiber

◆

STEAMED CAULIFLOWER WITH TOMATO-CURRY SAUCE

MAKES 4 SERVINGS

1 teaspoon olive oil
$\frac{1}{2}$ cup finely chopped onion
2 teaspoons grated fresh ginger root
2 teaspoons curry powder
$\frac{1}{2}$ teaspoon ground cumin
1 cup tomato purée
4 cups cauliflower florets, steamed until tender-crisp (hot)
1 tablespoon chopped fresh parsley

1. In large nonstick skillet, heat oil; add onion and ginger. Cook over medium heat, stirring frequently, 4–5 minutes, until onion is translucent. Stir in curry powder and cumin; cook 1 minute.

2. Stir in purée and $\frac{1}{2}$ cup water. Reduce heat to low; simmer, covered, stirring occasionally, 15 minutes. Remove from heat; let cool slightly. Transfer to blender or food processor; purée until smooth.

3. To serve, arrange florets in serving bowl; top with tomato-curry sauce and sprinkle with parsley.

EACH SERVING PROVIDES: $\frac{1}{4}$ Fat, $3\frac{1}{4}$ Vegetables
PER SERVING: 73 Calories, 3 g Protein, 2 g Fat, 14 g Carbohydrate, 266 mg Sodium, 0 mg Cholesterol, 5 g Dietary Fiber

◆

LEMON-SAUTÉED GREEN BEANS WITH PARSLEY

MAKES 4 SERVINGS

1 teaspoon olive oil
3 cups cut green beans (2" pieces)
2 tablespoons chopped fresh parsley
1 tablespoon fresh lemon juice

1. In large nonstick skillet, heat oil over medium-high heat; add beans. Sauté, stirring frequently, 3 minutes, until beans are bright green; add parsley. Cook, stirring frequently, 3 minutes.

2. Add juice and 2 tablespoons water; mix well. Reduce heat to medium; cook, covered, 2–3 minutes. Uncover; cook, stirring frequently, 2–3 minutes longer, until beans are tender-crisp.

EACH SERVING PROVIDES: $\frac{1}{4}$ Fat, $1\frac{1}{2}$ Vegetables
PER SERVING: 37 Calories, 2 g Protein, 1 g Fat, 6 g Carbohydrate, 6 mg Sodium, 0 mg Cholesterol, 2 g Dietary Fiber

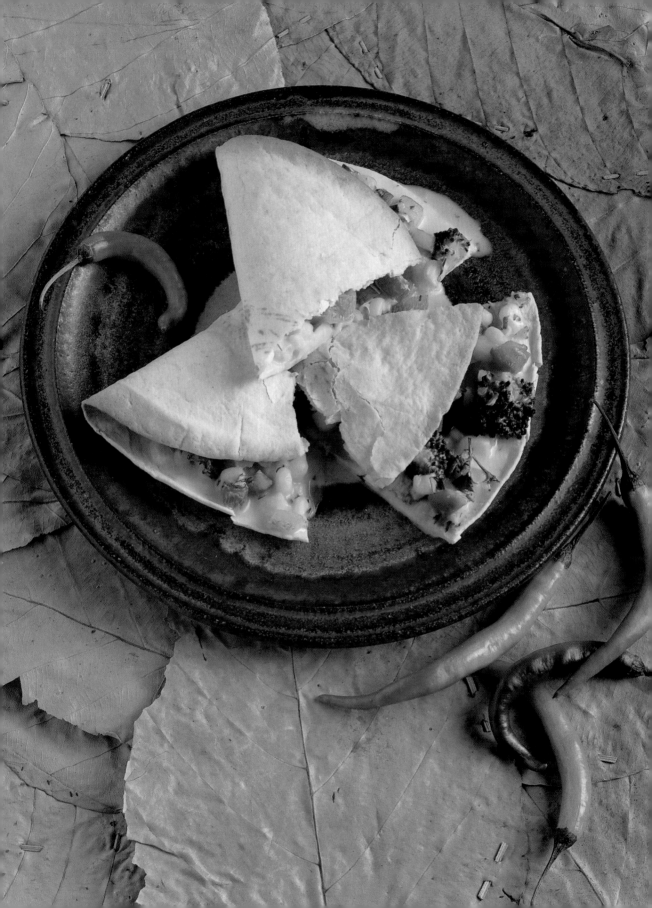

VEGETABLE QUESADILLAS

MAKES 4 SERVINGS

2 cups small broccoli florets
$1\frac{1}{2}$ cups skim milk
$\frac{1}{3}$ cup + 2 teaspoons all-purpose flour
$\frac{1}{2}$ cup thawed frozen whole-kernel corn
$\frac{1}{4}$ cup coarsely chopped red bell pepper
$\frac{1}{4}$ cup coarsely chopped green chilies
$\frac{1}{2}$ teaspoon salt
$\frac{1}{8}$ teaspoon ground red pepper
$\frac{1}{4}$ cup chopped fresh cilantro
4 flour tortillas (6" diameter)

1. In large pot of boiling water, cook broccoli 2 minutes; drain. Set aside; keep warm.

2. In small saucepan, whisk milk and flour; cook over medium heat, stirring frequently, 4–5 minutes. Stir in corn, bell pepper, chilies, salt and red pepper; remove from heat. Stir in cilantro.

3. Preheat oven to 425°F. Spray baking sheet with nonstick cooking spray.

4. Spoon one-fourth of the vegetable mixture over bottom half of one tortilla, leaving a $\frac{1}{2}$" border; fold top half over vegetable mixture and press to seal. Repeat procedure with remaining vegetable mixture and tortillas, making 4 quesadillas.

5. Arrange quesadillas on prepared baking sheet; bake 8 minutes, or until hot and bubbly. Serve immediately.

EACH SERVING PROVIDES: $\frac{1}{4}$ Milk, $1\frac{1}{4}$ Vegetables, $1\frac{3}{4}$ Breads, 10 Optional Calories
PER SERVING: 184 Calories, 9 g Protein, 2 g Fat, 33 g Carbohydrate, 436 mg Sodium, 2 mg Cholesterol, 4 g Dietary Fiber

OVEN-ROASTED LEEKS AND FENNEL PARMESAN

A harmonious pairing: the mildly onion taste of leek and licorice-flavored fennel are baked under a blanket of cheese.

MAKES 4 SERVINGS

1 large leek (6 ounces), trimmed and quartered
1 small fennel bulb (6 ounces), vertically sliced into 8 pieces
$\frac{1}{2}$ cup chicken broth
2 tablespoons grated Parmesan cheese
$\frac{1}{4}$ teaspoon freshly ground black pepper

1. Preheat oven to 350°F. In a 13 × 9" baking pan, arrange leek and fennel; add broth. Cover with foil; bake 30 minutes, until tender.

2. Uncover; sprinkle with cheese and pepper. Bake 5 minutes, until cheese is melted.

EACH SERVING PROVIDES: $4\frac{1}{2}$ Vegetables, 20 Optional Calories
PER SERVING: 47 Calories, 2 g Protein, 1 g Fat, 7 g Carbohydrate, 217 mg Sodium, 2 mg Cholesterol, 1 g Dietary Fiber

Broiled Eggplant

When eggplant is traditionally fried, it becomes an oil sponge! Here, it's baked with a fresh tomato sauce for just 33 calories a serving.

Makes 4 Servings

$\frac{1}{2}$ cup finely chopped plum tomato
3 tablespoons balsamic vinegar
2 tablespoons chopped fresh basil
1 small garlic clove, crushed
1 small eggplant (about 12 ounces), cut into $\frac{1}{2}$" slices
$\frac{1}{4}$ teaspoon salt
$\frac{1}{4}$ teaspoon freshly ground black pepper

1. Preheat broiler. Spray broiler rack with nonstick cooking spray.

2. In small bowl, whisk together tomato, vinegar, basil and garlic. Arrange eggplant slices on prepared rack; brush slices with some of the tomato mixture.

3. Broil 5–6" from heat 8 minutes, until lightly browned. Turn slices; brush with more of the tomato mixture. Broil 3–5 minutes, until lightly browned. Transfer slices to serving bowl; keep warm.

4. Add salt and pepper to remaining tomato mixture; stir to combine. To serve, pour remaining tomato mixture over eggplant slices.

EACH SERVING PROVIDES: 1$\frac{1}{4}$ Vegetables
PER SERVING: 33 Calories, 1 g Protein, 0 g Fat, 7 g Carbohydrate, 143 mg Sodium, 0 mg Cholesterol, 2 g Dietary Fiber

VARIATION

Eggplant slices can be prepared on a grill. Spray grill with nonstick cooking spray. Place grill rack 5–6" from coals. Prepare grill according to manufacturer's directions. Follow steps 2–4 above.

Steamed Kale with Balsamic Vinaigrette

Makes 4 Servings

2 teaspoons olive oil
$\frac{1}{2}$ cup finely chopped shallots
1 tablespoon balsamic vinegar
$\frac{1}{2}$ teaspoon Dijon-style mustard
4 cups chopped kale, steamed just until tender (hot)
$\frac{1}{8}$ teaspoon salt
$\frac{1}{8}$ teaspoon freshly ground black pepper

1. In large nonstick skillet, heat oil; add shallots. Sauté over medium heat, stirring frequently, 5 minutes, until transparent. Add $\frac{1}{4}$ cup water, the vinegar and mustard; bring to a boil. Cook, stirring constantly, 1 minute.

2. Add kale to skillet; toss to mix well. Sprinkle with salt and pepper.

EACH SERVING PROVIDES: $\frac{1}{2}$ Fat, 2$\frac{1}{4}$ Vegetables
PER SERVING: 70 Calories, 3 g Protein, 3 g Fat, 10 g Carbohydrate, 120 mg Sodium, 0 mg Cholesterol, 5 g Dietary Fiber

CREOLE-STYLE OKRA

MAKES 6 SERVINGS

2 teaspoons vegetable oil
$\frac{1}{2}$ cup chopped onion
$\frac{1}{2}$ cup chopped celery
$4\frac{1}{2}$ cups fresh or frozen okra, trimmed
2 cups canned crushed tomatoes
2 strips crisp cooked bacon, crumbled
$\frac{1}{8}$ teaspoon ground red pepper
$\frac{1}{8}$ teaspoon freshly ground black pepper
1 bay leaf
$\frac{1}{8}$ teaspoon filé powder

1. In large nonstick skillet, heat oil; add onion and celery. Cook over medium heat, stirring frequently, 6–8 minutes, until golden.

2. Stir in okra, tomatoes, $\frac{3}{4}$ cup water, bacon, red pepper, black pepper and bay leaf. Reduce heat to low; simmer, covered, 12–15 minutes, until okra is tender. Stir in filé powder.

EACH SERVING PROVIDES: $\frac{1}{4}$ Fat, $2\frac{1}{2}$ Vegetables, 15 Optional Calories
PER SERVING: 67 Calories, 3 g Protein, 3 g Fat, 9 g Carbohydrate, 177 mg Sodium, 2 mg Cholesterol, 3 g Dietary Fiber

BAKED ONIONS

MAKES 4 SERVINGS

Four 4-ounce onions, root ends trimmed
1 tablespoon + 1 teaspoon reduced-calorie tub margarine
1 tablespoon chopped fresh parsley
$\frac{1}{8}$ teaspoon freshly ground black pepper

1. Preheat oven to 400°F. In a 1-quart casserole combine onions and $\frac{1}{2}$ cup water; bake 1 hour, until tender. Let cool slightly. With cloth, carefully remove onion skins by pulling firmly from stem end; transfer to serving platter and keep warm.

2. Meanwhile, in small skillet, melt margarine over medium-high heat; stir in parsley and pepper. To serve, drizzle margarine mixture over onions.

EACH SERVING PROVIDES: $\frac{1}{2}$ Fat, $1\frac{1}{4}$ Vegetables
PER SERVING: 56 Calories, 1 g Protein, 2 g Fat, 9 g Carbohydrate, 40 mg Sodium, 0 mg Cholesterol, 2 g Dietary Fiber

---

Roasting Peppers

◆

Roasted peppers add wonderful flavor to salads, sandwiches, soups—or just eaten by themselves. Choose any color of pepper that you wish. Red peppers will give a slightly milder flavor than green.

- *Preheat broiler. On rack, broil peppers as close to heat source as possible, turning several times as top skin blackens and chars.*
- *When peppers are entirely blackened, remove from broiler and place in a paper bag for 5 minutes to cool. (Steam created by the cooling peppers will make skin easy to remove.)*
- *With a small, sharp knife, carefully scrape away the charred skin; run peppers under cold water to wash away any remaining bits of skin.*

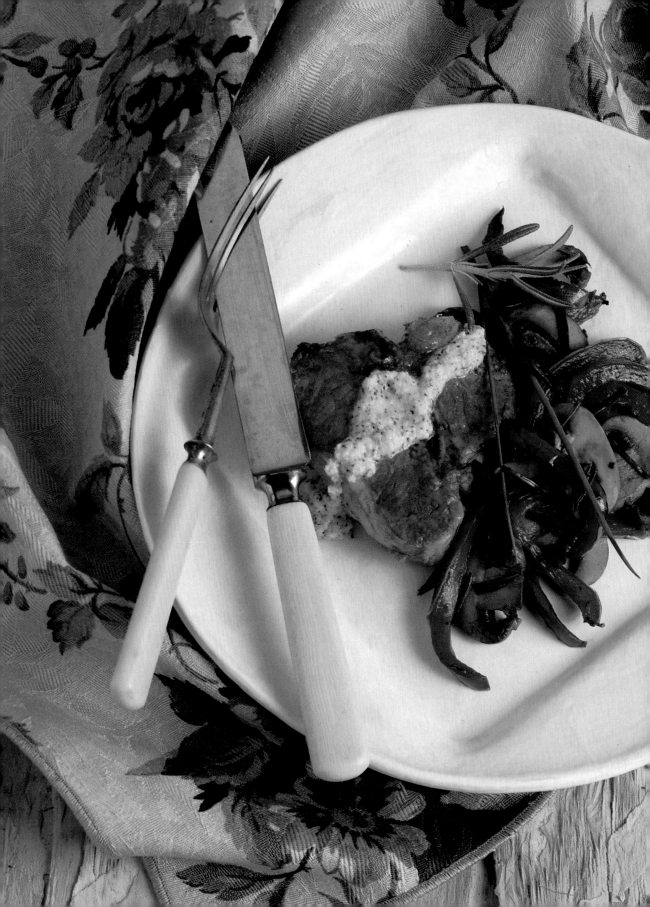

MUSHROOM AND RED BELL PEPPER SAUTÉ

MAKES 4 SERVINGS

1 teaspoon olive oil
4 cups sliced mushrooms
1 cup julienned red bell pepper
2 sun-dried tomato halves (not packed in oil), julienned
2 tablespoons dry white wine
1 tablespoon chopped fresh chives
1 teaspoon chopped fresh rosemary
$\frac{1}{8}$ teaspoon freshly ground black pepper

1. In large nonstick skillet, heat oil; add mushrooms and bell pepper. Sauté over high heat, stirring frequently, 4–5 minutes, until golden.

2. Add tomato, wine, chives, rosemary and black pepper to skillet; cook, covered, 2 minutes.

EACH SERVING PROVIDES: $\frac{1}{4}$ Fat, 2$\frac{3}{4}$ Vegetables, 5 Optional Calories
PER SERVING: 44 Calories, 2 g Protein, 2 g Fat, 6 g Carbohydrate, 5 mg Sodium, 0 mg Cholesterol, 2 g Dietary Fiber

OVEN-BAKED ONION RINGS

Pub-style onion rings inspired this baked instead of fried version; ground red pepper heats them up.

MAKES 6 SERVINGS

$\frac{1}{4}$ cup + 2 tablespoons all-purpose flour
$\frac{1}{2}$ teaspoon salt
$\frac{1}{8}$ teaspoon ground red pepper
1 large peeled Spanish onion, cut into $\frac{1}{4}$" slices
3 egg whites, lightly beaten
$\frac{3}{4}$ cup plain dried bread crumbs*

1. Preheat oven to 400°F. Spray nonstick baking sheet with nonstick cooking spray. On sheet of wax paper, combine flour, salt and red pepper.

2. Separate onion slices into rings; stack 2 rings together. Dredge each 2-ring stack in flour mixture; dip in egg white. Coat in bread crumbs; arrange on prepared baking sheet.

3. Bake on top oven rack 10 minutes, until browned. Turn and bake 5–10 minutes longer, until browned.

*Seasoned dried bread crumbs can be substituted for the plain.

EACH SERVING PROVIDES: $\frac{1}{2}$ Vegetable, 1 Bread, 10 Optional Calories
PER SERVING: 108 Calories, 5 g Protein, 1 g Fat, 20 g Carbohydrate, 330 mg Sodium, 0 mg Cholesterol, 1 g Dietary Fiber

SAUTÉED SUMMER SQUASH

MAKES 4 SERVINGS

2 teaspoons olive oil
3 cups diagonally sliced yellow squash ($\frac{1}{2}$" slices)
1 tablespoon fresh lemon juice
1 teaspoon chopped fresh thyme
$\frac{1}{2}$ teaspoon grated lemon zest
$\frac{1}{8}$ teaspoon salt
$\frac{1}{8}$ teaspoon freshly ground black pepper

1. In large nonstick skillet, heat oil; add half of the squash. Cook over medium-high heat, turning occasionally, until golden brown. Transfer to plate; set aside.

2. Add remaining squash to same skillet. Cook, turning occasionally, until golden brown. Add reserved squash to skillet; sprinkle with juice, thyme, lemon zest, salt and pepper. Cook 3 minutes, stirring occasionally, until heated through.

EACH SERVING PROVIDES: $\frac{1}{2}$ Fat, 1$\frac{1}{2}$ Vegetables
PER SERVING: 40 Calories, 1 g Protein, 2 g Fat, 4 g Carbohydrate, 71 mg Sodium, 0 mg Cholesterol, 1 g Dietary Fiber

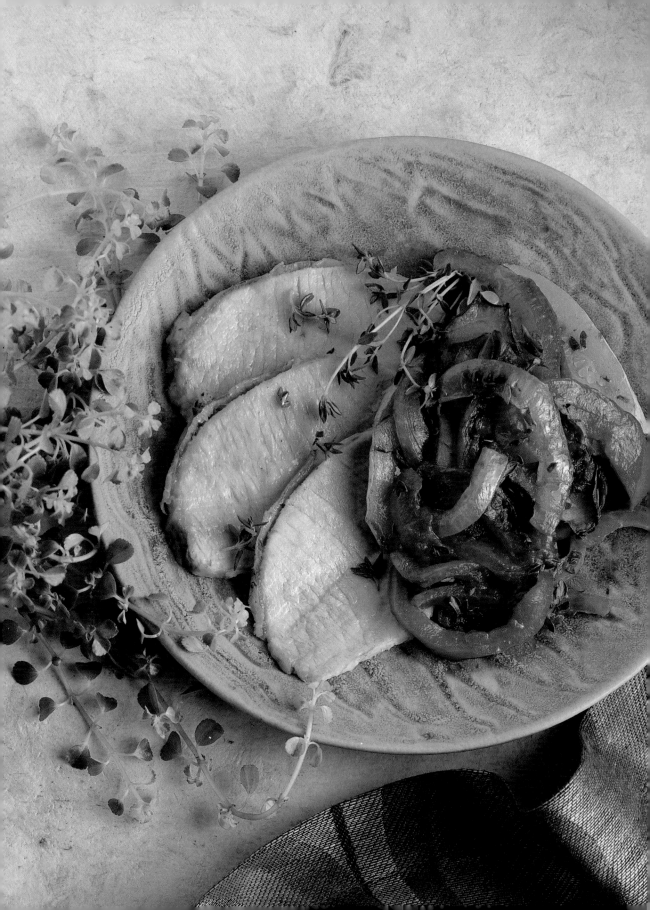

RATATOUILLE CASSEROLE

MAKES 6 SERVINGS

1 small eggplant (about 12 ounces), pared and cut
  into $\frac{1}{4}$" slices
1 tablespoon + 1 teaspoon olive oil
1 large yellow squash (about 8 ounces), cut into $\frac{1}{4}$"
  diagonal slices
1 medium zucchini, cut into $\frac{1}{4}$" diagonal slices
1 medium yellow onion, very thinly sliced
1 medium red bell pepper, julienned
3 garlic cloves, very thinly sliced
$\frac{1}{4}$ cup tomato paste
2 tablespoons chopped fresh parsley
2 tablespoons chopped fresh basil
2 teaspoons chopped fresh thyme
$\frac{1}{4}$ teaspoon salt
$\frac{1}{4}$ teaspoon freshly ground black pepper
1 medium tomato, thinly sliced

1. Preheat oven to 400°F. Spray nonstick baking sheet and a 1-quart casserole with nonstick cooking spray.

2. In medium bowl, combine eggplant and 1 teaspoon of the oil; toss to coat. On prepared baking sheet, arrange eggplant slices in a single layer. Repeat procedure with squash, then zucchini, tossing each with 1 teaspoon of the oil and arranging each separately in a single layer on the baking sheet. Bake 12 minutes; turn vegetables and bake 8 minutes longer. Reduce oven temperature to 350°F.

3. In large nonstick skillet, heat the remaining 1 teaspoon oil; add onion, bell pepper and garlic. Sauté over medium heat, 5 minutes, until onion is soft. Cook, covered, shaking pan occasionally, 5 minutes longer.

4. In small bowl, combine tomato paste and $\frac{1}{2}$ cup of water; set aside. In separate small bowl, combine parsley, basil, thyme, salt and pepper.

5. In prepared casserole, arrange half of the baked eggplant slices; sprinkle with 1 teaspoon of the herb mixture. Continue layering with half each of the sliced tomato, baked squash, onion mixture and baked zucchini, sprinkling 1 teaspoon of the herb mixture between each layer. Repeat procedure, ending with zucchini.

6. Pour tomato paste mixture over layered vegetables. Bake, covered with foil, 50 minutes. Uncover; bake 15 minutes longer.

EACH SERVING PROVIDES: $\frac{1}{2}$ Fat, 3 Vegetables, 5 Optional Calories
PER SERVING: 80 Calories, 2 g Protein, 4 g Fat, 12 g Carbohydrate, 184 mg Sodium, 0 mg Cholesterol, 3 g Dietary Fiber

◆

"CREAMED" SPINACH

Puréed cottage cheese, milk and Parmesan cheese double for the traditional cream sauce served on spinach; it's a delicious trade-off with only 1 gram of fat per serving.

MAKES 4 SERVINGS

$\frac{2}{3}$ cup low-fat (1%) cottage cheese
$\frac{1}{4}$ cup low-fat (1%) milk
1 tablespoon grated Parmesan cheese
$\frac{1}{2}$ garlic clove, minced
$\frac{1}{4}$ teaspoon salt
$\frac{1}{8}$ teaspoon freshly ground black pepper
20 ounces spinach leaves, steamed until tender and
  chopped

1. In food processor or blender, combine cottage cheese, milk, Parmesan cheese, garlic, salt and pepper; purée until smooth. Add one-fourth of the spinach; purée until smooth.

2. In large skillet, combine the remaining spinach and cottage cheese mixture. Cook over medium heat, stirring occasionally, 5 minutes, until heated through.

EACH SERVING PROVIDES: 5 Vegetables, $\frac{1}{2}$ Protein, 15 Optional Calories
PER SERVING: 71 Calories, 10 g Protein, 1 g Fat, 7 g Carbohydrate, 432 mg Sodium, 3 mg Cholesterol, 4 g Dietary Fiber

Ratatouille Casserole, Tuscan-style Pork Roast (page 208)

GINGERED PUMPKIN SOUFFLÉ

Almost a dessert, this light soufflé is touched with warm spices and sweetened with fruit. Make it with fresh pumpkin in the fall or canned purée anytime.

MAKES 4 SERVINGS

2 eggs, separated
$\frac{1}{4}$ cup dried currants
2 tablespoons orange juice
2 cups puréed cooked pumpkin
$\frac{1}{4}$ cup grated onion, squeezed dry
1 tablespoon + 1 teaspoon all-purpose flour
$1\frac{1}{2}$ teaspoons grated fresh ginger root
1 teaspoon ground coriander
$\frac{1}{4}$ teaspoon salt
Pinch ground red pepper
2 egg whites
Pinch cream of tartar

1. Preheat oven to 325°F. Spray a 5-cup soufflé dish with nonstick cooking spray. In small bowl, lightly beat egg yolks; set aside.

2. In small saucepan, bring currants and juice to a boil; remove from heat. Let stand 10 minutes.

3. In large bowl, thoroughly combine currant mixture, pumpkin, onion, flour, ginger, coriander, salt and red pepper. Add beaten egg yolks; stir to mix well.

4. In large bowl, with whisk or mixer on high speed, beat all of the egg whites until frothy; add cream of tartar. Continue beating until soft peaks form. Lightly stir one-fourth of the beaten whites into the pumpkin mixture; with rubber spatula, gently fold in the remaining whites. Spoon mixture into prepared dish.

5. Bake 45–50 minutes, until puffed and golden. Serve immediately.

EACH SERVING PROVIDES: $\frac{1}{2}$ Fruit, 1 Vegetable, $\frac{1}{2}$ Protein, 25 Optional Calories
PER SERVING: 115 Calories, 7 g Protein, 3 g Fat, 17 g Carbohydrate, 197 mg Sodium, 106 mg Cholesterol, 1 g Dietary Fiber

SPAGHETTI SQUASH

MAKES 4 SERVINGS

1 spaghetti squash (about 2 pounds)
2 teaspoons olive oil
3 tablespoons thinly sliced scallions
1 teaspoon minced garlic
$\frac{1}{2}$ cup chicken broth
$\frac{1}{2}$ teaspoon dried marjoram leaves
$\frac{1}{2}$ teaspoon grated lemon zest
$\frac{1}{4}$ teaspoon salt
12 small asparagus spears, cut into 2" diagonal pieces
1 cup thawed frozen peas
2 teaspoons fresh lemon juice

1. Preheat oven to 350°F.

2. Cut squash in half lengthwise; remove and discard seeds. Arrange squash, cut-side down, in an 11 × 7" baking dish; pour water into dish to a depth of about $\frac{1}{2}$"; bake, covered with foil, 45 minutes, until tender. Remove squash from water; let stand until cool enough to handle. With tines of a fork, scoop out pulp; transfer to medium bowl.

3. In large nonstick skillet heat oil; add scallions and garlic. Cook over low heat, stirring frequently, 1 minute. Add broth, marjoram, lemon zest and salt; bring to a boil. Add asparagus and peas. Reduce heat to low; simmer, covered, 2 minutes. Stir in cooked squash and juice. Cook, stirring occasionally, 3 minutes, until heated through.

EACH SERVING PROVIDES: $\frac{1}{2}$ Fat, 2 Vegetables, $\frac{1}{2}$ Bread, 3 Optional Calories
PER SERVING: 117 Calories, 5 g Protein, 4 g Fat, 19 g Carbohydrate, 328 mg Sodium, 0 mg Cholesterol, 2 g Dietary Fiber

BROILED TOMATOES

MAKES 4 SERVINGS

$\frac{1}{4}$ cup chopped fresh basil
2 garlic cloves, minced
1 teaspoon grated lemon zest
$\frac{1}{4}$ teaspoon freshly ground black pepper
1 teaspoon extra-virgin olive oil
$\frac{1}{8}$ teaspoon salt
2 large tomatoes (about 10 ounces each), halved
   crosswise

1. Preheat broiler. Spray broiler rack with nonstick cooking spray.

2. On cutting board, with knife, chop together basil, garlic, lemon zest and pepper, making a paste. Transfer to small bowl; stir in oil and salt.

3. Evenly spread one-fourth of the herb mixture on cut side of each tomato half; arrange tomatoes on prepared rack. Broil 5–6" from heat, 8–10 minutes, until lightly browned.

EACH SERVING PROVIDES: $\frac{1}{4}$ Fat, 1$\frac{1}{2}$ Vegetables
PER SERVING: 45 Calories, 1 g Protein, 2 g Fat, 7 g Carbohydrate, 82 mg Sodium, 0 mg Cholesterol, 2 g Dietary Fiber

◆

STEWED TOMATOES

MAKES 4 SERVINGS

4 ripe medium tomatoes, blanched, peeled, seeded
   and quartered
$\frac{1}{4}$ cup thinly sliced scallions
1 teaspoon chopped fresh basil
$\frac{1}{2}$ teaspoon granulated sugar
$\frac{1}{4}$ teaspoon paprika

1. In medium saucepan, combine tomatoes, scallions, 2 tablespoons water, the basil, sugar and paprika; bring to a boil.

2. Reduce heat to low; simmer, covered, 15 minutes, until tomatoes are very soft.

EACH SERVING PROVIDES: 2 Vegetables, 2 Optional Calories
PER SERVING: 37 Calories, 1 g Protein, 1 g Fat, 8 g Carbohydrate, 15 mg Sodium, 0 mg Cholesterol, 2 g Dietary Fiber

SWISS CHARD AU GRATIN

MAKES 4 SERVINGS

1 teaspoon salt
2 cups cut Swiss chard ribs (2" pieces)
4$\frac{1}{2}$ cups shredded Swiss chard leaves
1$\frac{1}{2}$ ounces coarsely grated light Jarlsberg cheese
1 tablespoon grated Parmesan cheese
1 garlic clove, minced
$\frac{1}{4}$ teaspoon freshly ground black pepper

1. Preheat oven to 400°F. Spray a 1-quart casserole with nonstick cooking spray.

2. In large saucepan, bring salt and 2 quarts water to a boil; add chard ribs. Boil 5 minutes; add chard leaves. Cook 3 minutes, until tender. Drain well; set aside.

3. In prepared casserole, arrange half of the chard mixture; top with half each of the Jarlsberg cheese, Parmesan cheese, garlic and pepper. Repeat procedure, ending with pepper.

4. Bake on top oven rack 20 minutes, until cheeses are melted and bubbly.

EACH SERVING PROVIDES: 3$\frac{1}{4}$ Vegetables, $\frac{1}{2}$ Protein, 10 Optional Calories
PER SERVING: 50 Calories, 5 g Protein, 2 g Fat, 3 g Carbohydrate, 736 mg Sodium, 7 mg Cholesterol, 0 g Dietary Fiber

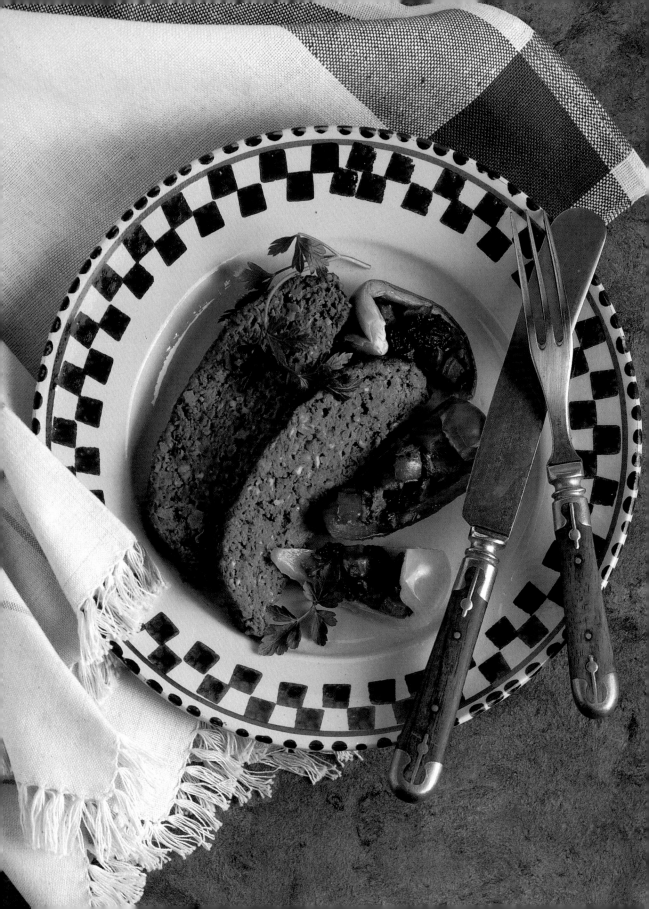

ROAST PEPPER WEDGES

MAKES 4 SERVINGS

1 large plum tomato, coarsely chopped
2 tablespoons chopped dark raisins
2 tablespoons chopped fresh parsley
1 tablespoon chopped fresh basil
3 anchovy fillets, mashed
2 teaspoons olive oil
2 garlic cloves, minced
$\frac{1}{8}$ teaspoon salt
$\frac{1}{8}$ teaspoon freshly ground black pepper
2 medium red bell peppers, halved, seeded and
   each half cut into 3 wedges

1. Preheat oven to 350°F. Line baking sheet with foil; spray foil with nonstick cooking spray.

2. In medium bowl, combine tomato, raisins, parsley, basil, anchovies, oil, garlic, salt and pepper; stir to mix well.

3. Arrange pepper wedges, cut-side up, on prepared baking sheet; spoon an equal amount of tomato mixture onto each pepper wedge; cover with foil.

4. Bake 30 minutes, or until peppers are tender. Carefully remove foil. Serve hot or at room temperature.

EACH SERVING PROVIDES: $\frac{1}{2}$ Fat, $\frac{1}{4}$ Fruit, $1\frac{1}{4}$ Vegetables, 5 Optional Calories
PER SERVING: 61 Calories, 2 g Protein, 3 g Fat, 8 g Carbohydrate, 183 mg Sodium, 2 mg Cholesterol, 1 g Dietary Fiber

HERBED ZUCCHINI FLAN

MAKES 4 SERVINGS

2 teaspoons olive oil
4 cups grated zucchini (about $1\frac{1}{4}$ pounds)
1 cup chopped onion
2 garlic cloves, minced
2 teaspoons white wine vinegar
$\frac{1}{4}$ cup chopped fresh parsley
1 teaspoon chopped fresh thyme
$\frac{1}{2}$ teaspoon chopped fresh rosemary
$\frac{1}{4}$ teaspoon freshly ground black pepper
1 cup egg substitute
$\frac{1}{3}$ cup + 2 teaspoons all-purpose flour
$\frac{1}{4}$ cup grated Parmesan cheese

1. Preheat oven to 300°F. Spray a 9" square baking pan with nonstick cooking spray.

2. In large nonstick skillet, heat oil; add zucchini, onion and garlic. Sauté over medium heat, 12 minutes, until vegetables are tender; add vinegar. Cook, stirring frequently, 2 minutes. Remove from heat; let cool slightly. Stir in parsley, thyme, rosemary and pepper.

3. In large bowl, whisk egg substitute, flour and cheese; stir in zucchini mixture. Transfer zucchini mixture to prepared pan. Bake 30–35 minutes, until set.

EACH SERVING PROVIDES: $\frac{1}{2}$ Fat, $2\frac{1}{2}$ Vegetables, 1 Protein, $\frac{1}{2}$ Bread, 30 Optional Calories
PER SERVING: 152 Calories, 11 g Protein, 4 g Fat, 19 g Carbohydrate, 181 mg Sodium, 4 mg Cholesterol, 2 g Dietary Fiber

Roast Pepper Wedges, Spicy Meatloaf with Herbs (page 191)

ROASTED ZUCCHINI PROVENÇALE

MAKES 4 SERVINGS

4 medium zucchini, cut into wedges
2 teaspoons olive oil
5 small Niçoise olives, pitted
3 anchovy fillets
1 large garlic clove, minced
$\frac{1}{2}$ teaspoon grated lemon zest
2 tablespoons plain dried bread crumbs
2 teaspoons chopped fresh thyme
$\frac{1}{8}$ teaspoon freshly ground black pepper

1. Preheat oven to 425°F. Spray nonstick baking sheet with nonstick cooking spray.

2. In medium bowl, combine zucchini and oil; toss to mix well. Arrange zucchini on prepared baking sheet. Roast 10 minutes, until golden; turn and roast 5 minutes longer, until golden. Transfer to a 2-cup baking dish.

3. Meanwhile, on cutting board, with knife, chop together olives, anchovies, garlic and lemon zest. Transfer to small bowl. Add bread crumbs, thyme and pepper; toss to mix well.

4. Sprinkle bread crumb mixture over zucchini; bake 8–10 minutes or until crumbs are browned.

EACH SERVING PROVIDES: $\frac{1}{2}$ Fat, 2 Vegetables, 25 Optional Calories
PER SERVING: 71 Calories, 3 g Protein, 4 g Fat, 8 g Carbohydrate, 175 mg Sodium, 2 mg Cholesterol, 1 g Dietary Fiber

VEGETABLE LOAF

MAKES 6 SERVINGS

1 tablespoon olive oil
1 cup chopped onion
4 garlic cloves, minced
2 cups broccoli florets, finely chopped
$1\frac{1}{2}$ cups finely chopped mushrooms
1 cup cauliflower, finely chopped
1 cup finely diced red bell pepper
$1\frac{1}{2}$ cups cooked regular long-grain rice
1 cup drained thawed frozen chopped spinach
2 sun-dried tomato halves (not packed in oil), soaked, drained and chopped
3 tablespoons finely chopped fresh basil
2 tablespoons grated Parmesan cheese
2 tablespoons cider vinegar
$\frac{1}{4}$ teaspoon grated lemon zest
$\frac{1}{2}$ teaspoon salt
$\frac{1}{2}$ teaspoon freshly ground black pepper
3 egg whites, lightly beaten
2 tablespoons tomato paste

1. Preheat oven to 350°F. Spray a 9 × 5" loaf pan with nonstick cooking spray.

2. In large nonstick skillet, heat oil; add onion and garlic. Cook over medium heat, stirring frequently, 6–7 minutes, until onion is translucent; add broccoli, mushrooms, cauliflower and bell pepper. Sauté 8–10 minutes, until broccoli is tender and most of the liquid has evaporated.

3. Add rice, spinach, tomatoes, basil, cheese, vinegar, lemon zest, salt and pepper; toss to mix well. Remove from heat; let cool slightly.

4. Add egg whites to skillet; stir to combine. Press vegetable mixture into prepared pan. Spread tomato paste evenly over the top of the loaf.

5. Bake 40–45 minutes, until firm. Let cool 10–15 minutes before slicing.

EACH SERVING PROVIDES: $\frac{1}{2}$ Fat, $2\frac{3}{4}$ Vegetables, $\frac{1}{2}$ Bread, 20 Optional Calories
PER SERVING: 160 Calories, 7 g Protein, 4 g Fat, 26 g Carbohydrate, 328 mg Sodium, 1 mg Cholesterol, 4 g Dietary Fiber

STIR-FRIED CHINESE VEGETABLES

MAKES 4 SERVINGS

¼ cup chicken broth
1 tablespoon reduced-sodium soy sauce
2 garlic cloves, minced
1½ teaspoons grated fresh ginger root
2 teaspoons vegetable oil
2 cups chopped bok choy cabbage
1 medium red bell pepper, cut into 1" squares
1 cup snow peas, stem ends and strings removed
½ cup diagonally sliced carrot (thin slices)
¼ cup drained canned sliced bamboo shoots
¼ cup drained canned sliced water chestnuts

1. In small bowl, combine broth, soy sauce, garlic and ginger; set aside.

2. In large nonstick skillet, heat oil; add cabbage and bell pepper. Stir-fry 3 minutes; add broth mixture, snow peas and carrot. Reduce heat to medium; cook, stirring frequently, 3 minutes, until vegetables are tender-crisp and sauce is thickened.

3. Add bamboo shoots and water chestnuts; cook, stirring frequently, 1 minute, until heated through.

EACH SERVING PROVIDES: ½ Fat, 2½ Vegetables, 10 Optional Calories
PER SERVING: 65 Calories, 3 g Protein, 3 g Fat, 9 g Carbohydrate, 243 mg Sodium, 0 mg Cholesterol, 2 g Dietary Fiber

TURNIP PURÉE

MAKES 4 SERVINGS

3 cups diced pared turnips (1" dice), steamed until tender, hot
8 ounces pared potato, cooked and diced, hot
2 tablespoons light sour cream
½ teaspoon salt
½ teaspoon freshly ground black pepper
⅛ teaspoon ground nutmeg

In food processor combine turnips, potato, sour cream, salt, pepper and nutmeg; purée until smooth. If using blender, blend in batches. Transfer to serving bowl; serve immediately.

EACH SERVING PROVIDES: 1½ Vegetables, ½ Bread, 10 Optional Calories
PER SERVING: 89 Calories, 2 g Protein, 1 g Fat, 18 g Carbohydrate, 342 mg Sodium, 3 mg Cholesterol, 3 g Dietary Fiber

◆

TENDER GREENS WITH LIGHT LEMON DRESSING

MAKES 4 SERVINGS

1 tablespoon + 2 teaspoons fresh lemon juice
1 tablespoon low-sodium chicken broth
2 teaspoons vegetable oil
¼ teaspoon salt
¼ teaspoon granulated sugar
Pinch freshly ground black pepper
4 cups torn Boston lettuce leaves (bite-size pieces)
¼ cup thinly sliced scallions
3 tablespoons chopped fresh dill

1. To prepare dressing, in small bowl, whisk juice, broth, oil, salt, sugar and pepper.

2. In large serving bowl, combine lettuce, scallions and dill. Add dressing; toss to mix well.

EACH SERVING PROVIDES: ½ Fat, 2 Vegetables, 1 Optional Calorie
PER SERVING: 36 Calories, 1 g Protein, 2 g Fat, 4 g Carbohydrate, 152 mg Sodium, 0 mg Cholesterol, 1 g Dietary Fiber

ROMAINE SALAD WITH CAESAR DRESSING

An updated version of the classic Caesar salad, this dressing contains no oil, and the entire dish is a mere 55 calories.

MAKES 4 SERVINGS

$\frac{1}{2}$ cup low-fat (1.5%) buttermilk
2 tablespoons part-skim ricotta cheese
2 tablespoons grated Parmesan cheese
2 anchovy fillets, mashed to a paste
1 garlic clove, crushed
$\frac{1}{4}$ teaspoon freshly ground black pepper
4 cups sliced romaine lettuce leaves
6 cherry tomatoes, quartered

1. To prepare dressing, in small bowl, combine buttermilk, ricotta cheese, Parmesan cheese, anchovies, garlic and pepper; stir to mix well.

2. In large serving bowl, combine lettuce and tomatoes. Add dressing; toss to mix well.

EACH SERVING PROVIDES: $2\frac{1}{4}$ Vegetables, 40 Optional Calories
PER SERVING: 55 Calories, 5 g Protein, 2 g Fat, 4 g Carbohydrate, 167 mg Sodium, 7 mg Cholesterol, 1 g Dietary Fiber

---

All Dressed Up

◆

Salad dressings add zest to salads and give them their finishing touch. For many people, salad dressings used to be fat traps, where great taste came at the price of a high percentage of calories from fat. Not anymore! The dressings here pack great flavor, without a high fat content.

An easy way to vary the flavor of your salad dressing is to experiment with different vinegars, such as red or white wine vinegar; rice, cider or malt varieties; or herb-flavored vinegars such as tarragon or dill.

Dressings can be prepared in advance and stored in a covered container in the refrigerator for 2 to 3 days. Shake well or blend before serving.

GREEK SALAD WITH OREGANO-FETA DRESSING

Feta, oregano and Greek olives provide the authentic seasonings in this salad. Grilled lamb and steamed orzo would be its perfect partners.

MAKES 4 SERVINGS

3 ounces feta cheese
2 tablespoons fresh lemon juice
1 teaspoon olive oil
1 garlic clove, crushed
$\frac{1}{2}$ teaspoon dried oregano leaves, crushed
$\frac{1}{4}$ teaspoon freshly ground black pepper
2 tablespoons chopped green bell pepper
3 cups torn romaine lettuce leaves
1 medium tomato, cut into wedges
1 cup sliced cucumber semicircles ($\frac{1}{4}$" thick slices)
$\frac{1}{2}$ cup sliced red onion
6 large Greek olives

1. To prepare dressing, in food processor or blender, combine feta cheese, juice, 2 tablespoons water, oil, garlic, oregano and pepper; purée until smooth. Add bell pepper; purée 3 seconds.

2. In large serving bowl, combine lettuce, tomato, cucumber and onion; toss to mix well. Add dressing; toss to coat. Sprinkle with olives.

EACH SERVING PROVIDES: $\frac{1}{2}$ Fat, $2\frac{3}{4}$ Vegetables, 1 Protein
PER SERVING: 121 Calories, 5 g Protein, 9 g Fat, 8 g Carbohydrate, 480 mg Sodium, 19 mg Cholesterol, 2 g Dietary Fiber

Greek Salad with Oregano-Feta Dressing

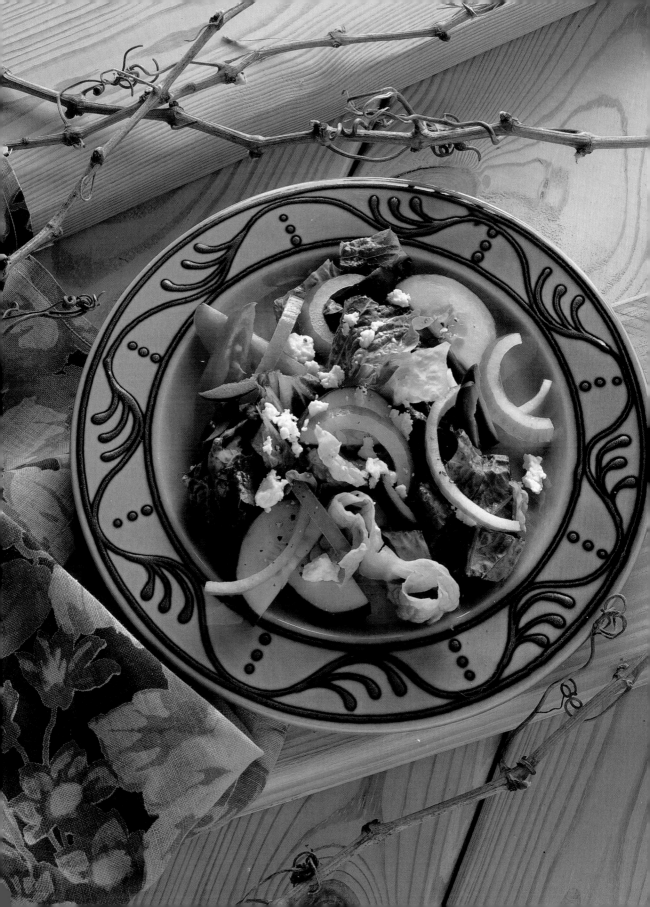

WILTED SPINACH SALAD WITH SPICY ONION DRESSING

Onions cooked in cider vinegar and orange juice add just the right sweet-sour touch to the greens and mushrooms.

MAKES 4 SERVINGS

4 cups spinach leaves
1 cup thinly sliced mushrooms
2 teaspoons olive oil
$\frac{3}{4}$ cup thinly sliced onions
2 cups reduced-sodium chicken broth
$\frac{1}{3}$ cup + 2 teaspoons cider vinegar
$\frac{1}{3}$ cup + 2 teaspoons orange juice
1 teaspoon grated orange zest
$\frac{1}{8}$ teaspoon red pepper flakes

1. Thoroughly wash spinach leaves; drain on paper towels. On large serving platter arrange spinach; sprinkle with mushrooms; set aside.

2. To prepare dressing, in large nonstick skillet, heat oil; add onions. Sauté over medium-high heat, stirring occasionally, 4 minutes, until tender; add broth, vinegar, juice, orange zest and pepper flakes and bring to a boil. Reduce heat to low; simmer, stirring occasionally, 15–20 minutes, until thickened.

3. To serve, pour hot dressing evenly over spinach and mushrooms; serve immediately.

EACH SERVING PROVIDES: $\frac{1}{2}$ Fat, 3 Vegetables, 20 Optional Calories
PER SERVING: 73 Calories, 4 g Protein, 3 g Fat, 10 g Carbohydrate, 366 mg Sodium, 0 mg Cholesterol, 2 g Dietary Fiber

WINTER GREENS WITH BALSAMIC VINAIGRETTE

The red and green hues of this salad earn it a place on your holiday table. Nonfat yogurt stands in for some of the oil, making it a smart choice as well.

MAKES 4 SERVINGS

3 tablespoons plain nonfat yogurt
1 tablespoon + 1 teaspoon balsamic vinegar
2 teaspoons olive oil
$\frac{1}{2}$ teaspoon Dijon-style mustard
$\frac{1}{4}$ teaspoon salt
$\frac{1}{4}$ teaspoon freshly ground black pepper
1 cup shredded radicchio leaves
1 cup torn arugula leaves
1 cup torn watercress
8 ounces Belgian endive, separated and sliced crosswise
$\frac{1}{2}$ cup thinly sliced red onion

1. To prepare dressing, in small bowl, combine yogurt, vinegar, oil, mustard, salt and pepper; stir to mix well.

2. In large serving bowl, combine radicchio, arugula, watercress, endive and red onion. Add dressing; toss to coat.

EACH SERVING PROVIDES: $\frac{1}{2}$ Fat, $2\frac{1}{4}$ Vegetables, 5 Optional Calories
PER SERVING: 49 Calories, 2 g Protein, 2 g Fat, 5 g Carbohydrate, 176 mg Sodium, 0 mg Cholesterol, 2 g Dietary Fiber

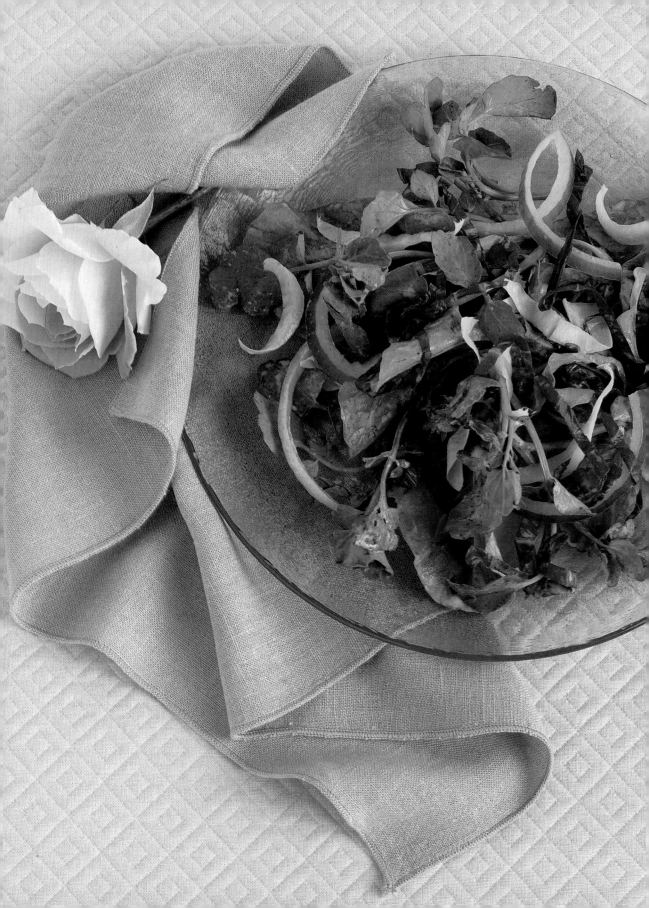

CHICORY WITH MUSTARD AND CAPER DRESSING

Sturdy and slightly bitter chicory stands up well to the tangy dressing with a piquant touch of capers.

MAKES 4 SERVINGS

2 tablespoons plain nonfat yogurt
1 tablespoon white wine vinegar
2 teaspoons olive oil
2 teaspoons Dijon-style mustard
$\frac{1}{2}$ teaspoon grated lemon zest
$\frac{1}{4}$ teaspoon granulated sugar
2 tablespoons + 1 teaspoon capers, drained
2 teaspoons chopped fresh thyme
4 cups torn chicory leaves
5 small pitted black olives, julienned

1. To prepare dressing, in medium bowl with tight-fitting cover, whisk yogurt, vinegar, oil, mustard, lemon zest and sugar; stir in capers and thyme. Refrigerate, covered, 2–3 hours.

2. In large bowl, combine chicory and dressing; toss to mix well. Sprinkle with olives.

EACH SERVING PROVIDES: $\frac{1}{2}$ Fat, 2 Vegetables, 10 Optional Calories
PER SERVING: 75 Calories, 3 g Protein, 3 g Fat, 10 g Carbohydrate, 321 mg Sodium, 0 mg Cholesterol, 3 g Dietary Fiber

◆

CUCUMBER WITH DILLED BUTTERMILK DRESSING

MAKES 4 SERVINGS

$\frac{1}{2}$ cup low-fat (1.5%) buttermilk
$\frac{1}{3}$ cup chopped fresh dill
$\frac{1}{2}$ teaspoon white wine vinegar
$\frac{1}{4}$ teaspoon powdered mustard
$\frac{1}{4}$ teaspoon salt
Pinch white pepper
$\frac{1}{8}$ teaspoon freshly ground black pepper (optional)
2 cups thinly sliced cucumbers

1. To prepare dressing, in small bowl with tight-fitting cover, combine buttermilk, dill, vinegar, mustard, salt, white pepper and black pepper if using; refrigerate, covered, 2–3 hours.

2. In medium bowl, combine cucumbers with dressing; toss to mix well. Serve immediately.

EACH SERVING PROVIDES: 1 Vegetable, 10 Optional Calories
PER SERVING: 26 Calories, 2 g Protein, 1 g Fat, 4 g Carbohydrate, 170 mg Sodium, 2 mg Cholesterol, 1 g Dietary Fiber

◆

TOMATO SALAD WITH RED ONION AND BASIL

The showcase for summer's trio, best enjoyed at the height of the season, when tomatoes are ripe and juicy and fresh basil is plentiful.

MAKES 4 SERVINGS

3 tablespoons red wine vinegar
1 tablespoon + 1 teaspoon olive oil
$\frac{1}{2}$ teaspoon granulated sugar
$\frac{1}{2}$ teaspoon salt
$\frac{1}{2}$ teaspoon prepared mustard
$\frac{1}{4}$ teaspoon freshly ground black pepper
4 medium tomatoes, cut into wedges
$\frac{3}{4}$ cup thinly sliced red onions
$\frac{1}{3}$ cup tightly packed fresh basil leaves, shredded

1. To prepare dressing, in small bowl, whisk vinegar, oil, sugar, salt, mustard and pepper; set aside.

2. In large bowl, combine tomatoes, onions and basil. Add dressing; toss to coat.

3. Refrigerate, covered, 1 hour, tossing once.

EACH SERVING PROVIDES: 1 Fat, $2\frac{1}{2}$ Vegetables, 2 Optional Calories
PER SERVING: 92 Calories, 2 g Protein, 5 g Fat, 12 g Carbohydrate, 299 mg Sodium, 0 mg Cholesterol, 3 g Dietary Fiber

ZUCCHINI-CARROT SALAD WITH CUMIN DRESSING

MAKES 4 SERVINGS

1 teaspoon ground cumin
2 tablespoons + 2 teaspoons reduced-calorie mayonnaise
1 tablespoon chopped cilantro
1 tablespoon lime juice
$\frac{1}{2}$ teaspoon grated lime zest
$\frac{1}{4}$ teaspoon salt
$\frac{1}{8}$ teaspoon freshly ground black pepper
2 medium carrots, julienned
1 medium zucchini, julienned

1. To prepare dressing, in small skillet, heat cumin; cook over low heat, stirring frequently, 1 minute, until fragrant.

2. In small bowl, combine warm cumin, mayonnaise, cilantro, juice, lime zest, salt and pepper; stir to mix well.

3. In medium bowl, combine carrots and zucchini. Add dressing; toss to mix well.

EACH SERVING PROVIDES: 1 Fat, 1½ Vegetables
PER SERVING: 58 Calories, 1 g Protein, 3 g Fat, 8 g Carbohydrate, 210 mg Sodium, 3 mg Cholesterol, 2 g Dietary Fiber

BROCCOLI AND BULGUR IN SPICY PEANUT SAUCE

With definite Asian ancestry, this is a hearty and filling salad best served warm.

MAKES 6 SERVINGS

6 ounces uncooked bulgur
$\frac{1}{2}$ cup cilantro
$\frac{1}{4}$ cup reduced-sodium soy sauce
3 tablespoons chunky-style peanut butter
1 tablespoon white wine vinegar
1 teaspoon granulated sugar
$\frac{1}{8}$ teaspoon ground red pepper
3 cups small broccoli florets, steamed until tender-crisp

1. In large saucepan, bring 3 cups water to a boil; stir in bulgur. Reduce heat to low; simmer 10–15 minutes, or until all liquid is absorbed.

2. In food processor or blender, combine cilantro, soy sauce, peanut butter, vinegar, sugar and red pepper; purée until smooth.

3. Pour peanut sauce into bulgur; stir to combine. Add broccoli; gently stir to mix well. Cook over medium heat, stirring occasionally, 5 minutes, until heated through.

EACH SERVING PROVIDES: ½ Fat, 1 Vegetable, ½ Protein, 1 Bread, 3 Optional Calories
PER SERVING: 174 Calories, 8 g Protein, 5 g Fat, 29 g Carbohydrate, 460 mg Sodium, 0 mg Cholesterol, 8 g Dietary Fiber

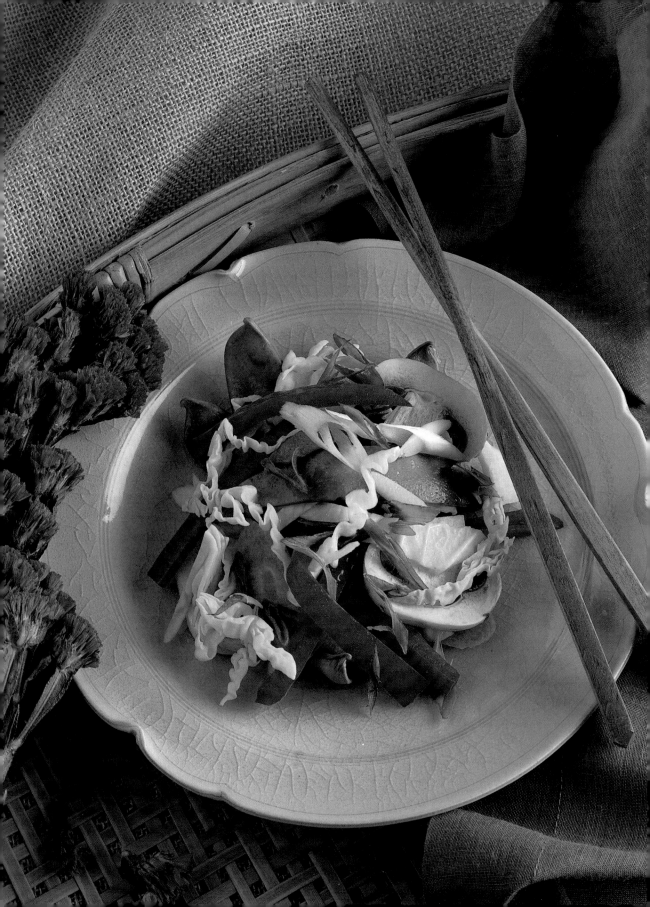

ORIENTAL VEGETABLE SALAD

MAKES 4 SERVINGS

1 tablespoon orange juice
2 teaspoons white wine vinegar
2 teaspoons soy sauce
1 teaspoon grated fresh ginger root
1 teaspoon sesame oil
1 teaspoon vegetable oil
1 garlic clove, minced
$\frac{1}{8}$ teaspoon Oriental hot pepper oil
1 cup snow peas, stem ends and strings removed, blanched
$\frac{1}{2}$ cup diagonally sliced Chinese cabbage
$\frac{1}{2}$ cup sliced mushrooms
$\frac{1}{2}$ cup thinly sliced red bell pepper
$\frac{1}{2}$ cup diagonally sliced carrot (thin slices)
$\frac{1}{4}$ cup diagonally sliced scallions (thin slices)

1. To prepare dressing, in small bowl, combine juice, vinegar, soy sauce, ginger, sesame oil, vegetable oil, garlic and hot pepper oil; stir to mix well. Set aside.

2. In medium bowl, combine snow peas, cabbage, mushrooms, bell pepper, carrot and scallions. Add dressing; toss to coat.

EACH SERVING PROVIDES: $\frac{1}{2}$ Fat, 1$\frac{1}{2}$ Vegetables, 3 Optional Calories
PER SERVING: 57 Calories, 2 g Protein, 3 g Fat, 7 g Carbohydrate, 181 mg Sodium, 0 mg Cholesterol, 2 g Dietary Fiber

COLD BARLEY SALAD WITH CURRIED CAULIFLOWER

MAKES 6 SERVINGS

$\frac{1}{3}$ cup white-wine vinegar
1 tablespoon granulated sugar
1 tablespoon olive oil
2 teaspoons curry powder
$\frac{1}{8}$ teaspoon freshly ground black pepper
4$\frac{1}{2}$ cups cauliflower florets, steamed until tender-crisp
4$\frac{1}{2}$ ounces uncooked pearl barley
1$\frac{1}{2}$ cups red bell pepper strips (3" strips)
12 red leaf lettuce leaves

1. To prepare marinade, in gallon-size sealable plastic bag, combine vinegar, sugar, oil, curry powder and black pepper; add cauliflower. Seal bag, squeezing out air; turn to coat cauliflower. Let stand at room temperature 1 hour, turning bag occasionally.

2. Meanwhile, in medium saucepan bring 1$\frac{1}{2}$ cups water to a boil; add barley. Reduce heat to low; simmer, covered, 30–45 minutes, or until barley is tender and liquid is absorbed.

3. In medium bowl, combine marinated cauliflower mixture, cooked barley and bell pepper strips. Refrigerate, covered, 2–3 hours.

4. To serve, line 6 plates with 2 lettuce leaves each; top each with an equal amount of the barley mixture.

EACH SERVING PROVIDES: $\frac{1}{2}$ Fat, 2$\frac{1}{2}$ Vegetables, 1 Bread, 10 Optional Calories
PER SERVING: 133 Calories, 4 g Protein, 3 g Fat, 25 g Carbohydrate, 15 mg Sodium, 0 mg Cholesterol, 6 g Dietary Fiber

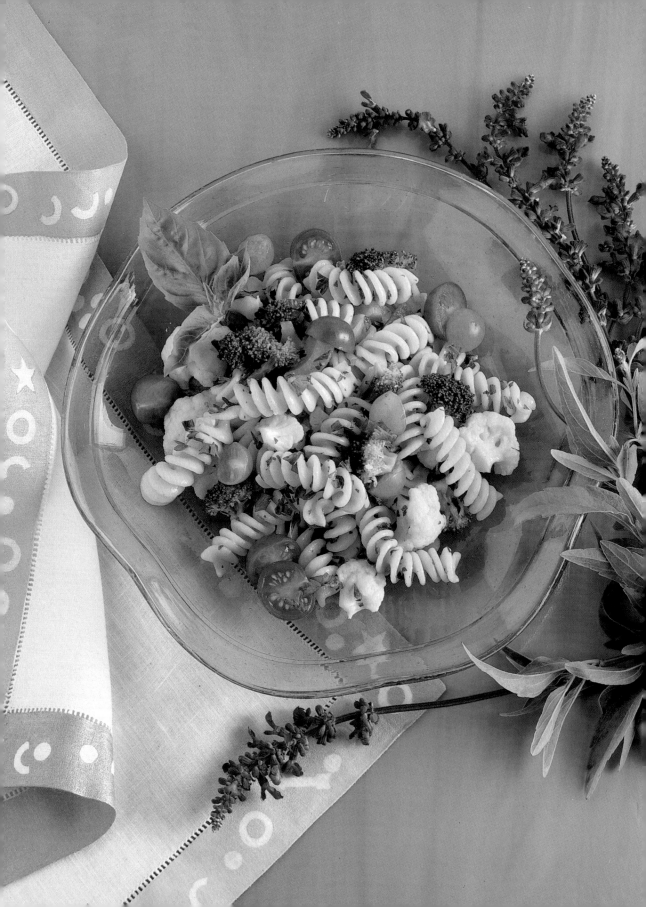

PASTA SALAD PRIMAVERA

A low-in-fat yet rich-tasting pasta salad studded with vibrant vegetables and tossed with a yogurt-based dressing.

MAKES 4 SERVINGS

⅓ cup plain nonfat yogurt

2 tablespoons grated Parmesan cheese

1 tablespoon + 1 teaspoon red wine vinegar

1 teaspoon grated lemon zest

1 teaspoon olive oil

1 garlic clove, minced

¼ teaspoon freshly ground black pepper

2 cups cooked rotelle (spiral pasta)

1 cup small broccoli florets, steamed until tender-crisp

1 cup small cauliflower florets, steamed until tender-crisp

12 cherry tomatoes, halved

¼ cup shredded fresh basil leaves

¼ cup chopped red onion

1. To prepare dressing, in small bowl, combine yogurt, cheese, vinegar, lemon zest, oil, garlic and pepper; stir to mix well.

2. In large bowl, combine pasta, broccoli, cauliflower, tomatoes, basil and onion. Pour yogurt mixture over pasta mixture; toss to coat.

3. Refrigerate, covered, at least 1 hour, until well chilled.

EACH SERVING PROVIDES: ¼ Fat, 1¾ Vegetables, 1 Bread, 25 Optional Calories
PER SERVING: 158 Calories, 7 g Protein, 3 g Fat, 27 g Carbohydrate, 77 mg Sodium, 2 mg Cholesterol, 3 g Dietary Fiber

COLE SLAW WITH CARAWAY-MINT DRESSING

MAKES 4 SERVINGS

2 tablespoons + 2 teaspoons reduced-calorie mayonnaise

2 tablespoons cider vinegar

1 tablespoon caraway seeds

1 teaspoon granulated sugar

¼ teaspoon freshly ground black pepper

3 cups shredded green cabbage

1 cup grated carrots

⅓ cup grated onion

2 tablespoons chopped fresh mint

1. To prepare dressing, in small bowl, combine mayonnaise, vinegar, caraway seeds, sugar and pepper; stir to mix well.

2. In large bowl, combine cabbage, carrots, onion and mint. Add dressing; toss to mix well.

3. Refrigerate, covered, 2–3 hours.

EACH SERVING PROVIDES: 1 Fat, 2¼ Vegetables, 15 Optional Calories
PER SERVING: 68 Calories, 2 g Protein, 3 g Fat, 10 g Carbohydrate, 74 mg Sodium, 3 mg Cholesterol, 2 g Dietary Fiber

GERMAN POTATO SALAD

MAKES 4 SERVINGS

1 pound diced cooked potatoes
$\frac{1}{2}$ cup chopped onion
$\frac{1}{2}$ cup chopped celery
$\frac{1}{2}$ cup chopped green bell pepper
3 slices crisp cooked bacon, crumbled
$\frac{1}{2}$ cup apple juice
$\frac{1}{4}$ cup cider vinegar
1 tablespoon all-purpose flour
$\frac{1}{2}$ teaspoon salt
$\frac{1}{4}$ teaspoon freshly ground black pepper

1. In large bowl, combine potatoes, onion, celery, bell pepper and bacon; set aside.

2. In small saucepan, whisk juice, vinegar and flour; stirring constantly, bring mixture to a boil. Boil, whisking constantly, 4 minutes, until thickened; stir in salt and pepper.

3. Pour juice mixture over potato mixture; toss gently to combine. Serve immediately.

EACH SERVING PROVIDES: $\frac{1}{4}$ Fruit, $\frac{3}{4}$ Vegetable, 1 Bread, 35 Optional Calories
PER SERVING: 163 Calories, 4 g Protein, 3 g Fat, 32 g Carbohydrate, 370 mg Sodium, 4 mg Cholesterol, 3 g Dietary Fiber

◆

MARINATED THREE-BEAN SALAD

MAKES 4 SERVINGS

2 tablespoons cider vinegar
2 tablespoons apple juice
2 teaspoons grated fresh ginger root
1 cup cut green beans (2" pieces), steamed until tender-crisp (hot)
1 cup cut wax beans (2" pieces), steamed until tender-crisp (hot)
4 ounces drained cooked kidney beans
$\frac{1}{4}$ cup minced onion
$\frac{1}{4}$ cup finely diced red bell pepper
2 tablespoons chopped fresh basil

1. To prepare dressing, in large bowl, combine vinegar, juice and ginger; stir to mix well.

2. Add green beans, wax beans, kidney beans, onion, bell pepper and basil; toss to mix well.

3. Refrigerate, covered, at least 3 hours.

EACH SERVING PROVIDES: $1\frac{1}{4}$ Vegetables, $\frac{1}{2}$ Bread, 5 Optional Calories
PER SERVING: 65 Calories, 4 g Protein, 0 g Fat, 13 g Carbohydrate, 5 mg Sodium, 0 mg Cholesterol, 2 g Dietary Fiber

◆

YUCATAN SALAD

Jicama, a knobby root vegetable frequently found in Mexican dishes, has the texture of a turnip with a milder flavor. It is delicious raw, as in this salad, and turns sweeter when cooked.

MAKES 4 SERVINGS

8 ounces pared jicama
$\frac{3}{4}$ cup fresh orange juice
1 small navel orange, peeled and sectioned
$\frac{1}{2}$ cup sliced scallions, including some green stems
$\frac{1}{2}$ cup finely diced red bell pepper
2 tablespoons fresh lime juice
1 teaspoon chili powder
$\frac{1}{2}$ teaspoon salt
2 cups soft lettuce leaves such as Bibb or butter lettuce

1. Cut jicama into $\frac{1}{8}$" slices, then cut each slice into $\frac{1}{8}$" strips.

2. In nonreactive bowl, combine jicama with remaining ingredients except lettuce. Cover with plastic wrap and refrigerate, stirring several times, at least 4 hours or overnight.

3. Line each of four salad plates with $\frac{1}{4}$ of the lettuce leaves; top evenly with jicama mixture.

EACH SERVING PROVIDES: $\frac{1}{2}$ Fruit, $2\frac{1}{2}$ Vegetables, 10 Optional Calories
PER SERVING: 75 Calories, 2 g Protein, 0 g Fat, 17 g Carbohydrate, 289 mg Sodium, 0 mg Cholesterol, 3 g Dietary Fiber

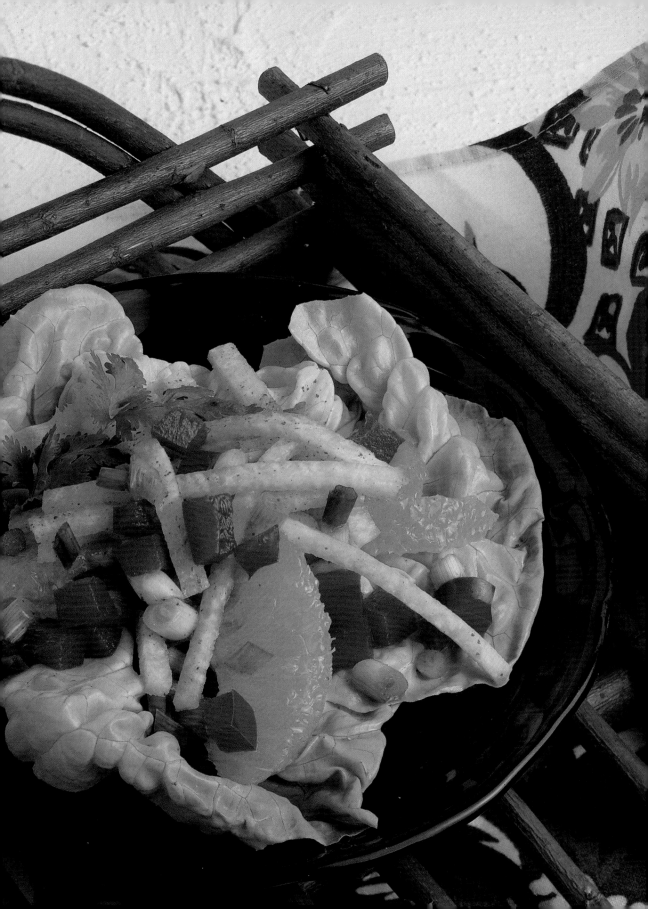

ZUCCHINI AND MUSHROOM GRAIN SALAD

MAKES 6 SERVINGS

$2\frac{1}{4}$ ounces uncooked wheat berries
3 ounces uncooked quinoa
$\frac{1}{4}$ cup tahini (sesame paste)
2 tablespoons reduced-sodium soy sauce
2 tablespoons fresh lemon juice
1 tablespoon cornstarch
1 cup minced onion
3 cups sliced zucchini
2 teaspoons low-sodium chicken bouillon granules
$\frac{1}{8}$ teaspoon pepper
2 cups sliced mushrooms

1. In small saucepan, bring 1 cup water to a boil; add wheat berries. Reduce heat to low; simmer 2 hours, stirring occasionally, until plump and tender. Set aside.

2. In separate small saucepan, bring $\frac{1}{2}$ cup water to a boil; add quinoa. Reduce heat to low; simmer 15 minutes, until quinoa is translucent. Set aside.

3. Meanwhile, in food processor or blender, combine tahini, soy sauce, juice and cornstarch; purée until smooth. Set aside.

4. Heat large nonstick skillet sprayed with nonstick cooking spray; add onion. Cook over medium-high heat, stirring constantly, 3 minutes, or until onions are browned. Stir in zucchini, 1 cup water, bouillon granules and pepper. Reduce heat to low; simmer 3–4 minutes, until zucchini is tender-crisp.

5. Add mushrooms to skillet; stir to combine. Bring zucchini mixture to a boil; add tahini mixture. Cook, stirring constantly, 2 minutes, until thickened; add cooked wheat berries and cooked quinoa. Cook, stirring occasionally, until heated through.

EACH SERVING PROVIDES: $\frac{1}{2}$ Fat, 2 Vegetables, $\frac{1}{4}$ Protein, 1 Bread, 10 Optional Calories
PER SERVING: 190 Calories, 7 g Protein, 7 g Fat, 27 g Carbohydrate, 227 mg Sodium, 0 mg Cholesterol, 4 g Dietary Fiber

SWEET AND SAVORY SALAD

MAKES 4 SERVINGS

2 cups sugar snap peas, trimmed and steamed until bright green
2 cups broccoli, stems pared, cut into bite-size pieces and steamed until bright green
2 cups asparagus, cut diagonally into 2-inch pieces and steamed until bright green
1 tablespoon + 1 teaspoon olive oil
$\frac{1}{4}$ cup thinly sliced scallions
1 tablespoon finely chopped fresh mint
1 tablespoon finely chopped flat-leafed parsley
1 garlic clove, finely chopped
1 teaspoon finely chopped fresh ginger root
Salt and freshly ground black pepper to taste
Juice of $\frac{1}{2}$ lemon (optional)
2 teaspoons toasted sesame seeds

In large bowl, toss sugar snap peas, broccoli and asparagus with oil. Add scallions, mint, parsley, garlic, ginger, salt and pepper. Mix in juice, if using, just before serving. Sprinkle with sesame seeds and serve.

EACH SERVING ($1\frac{1}{2}$ cups) PROVIDES: 1 Fat, $3\frac{1}{4}$ Vegetables, 10 Optional Calories
PER SERVING: 131 Calories, 6 g Protein, 6 g Fat, 16 g Carbohydrate, 21 mg Sodium, 0 mg Cholesterol, 7 g Dietary Fiber

MESCLUN, ORANGE AND WALNUT SALAD

Mesclun, meaning a mixture of small, tender young lettuce leaves, includes frisée or curly endive; mâche or lamb's lettuce; and arugula and radicchio, along with bibb and red and green oak leaf.

MAKES 4 SERVINGS

2 tablespoons orange juice
2 teaspoons walnut oil
$\frac{1}{4}$ teaspoon salt
Pinch ground red pepper
6 cups torn mesclun leaves
1 cup peeled orange sections, membrane removed
$\frac{1}{4}$ cup julienned red onion
1 ounce chopped walnuts, lightly toasted

1. To prepare dressing, in small bowl, whisk juice, walnut oil, salt and red pepper; stir to mix well.

2. In large bowl, combine mesclun, orange sections, onion and walnuts. Add dressing; toss to mix well. Serve immediately.

EACH SERVING PROVIDES: 1 Fat, $\frac{1}{2}$ Fruit, $3\frac{1}{4}$ Vegetables, $\frac{1}{4}$ Protein, 5 Optional Calories
PER SERVING: 109 Calories, 3 g Protein, 7 g Fat, 11 g Carbohydrate, 144 mg Sodium, 0 mg Cholesterol, 2 g Dietary Fiber

TARRAGON-ORANGE WALDORF SALAD

MAKES 4 SERVINGS

2 tablespoons orange juice
1 tablespoon reduced-calorie mayonnaise
1 tablespoon slivered orange peel
2 teaspoons chopped fresh tarragon
1 medium tart red apple (6 ounces), cored and diced
1 medium tart green apple (6 ounces), cored and diced
1 cup diced celery
3 tablespoons chopped red onion
3 tablespoons dried currants
$\frac{1}{2}$ ounce chopped walnuts, toasted

1. To prepare dressing, in small bowl, combine juice, mayonnaise, orange peel and tarragon; stir to mix well.

2. In large bowl, combine red apple, green apple, celery, onion, currants and walnuts. Add dressing; toss to coat.

EACH SERVING PROVIDES: $\frac{1}{2}$ Fat, 1 Fruit, $\frac{1}{2}$ Vegetable, 25 Optional Calories
PER SERVING: 112 Calories, 1 g Protein, 4 g Fat, 21 g Carbohydrate, 48 mg Sodium, 1 mg Cholesterol, 3 g Dietary Fiber

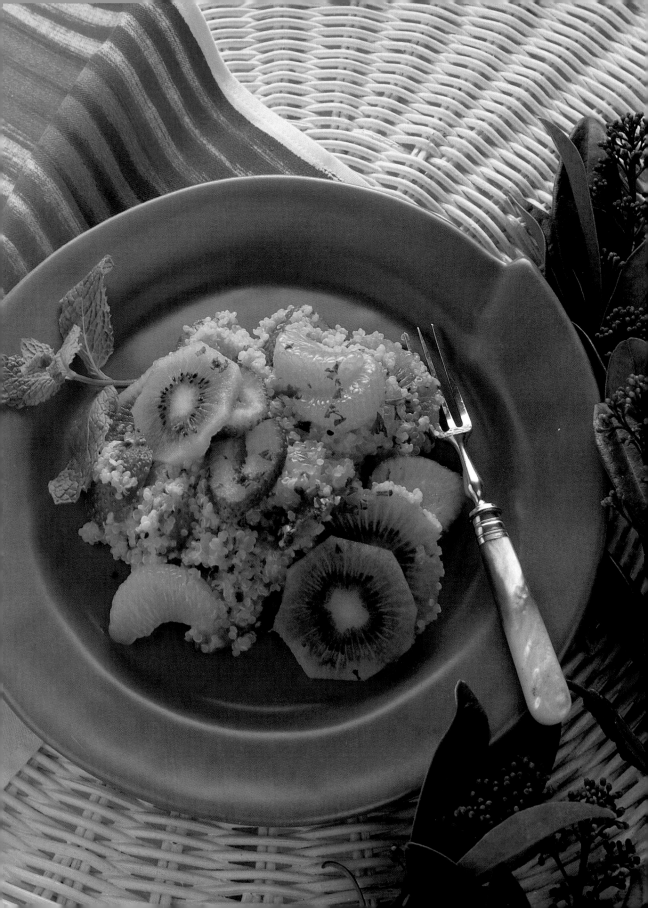

MINTED QUINOA FRUIT SALAD

Pronounced "keen-wa," this grain was discovered by the ancient Incas. Newly embraced as a rich source of nutrients, this sweet and nutty grain is easy to prepare and can be used in recipes calling for rice or pasta.

MAKES 6 SERVINGS

¼ teaspoon salt
6 ounces uncooked quinoa
⅓ cup chopped mint
¼ cup vanilla-flavored nonfat yogurt, sweetened with aspartame
2 tablespoons orange juice
1½ cups sliced strawberries
2 medium kiwi fruits, pared and sliced
1 cup drained canned mandarin orange sections

1. In medium saucepan, bring 2 cups water and the salt to a boil; add quinoa. Reduce heat to low; simmer 15 minutes, until quinoa is translucent.

2. In food processor or blender, combine mint, yogurt and juice; purée until smooth. Set aside.

3. Set aside six strawberry slices and three kiwi slices for garnish. In large serving bowl, combine the remaining strawberries, the remaining kiwi and the mandarin orange sections.

4. Pour yogurt sauce over fruit mixture; toss to coat. Add cooked quinoa; toss gently to mix well.

5. Garnish with reserved strawberry and kiwi slices. Refrigerate, covered, 1–2 hours, until thoroughly chilled.

EACH SERVING PROVIDES: 1 Fruit, 1 Bread, 5 Optional Calories
PER SERVING: 160 Calories, 5 g Protein, 2 g Fat, 32 g Carbohydrate, 117 mg Sodium, 0 mg Cholesterol, 6 g Dietary Fiber

PEAR SALAD WITH BLUE CHEESE DRESSING

Unusual and refreshing, the cheese is in the dressing, coating the pears with a creamy tang.

MAKES 4 SERVINGS

¼ cup part-skim ricotta cheese
1½ ounces blue cheese, crumbled
2 large pears, cut into thin wedges
4 medium celery stalks, cut into 3" sticks
2 teaspoons white wine vinegar
¼ cup golden raisins

1. To prepare dressing, in processor or blender, combine ricotta cheese and 2 tablespoons water; purée until smooth. Transfer to small bowl; add blue cheese. Stir, pressing cheese against sides of bowl, mixing thoroughly.

2. To serve, on each of four plates, evenly arrange pear wedges and celery stalks; sprinkle each evenly with vinegar. Drizzle each with one-fourth of the dressing; top each with 1 tablespoon of the raisins.

EACH SERVING PROVIDES: 1½ Fruits, ½ Vegetable, ¾ Protein
PER SERVING: 184 Calories, 5 g Protein, 5 g Fat, 33 g Carbohydrate, 195 mg Sodium, 13 mg Cholesterol, 5 g Dietary Fiber

ITALIAN DRESSING

MAKES 4 SERVINGS

$\frac{1}{4}$ cup low-sodium chicken broth
1 tablespoon finely diced red bell pepper
1 tablespoon chopped fresh basil
1 tablespoon white wine vinegar
2 teaspoons olive oil
$\frac{1}{2}$ teaspoon grated lemon zest
$\frac{1}{2}$ teaspoon salt
$\frac{1}{2}$ garlic clove, minced
$\frac{1}{4}$ teaspoon oregano leaves, crumbled
$\frac{1}{8}$ teaspoon freshly ground black pepper

1. In small bowl or jar with tight-fitting cover, combine broth, bell pepper, basil, vinegar, oil, lemon zest, salt, garlic, oregano and pepper; whisk or cover and shake to mix well.

2. Refrigerate, covered, overnight. Whisk or shake before serving.

EACH SERVING (2 tablespoons) PROVIDES: $\frac{1}{2}$ Fat, 1 Optional Calorie
PER SERVING: 24 Calories, 0 g Protein, 2 g Fat, 1 g Carbohydrate, 314 mg Sodium, 0 mg Cholesterol, 0 g Dietary Fiber

"RUSSIAN" DRESSING

MAKES 4 SERVINGS

3 tablespoons orange juice
2 tablespoons + 2 teaspoons reduced-calorie mayonnaise
2 tablespoons minced green bell pepper
2 tablespoons minced red bell pepper
2 tablespoons tomato paste
2 tablespoons plain nonfat yogurt
1 tablespoon drained horseradish
1 tablespoon grated onion
1 teaspoon prepared mustard
$\frac{1}{2}$ teaspoon chili powder
$\frac{1}{4}$ teaspoon freshly ground black pepper

1. In small bowl or jar with tight-fitting cover, combine juice, mayonnaise, green bell pepper, red bell pepper, tomato paste, yogurt, horseradish, onion, mustard, chili powder and pepper; whisk or cover and shake to mix well.

2. Refrigerate, covered, 2–3 hours. Whisk or shake before serving.

EACH SERVING (3 tablespoons) PROVIDES: 1 Fat, $\frac{1}{2}$ Vegetable, 10 Optional Calories
PER SERVING: 49 Calories, 1 g Protein, 3 g Fat, 5 g Carbohydrate, 148 mg Sodium, 3 mg Cholesterol, 1 g Dietary Fiber

HONEY-MUSTARD DRESSING

MAKES 4 SERVINGS

$\frac{1}{2}$ cup plain nonfat yogurt
1 tablespoon + 1 teaspoon prepared mustard
1 tablespoon + 1 teaspoon honey
1 tablespoon chopped fresh dill
2 teaspoons white wine vinegar
$\frac{1}{2}$ teaspoon granulated sugar
$\frac{1}{8}$ teaspoon white pepper

1. In small bowl with tight-fitting cover, combine yogurt, mustard, honey, dill, vinegar, sugar and white pepper; stir to mix well.

2. Refrigerate, covered, 2–3 hours before serving.

EACH SERVING (2 tablespoons) PROVIDES: 35 Optional Calories
PER SERVING: 44 Calories, 2 g Protein, 0 g Fat, 9 g Carbohydrate, 87 mg Sodium, 1 mg Cholesterol, 0 g Dietary Fiber

PESTO DRESSING

MAKES 4 SERVINGS

2 cups fresh basil leaves
$\frac{1}{2}$ cup flat-leaf parsley
$\frac{1}{4}$ cup part-skim ricotta cheese
3 tablespoons grated Parmesan cheese
3 garlic cloves, minced
$\frac{1}{2}$ teaspoon freshly ground black pepper
2 tablespoons plain nonfat yogurt

1. In blender or food processor, combine basil, parsley, ricotta cheese, Parmesan cheese, garlic and pepper; purée until smooth. Transfer to small bowl with tight-fitting cover; stir in yogurt.

2. Refrigerate, covered, at least 2 hours. Stir before serving.

EACH SERVING (3 tablespoons) PROVIDES: $\frac{1}{4}$ Protein, 25 Optional Calories
PER SERVING: 69 Calories, 5 g Protein, 3 g Fat, 8 g Carbohydrate, 99 mg Sodium, 8 mg Cholesterol, 0 g Dietary Fiber

CREAMY GARLIC AND CHIVE DRESSING

MAKES 4 SERVINGS

10 garlic cloves, peeled
½ cup part-skim ricotta cheese
¼ cup plain nonfat yogurt
2 tablespoons chopped chives
½ teaspoon salt
¼ teaspoon freshly ground black pepper

1. In small saucepan, combine garlic and 1 cup water; bring to a boil. Reduce heat to low; simmer 10 minutes. With slotted spoon, transfer garlic to paper towel, reserving 2 tablespoons of the cooking liquid.

2. In blender or food processor, combine cooked garlic, reserved liquid, ricotta cheese and yogurt; purée until smooth. Transfer to bowl with tight-fitting cover; stir in chives, salt and pepper.

3. Refrigerate, covered, at least 2 hours. Stir before serving.

EACH SERVING (3 tablespoons) PROVIDES: ½ Protein, 10 Optional Calories
PER SERVING: 62 Calories, 5 g Protein, 2 g Fat, 5 g Carbohydrate, 324 mg Sodium, 10 mg Cholesterol, 0 g Dietary Fiber

---

Grilling Tips

Vegetables have come into their own, leaping from the maligned to the sublime, and one of the most popular ways to enjoy them is on the grill. Grill up your favorite vegetables for a fat-free flavor sensation!

- *Use a hinged grilling basket for soft vegetables to make turning easier.*
- *When grilling root vegetables such as potatoes, yams or turnips, shorten cooking time by parboiling or precooking them in the microwave for a few minutes.*
- *Cooking time will vary according to the vegetables and the intensity of the heat. Test with a skewer to determine doneness—it should be easy to insert when vegetables are done.*

Garlic Roasted Chicken with Herb-Lemon Gravy (page 140), Cornbread Cranberry Dressing (page 183)

CHAPTER SEVEN

POULTRY

GARLIC ROASTED CHICKEN WITH HERB-LEMON GRAVY

Stuffing the chicken cavity with lemon, onion, garlic and herbs infuses the meat with wonderful flavor, which is echoed in both the basting liquid and the gravy.

MAKES 6 SERVINGS

One 3-pound, 8-ounce chicken, skinned
1 medium lemon, halved
1 medium onion, halved
4 rosemary sprigs
4 thyme sprigs
6 garlic cloves, peeled
1 cup low-sodium chicken broth
2 tablespoons lemon juice
1 tablespoon cornstarch
2 tablespoons dry white wine
1 tablespoon minced scallion
1 tablespoon reduced-sodium soy sauce
¼ teaspoon dried sage leaves

1. Preheat oven to 400°F. Spray broiler rack in roasting pan with nonstick cooking spray. Remove chicken giblets and neck from body cavity; refrigerate or freeze for another use. Rinse chicken with cold running water inside and out; pat dry with paper towels.

2. Arrange lemon halves, onion, rosemary, thyme and garlic in body cavity; with poultry string, tie legs together. Transfer chicken, breast-side up, to rack in roasting pan. Roast 30 minutes; pour broth and lemon juice over chicken. Reduce heat to 325°F. Make a foil tent over chicken; roast about 1 hour longer, basting frequently, until meat thermometer, inserted into center of inner thigh muscle (not touching bone), reaches 180–185°F. Transfer chicken to carving board; let stand 15 minutes.

3. Meanwhile, pour pan juices into medium saucepan, reserving 1 tablespoon liquid. In small bowl, with whisk, dissolve cornstarch in reserved liquid. Add ¼ cup water, wine, scallion, soy sauce and sage to saucepan; bring to a boil, boiling for 5 minutes. Reduce heat to low; whisk in dissolved cornstarch. Cook, stirring constantly, about 1 minute, until gravy thickens.

4. Carve chicken and serve with gravy.

EACH SERVING PROVIDES: 3 Proteins, 15 Optional Calories
PER SERVING: 195 Calories, 26 g Protein, 7 g Fat, 6 g Carbohydrate, 185 mg Sodium, 76 mg Cholesterol, 0 g Dietary Fiber

SOUTHERN OVEN-"FRIED" CHICKEN

MAKES 4 SERVINGS

½ cup skim buttermilk
2–3 drops hot red pepper sauce
¾ ounce corn flakes, crushed
3 tablespoons all-purpose flour
¼ teaspoon salt
¼ teaspoon freshly ground black pepper
One 1-pound, 14-ounce chicken, skinned and
    quartered
1 tablespoon + 1 teaspoon canola oil

1. Preheat oven to 400°F. Spray large baking sheet with nonstick cooking spray.

2. In large shallow bowl, combine buttermilk and red pepper sauce. On sheet of wax paper combine corn flake crumbs, flour, salt and black pepper. Dip chicken pieces in buttermilk mixture; dredge, coating completely, with corn flake mixture.

3. Arrange chicken on prepared baking sheet; drizzle evenly with oil. Bake 30 minutes; turn pieces over and bake 15–20 minutes longer, until cooked through.

EACH SERVING PROVIDES: 1 Fat, 2½ Proteins, ½ Bread, 10 Optional Calories
PER SERVING: 229 Calories, 23 g Protein, 10 g Fat, 11 g Carbohydrate, 295 mg Sodium, 64 mg Cholesterol, 0 g Dietary Fiber

Southern Oven-"Fried" Chicken,
Garlic Mashed Potatoes (page 302)

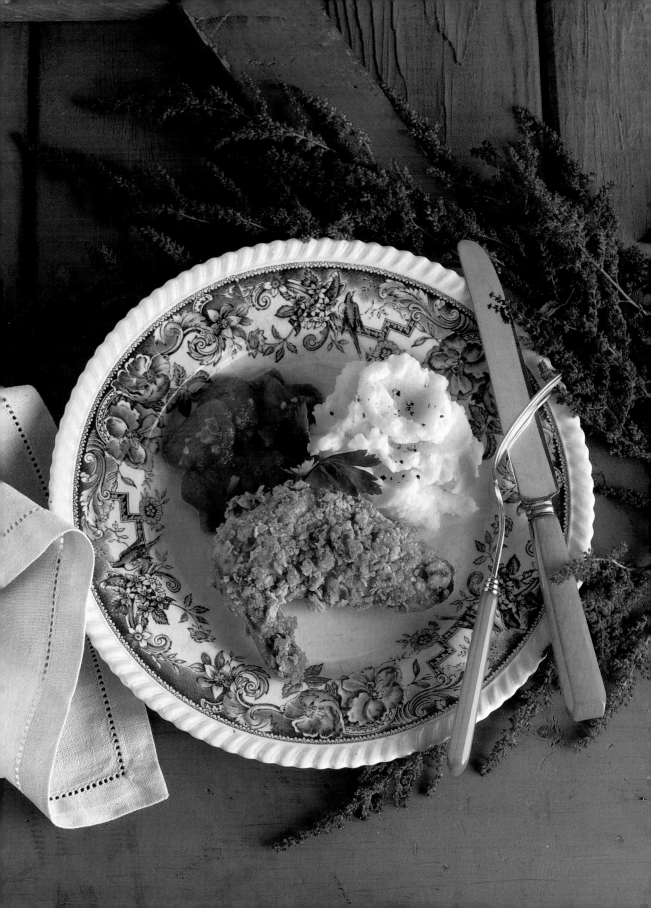

CHICKEN STUFFED WITH ORANGE-TARRAGON RICE

MAKES 6 SERVINGS

3 cups cooked regular long-grain rice
$\frac{1}{2}$ cup dark raisins
Three 5-ounce skinless boneless chicken breasts,
   pounded to $\frac{1}{4}$" thickness
3 tarragon sprigs or $\frac{1}{2}$ teaspoon dried leaves
2 tablespoons stick margarine
2 garlic cloves, minced
1 cup dry white wine
1 cup orange juice
2 teaspoons tarragon leaves
2 tablespoons cornstarch, dissolved in $\frac{1}{4}$ cup water

1. In small bowl, combine $\frac{1}{3}$ cup + 2 teaspoons of the rice and the raisins; stir to mix well. Keep remaining rice warm.

2. Place chicken on clean, flat work surface; spoon one-third of the rice-raisin mixture on each chicken breast. Top each with 1 tarragon sprig. Starting from narrow end, roll each chicken breast jelly-roll style, enclosing stuffing. Secure ends with toothpicks.

3. In large skillet melt margarine over medium heat; add garlic. Sauté 2 minutes; add stuffed chicken breasts and brown on all sides. Transfer to plate.

4. Add wine, orange juice and tarragon leaves to same skillet; stir to mix well. Return chicken to skillet. Reduce heat to low; simmer 30 minutes. With slotted spoon, transfer chicken to cutting board; remove and discard toothpicks. Slice each breast into thirds; set aside and keep warm.

5. Add dissolved cornstarch to same skillet; stir to mix well. Cook over medium heat, stirring frequently, until sauce thickens.

6. To serve, arrange remaining rice on serving platter; top with sliced stuffed chicken. Spoon sauce evenly over chicken.

EACH SERVING PROVIDES: 1 Fat, 1 Fruit, 2 Proteins, 1 Bread, 45 Optional Calories
PER SERVING: 341 Calories, 20 g Protein, 5 g Fat, 46 g Carbohydrate, 98 mg Sodium, 41 mg Cholesterol, 1 g Dietary Fiber

CREOLE POACHED CHICKEN BREASTS

MAKES 4 SERVINGS

2 teaspoons olive oil
1 cup chopped onion
1 cup chopped green bell pepper
$\frac{1}{2}$ cup chopped celery
$\frac{1}{2}$ cup chopped carrot
Four 3-ounce skinless boneless chicken breasts
2 cups canned stewed tomatoes
$\frac{1}{2}$ cup low-sodium chicken broth
2 tablespoons chopped fresh parsley
1 teaspoon ground thyme
$\frac{1}{4}$ teaspoon salt
$\frac{1}{8}$ teaspoon ground red pepper

1. In large nonstick skillet, heat oil; add onion, bell pepper, celery and carrot. Cook over medium-high heat, stirring frequently, 4–5 minutes, until tender. Stir in chicken, tomatoes, broth, parsley, thyme, salt and red pepper; bring to a boil. Reduce heat to low; poach, partially covered, 8–10 minutes, until chicken is cooked through.

2. With slotted spoon, transfer chicken to serving platter and keep warm. Simmer sauce, uncovered, 4–5 minutes, until reduced by half.

3. To serve, spoon sauce evenly over chicken.

EACH SERVING PROVIDES: $\frac{1}{2}$ Fat, $2\frac{1}{2}$ Vegetables, 2 Proteins, 3 Optional Calories
PER SERVING: 182 Calories, 22 g Protein, 4 g Fat, 16 g Carbohydrate, 541 mg Sodium, 49 mg Cholesterol, 5 g Dietary Fiber

SWEET AND SOUR ZUCCHINI CHICKEN

MAKES 4 SERVINGS

1 large egg white, lightly beaten
2 tablespoons reduced-sodium soy sauce
1 tablespoon low-sodium chicken broth
1 tablespoon firmly packed dark brown sugar
$\frac{1}{4}$ teaspoon white pepper
10 ounces skinless boneless chicken breast, cut into 1" pieces
$\frac{1}{3}$ cup pineapple juice
2 tablespoons cornstarch
2 tablespoons ketchup
2 tablespoons rice-wine vinegar
1 tablespoon all-purpose flour
1 tablespoon + 1 teaspoon peanut oil
2 cups coarsely chopped zucchini
1 medium red bell pepper, cut into 1" pieces
1$\frac{1}{2}$ cups sliced drained canned water chestnuts
1 cup chopped scallions
1 tablespoon grated fresh ginger root
1$\frac{1}{2}$ cups drained canned pineapple chunks

1. To prepare marinade, in gallon-size sealable plastic bag, combine egg white, soy sauce, broth, $\frac{1}{4}$ teaspoon of the brown sugar and the white pepper; add chicken. Seal bag, squeezing out air; turn to coat chicken. Refrigerate at least 1 hour, turning bag once. Drain and discard marinade.

2. In small bowl, combine juice, 1 teaspoon of the cornstarch, the ketchup, vinegar, and the remaining 2$\frac{3}{4}$ teaspoons sugar; set aside.

3. On sheet of wax paper, combine flour and the remaining 1 tablespoon + 2 teaspoons of cornstarch. Dredge chicken in flour mixture, coating completely.

4. In large nonstick skillet, heat 2 teaspoons of the oil; add chicken. Stir-fry, 6–8 minutes, until golden and cooked through; transfer to plate and set aside. Add the remaining 2 teaspoons oil to skillet and heat; add zucchini, bell pepper, water chestnuts, scallions and ginger. Stir-fry, 2 minutes, until tender. Stir in pineapple chunks; cook 1 minute.

5. Add juice mixture to skillet; cook, stirring constantly, until mixture comes to a boil. Return chicken to skillet; cook, stirring, 2 minutes, until heated through.

EACH SERVING PROVIDES: 1 Fat, 1 Fruit, 2 Vegetables, 2 Proteins, $\frac{1}{2}$ Bread, 45 Optional Calories
PER SERVING: 290 Calories, 20 g Protein, 6 g Fat, 41 g Carbohydrate, 465 mg Sodium, 41 mg Cholesterol, 2 g Dietary Fiber

Food Safety Tips

It's important to store and handle chicken properly, and with these tips you'll find it easy to serve wholesome chicken.

- *Wash your hands, countertops and utensils in hot, soapy water after handling raw chicken. Never transfer cooked chicken to a plate or bowl that has held raw chicken, unless it has been cleaned. For example, if grilling chicken, clean the platter on which you placed the raw chicken before placing the cooked chicken on it.*
- *Defrost chicken in the refrigerator or in a microwave, not on the counter.*
- *Cook chicken thoroughly. For chicken with bones, a meat thermometer should register 180°F; boneless parts should be cooked to an internal temperature of 160°F. When done, the juices of the chicken will be clear, not pink.*
- *Never leave raw or cooked chicken at room temperature for longer than 2 hours.*

SESAME CHICKEN AND ASPARAGUS STIR-FRY

MAKES 4 SERVINGS

2 tablespoons low-sodium chicken broth
1 tablespoon grated fresh ginger root
1 tablespoon reduced-sodium soy sauce
1 tablespoon Worcestershire sauce
2 teaspoons firmly packed brown sugar
1 teaspoon cornstarch
1 teaspoon sesame oil
$\frac{1}{4}$ teaspoon baking soda
10 ounces skinless boneless chicken breast, cut into strips
2 tablespoons sesame seeds
1 tablespoon peanut oil
1 cup chopped scallions, cut into 1" pieces
2 garlic cloves, minced
$\frac{1}{4}$ teaspoon red pepper flakes
12 asparagus spears, cut into 2" pieces
1 cup trimmed watercress

1. To prepare marinade, in gallon-size sealable plastic bag, combine broth, ginger, soy sauce, Worcestershire sauce, brown sugar, cornstarch, sesame oil and baking soda; add chicken. Seal bag, squeezing out air; turn to coat chicken. Refrigerate at least 2 hours or overnight, turning bag occasionally. Drain and discard marinade.

2. Heat large nonstick skillet until very hot; add sesame seeds. Cook over medium heat, stirring constantly, 2–3 minutes, until golden. Transfer to small bowl; set aside.

3. Heat peanut oil in skillet; add scallions, garlic and pepper flakes. Cook over high heat, stirring constantly, 2 minutes. Add asparagus and stir-fry, 4–5 minutes, until tender. Add marinated chicken and the watercress; stir-fry 6–8 minutes, until cooked through. Sprinkle with seeds before serving.

EACH SERVING PROVIDES: 1 Fat, 1$\frac{1}{2}$ Vegetables, 2 Proteins, 35 Optional Calories
PER SERVING: 184 Calories, 20 g Protein, 8 g Fat, 9 g Carbohydrate, 327 mg Sodium, 41 mg Cholesterol, 1 g Dietary Fiber

PROSCIUTTO AND LEEK-ROLLED CHICKEN BREASTS

MAKES 4 SERVINGS

2 teaspoons olive oil
1 cup thinly sliced leeks, white part only
1 cup thinly sliced mushrooms
2 garlic cloves, minced
$\frac{1}{2}$ cup chopped fresh basil
1 tablespoon grated Parmesan cheese
1 tablespoon grated lemon zest
$\frac{1}{4}$ teaspoon freshly ground black pepper
Four 3-ounce skinless boneless chicken breasts
2 ounces thinly sliced prosciutto
1 cup low-sodium chicken broth

1. Preheat oven to 350°F. Spray an 8 × 8" baking pan with nonstick cooking spray; set aside.

2. In medium nonstick skillet, heat oil; add leeks, mushrooms and garlic. Cook over medium-high heat, stirring frequently, 4–5 minutes, until tender. Set aside.

3. In small bowl, combine basil, cheese, lemon zest and pepper. Place chicken on clean, flat work surface; arrange one-fourth of the prosciutto on each chicken breast. Top each with one-fourth of the leek mixture; starting from the narrow end, roll each chicken breast jelly-roll style, enclosing filling.

4. Arrange rolls, seam-side down, in prepared pan; pour broth over rolls. Bake 30–35 minutes, basting frequently with broth, until golden.

5. To serve, cut rolls into $\frac{1}{2}$" slices; spoon any remaining juices evenly over rolls.

EACH SERVING PROVIDES: $\frac{1}{2}$ Fat, 1 Vegetable, 2$\frac{1}{2}$ Proteins, 15 Optional Calories
PER SERVING: 191 Calories, 26 g Protein, 7 g Fat, 7 g Carbohydrate, 361 mg Sodium, 62 mg Cholesterol, 1 g Dietary Fiber

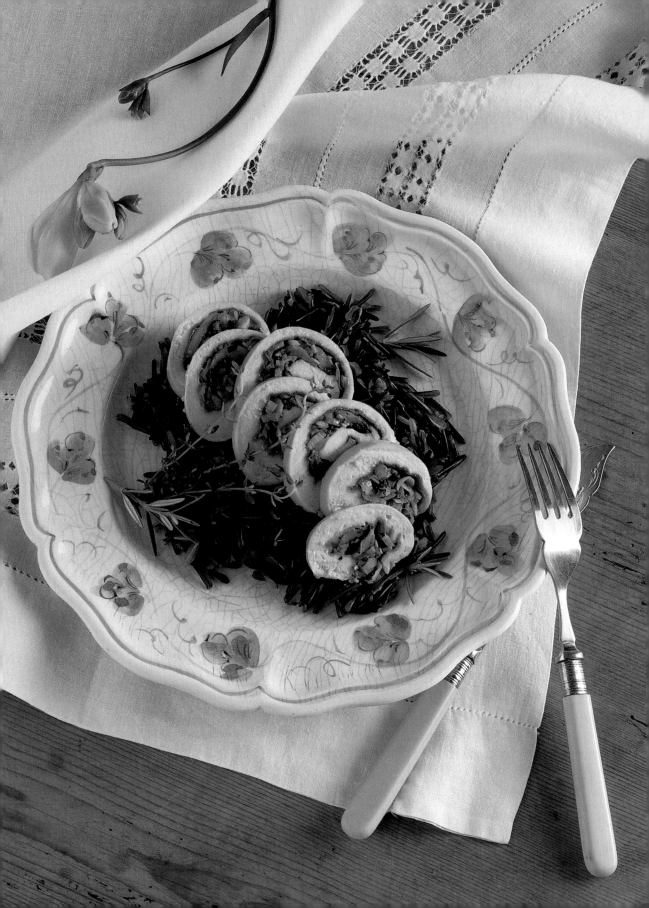

CHICKEN WITH OREGANO-FETA SAUCE

A lesson from the Greeks is learned in this fortuitous pairing of olive oil, oregano and feta cheese. Nostimo!

MAKES 4 SERVINGS

Four 3-ounce skinless boneless chicken breasts
2 tablespoons balsamic vinegar
$\frac{1}{2}$ teaspoon ground thyme
2 teaspoons olive oil
1 tablespoon + $1\frac{1}{2}$ teaspoons all-purpose flour
$\frac{1}{2}$ teaspoon ground oregano
1 cup skim milk
1 cup thawed frozen broccoli, carrots and cauliflower medley
$1\frac{1}{2}$ ounces crumbled peppercorn-flavored or regular feta cheese
1 teaspoon lemon juice
2 cups cooked regular long-grain white rice (hot)

1. On sheet of wax paper, sprinkle chicken with vinegar and thyme. In large nonstick skillet, heat oil; add chicken. Cook over medium-high heat, 4–5 minutes on each side, until browned and cooked through. Transfer to plate; keep warm.

2. To same skillet, sprinkle in flour and oregano; cook, stirring constantly, 1 minute. Gradually whisk in milk; cook, whisking constantly, 2–3 minutes, until thick and bubbly. Stir in vegetables, cheese and lemon juice; reduce heat to low. Simmer 2 minutes, until cheese melts.

3. To serve, spoon rice onto large serving platter; arrange chicken on rice. Spoon sauce evenly over chicken.

EACH SERVING PROVIDES: $\frac{1}{4}$ Milk, $\frac{1}{2}$ Fat, $\frac{1}{2}$ Vegetable, $2\frac{1}{2}$ Proteins, 1 Bread, 10 Optional Calories
PER SERVING: 319 Calories, 27 g Protein, 6 g Fat, 37 g Carbohydrate, 219 mg Sodium, 60 mg Cholesterol, 1 g Dietary Fiber

ITALIAN CHICKEN WITH SAUSAGE AND CAPERS

MAKES 4 SERVINGS

2 teaspoons olive oil
10 ounces skinless boneless chicken breast, cut into 1" pieces
5 ounces hot Italian turkey sausage (90% or more fat free), cut into $\frac{1}{2}$"-thick slices
2 tablespoons red wine vinegar
2 medium green bell peppers, cut into strips
1 medium red onion, chopped
2 garlic cloves, minced
$\frac{1}{2}$ teaspoon dried basil leaves
$\frac{1}{2}$ teaspoon dried Italian seasoning
$2\frac{1}{2}$ cups canned crushed tomatoes
$\frac{1}{2}$ cup low-sodium chicken broth
2 tablespoons grated Parmesan cheese
2 tablespoons rinsed drained capers

1. In large nonstick skillet, heat oil; add chicken. Cook over medium-high heat, stirring frequently, 6–8 minutes, until golden and cooked through. With slotted spoon, transfer chicken to bowl; set aside.

2. Add sausage to skillet; cook, stirring frequently, 8–10 minutes, until browned. Pour in vinegar; cook 1–2 minutes, until liquid evaporates. Add peppers, onion, garlic, basil and Italian seasoning; cook, stirring frequently, 4–5 minutes, until tender.

3. Stir in tomatoes, broth, cheese and capers; bring to a boil. Return chicken to skillet; reduce heat to low. Simmer, stirring occasionally, 5–10 minutes, until sauce thickens slightly.

EACH SERVING PROVIDES: $\frac{1}{2}$ Fat, $2\frac{1}{2}$ Vegetables, 3 Proteins, 20 Optional Calories
PER SERVING: 220 Calories, 24 g Protein, 8 g Fat, 13 g Carbohydrate, 633 mg Sodium, 73 mg Cholesterol, 2 g Dietary Fiber

CHICKEN WITH APPLES AND CIDER

MAKES 4 SERVINGS

2 tablespoons + 2 teaspoons reduced-calorie tub
   margarine
1 small Granny Smith apple (4 ounces), cored and
   cut into $\frac{1}{4}$" slices
1 tablespoon firmly packed dark brown sugar
Four 3-ounce skinless boneless chicken breasts
$\frac{1}{4}$ teaspoon cinnamon
$\frac{1}{4}$ teaspoon salt
$\frac{1}{4}$ teaspoon freshly ground black pepper
1 medium onion, thinly sliced and separated into
   rings
$\frac{1}{2}$ cup apple cider
$\frac{1}{4}$ cup cider vinegar
2 cups cooked wide noodles (hot)

1. In large nonstick skillet, melt 1 tablespoon + 1 teaspoon of the margarine over medium-high heat; add apple slices. Cook, stirring frequently, 5 minutes. Sprinkle with brown sugar; cook over high heat, stirring frequently, until golden on both sides. Transfer to plate; set aside.

2. On sheet of wax paper, sprinkle chicken with cinnamon, salt and pepper. Melt the remaining 1 tablespoon + 1 teaspoon margarine over medium-high heat; add chicken. Cook, 4–5 minutes on each side, until browned. Transfer to plate; set aside.

3. Add onion to skillet; reduce heat to medium. Cook, covered, 6–8 minutes, until tender. Uncover; stir in cider and vinegar. Reduce heat to low; simmer 2 minutes. Return chicken to skillet; simmer, spooning sauce over chicken, 4–5 minutes, until chicken is cooked through and liquid is reduced by half.

4. Spoon apple slices over chicken; cook, about 2 minutes, until heated through. To serve, arrange noodles on serving platter; top with chicken mixture, pouring any remaining juices over chicken.

EACH SERVING PROVIDES: 1 Fat, $\frac{1}{2}$ Fruit, $\frac{1}{4}$ Vegetable, 2 Proteins, 1 Bread, 10 Optional Calories
PER SERVING: 287 Calories, 24 g Protein, 6 g Fat, 34 g Carbohydrate, 273 mg Sodium, 76 mg Cholesterol, 3 g Dietary Fiber

CHICKEN SAUTÉ WITH MUSHROOMS AND ESCAROLE

The slightly bitter edge of escarole adds piquant flavor to this quick but elegant sauté.

MAKES 4 SERVINGS

3 tablespoons all-purpose flour
1 tablespoon grated Parmesan cheese
$\frac{1}{4}$ teaspoon white pepper
Four 3-ounce skinless boneless chicken breasts
1 tablespoon + 1 teaspoon olive oil
2 cups sliced mushrooms
1 cup chopped scallions
$\frac{1}{4}$ cup dry white wine
4 cups coarsely chopped escarole

1. On sheet of wax paper, combine flour, cheese and white pepper. Dredge chicken in flour mixture, coating both sides.

2. In large nonstick skillet, heat 2 teaspoons of the oil; add chicken. Cook over medium-high heat, 4–5 minutes on each side, until golden and cooked through. Transfer to plate; keep warm.

3. Heat the remaining 2 teaspoons of oil in skillet; add mushrooms and scallions. Cook, stirring constantly, 2–3 minutes. Pour in wine; cook 1–2 minutes, until liquid evaporates. Add escarole; cook, stirring occasionally, 2 minutes, until escarole wilts and is tender.

4. To serve, arrange chicken on serving platter. Spoon escarole mixture over chicken.

EACH SERVING PROVIDES: 1 Fat, $3\frac{1}{2}$ Vegetables, 2 Proteins, $\frac{1}{4}$ Bread, 20 Optional Calories
PER SERVING: 196 Calories, 23 g Protein, 6 g Fat, 10 g Carbohydrate, 96 mg Sodium, 50 mg Cholesterol, 2 g Dietary Fiber

CHICKEN WITH SPINACH AND NOODLES

In this hearty pasta dish with colorful vegetables, you toss the cheese in with the hot noodle mixture to melt.

MAKES 4 SERVINGS

6 ounces uncooked wide noodles
2 teaspoons olive oil
10 ounces skinless boneless chicken breast, cubed
$\frac{1}{4}$ teaspoon salt
$\frac{1}{4}$ teaspoon freshly ground black pepper
2 garlic cloves, minced
2 cups chopped plum tomatoes
1 cup roasted red bell pepper strips
2 tablespoons chopped fresh parsley
2 cups julienned spinach leaves
2 tablespoons balsamic vinegar
$\frac{1}{2}$ teaspoon dried basil leaves
$\frac{1}{4}$ teaspoon red pepper flakes
1$\frac{1}{2}$ ounces part-skim mozzarella cheese, cut into pieces

1. In large pot of boiling water, cook noodles 9–11 minutes, until tender; drain and keep warm.

2. Meanwhile, in large nonstick skillet, heat oil; add chicken. Sprinkle with salt and pepper. Cook over medium-high heat, stirring frequently, 4–5 minutes, until browned and cooked through. With slotted spoon, transfer chicken to plate.

3. Add garlic to skillet; cook, stirring frequently, 2 minutes. Stir in tomatoes, bell pepper and parsley; reduce heat to low. Simmer, 2–3 minutes, until liquid evaporates. Stir in spinach, vinegar, basil and pepper flakes; cook 1 minute. Add chicken and noodles; toss to mix well.

4. In large serving bowl, arrange mozzarella cheese; add chicken mixture. Toss until cheese is melted.

EACH SERVING PROVIDES: $\frac{1}{2}$ Fat, 2$\frac{1}{2}$ Vegetables, 2$\frac{1}{2}$ Proteins, 2 Breads
PER SERVING: 327 Calories, 27 g Protein, 7 g Fat, 39 g Carbohydrate, 273 mg Sodium, 88 mg Cholesterol, 4 g Dietary Fiber

CHICKEN FETTUCCINE WITH BROCCOLI RABE

MAKES 4 SERVINGS

2 cups uncooked broccoli rabe
6 ounces uncooked spinach fettuccine
1 tablespoon + 1 teaspoon olive oil
Four 3-ounce skinless boneless chicken breasts
$\frac{1}{2}$ teaspoon salt-free garlic and herb seasoning
1 medium red onion, thinly sliced and separated into rings
4 garlic cloves, minced
2 cups shredded radicchio
2 tablespoons grated Parmesan cheese
$\frac{1}{4}$ teaspoon freshly ground black pepper
$\frac{1}{4}$ cup chopped fresh basil

1. In large pot of boiling water, cook broccoli rabe 2 minutes. With slotted spoon, transfer broccoli rabe to bowl; set aside. Return water to a boil; add fettuccine. Cook 9–11 minutes, until tender; drain.

2. In large nonstick skillet, heat 2 teaspoons of the oil; add chicken and sprinkle with herb seasoning. Cook over medium-high heat 4–5 minutes, until cooked through; transfer to plate and keep warm.

3. Add the remaining 2 teaspoons oil to skillet and heat; add onion and garlic. Cook, stirring frequently, 3–4 minutes, until tender. Stir in cooked broccoli rabe and radicchio. Cook, stirring frequently, 4–5 minutes, until tender; add cooked fettuccine to skillet. Sprinkle with cheese and pepper; toss to mix well.

4. To serve, arrange one-fourth of the pasta onto each of 4 plates. Top each with a chicken breast; sprinkle each with 1 tablespoon basil.

EACH SERVING PROVIDES: 1 Fat, 2$\frac{1}{4}$ Vegetables, 2 Proteins, 2 Breads, 15 Optional Calories
PER SERVING: 339 Calories, 29 g Protein, 8 g Fat, 37 g Carbohydrate, 156 mg Sodium, 92 mg Cholesterol, 5 g Dietary Fiber

RED PEPPER CHICKEN WITH NOODLES

MAKES 4 SERVINGS

2 teaspoons olive oil
10 ounces skinless boneless chicken breast
1 teaspoon dried basil leaves
$\frac{1}{2}$ teaspoon crushed dried rosemary leaves
$\frac{1}{4}$ teaspoon salt
$\frac{1}{4}$ teaspoon freshly ground black pepper
1 cup chopped scallions
1 cup roasted chopped red bell peppers
8 ounces cooked red kidney beans
2 cups cooked wide egg noodles (hot)
$1\frac{1}{2}$ ounces part-skim mozzarella cheese, shredded

1. In large nonstick skillet, heat oil; add chicken. Sprinkle with basil, rosemary, salt and pepper; cook over medium-high heat, stirring frequently, 4–5 minutes. Stir in scallions; cook, 2–3 minutes, until chicken is lightly browned.

2. Add bell peppers and beans to skillet; stir to combine. Reduce heat to low; simmer 5 minutes, until sauce thickens slightly. Add noodles; toss to mix well. Sprinkle with cheese.

EACH SERVING PROVIDES: $\frac{1}{2}$ Fat, 1 Vegetable, $2\frac{1}{2}$ Proteins, 2 Breads
PER SERVING: 323 Calories, 28 g Protein, 6 g Fat, 38 g Carbohydrate, 242 mg Sodium, 74 mg Cholesterol, 5 g Dietary Fiber

CHICKEN BREASTS WITH CREAMY SHELLS

MAKES 4 SERVINGS

6 ounces uncooked medium shell pasta
1 tablespoon + 1 teaspoon reduced-calorie tub margarine
$\frac{1}{2}$ cup chopped fennel
$\frac{1}{2}$ cup chopped shallots
Four 3-ounce skinless boneless chicken breasts
$\frac{1}{4}$ teaspoon paprika
$\frac{1}{4}$ teaspoon salt
2 cups thawed frozen chopped spinach, squeezed dry
1 cup skim milk
$\frac{1}{4}$ cup grated Parmesan cheese
1 tablespoon balsamic vinegar

1. In large pot of boiling water, cook pasta 8–10 minutes, until tender. Drain.

2. Meanwhile, in large nonstick skillet, melt margarine over medium-high heat; add fennel and shallots. Cook, stirring frequently, 4–5 minutes, until tender. Add chicken; sprinkle with paprika and salt. Cook 4–5 minutes on each side, until golden and cooked through. Transfer to plate; keep warm.

3. Add spinach to same skillet; cook, stirring, 2 minutes. Stir in milk, cheese and vinegar. Reduce heat to low; simmer 5 minutes, until liquid is reduced by half. Add pasta to skillet; toss to mix well.

4. To serve, arrange each chicken breast on plate with one-fourth of the pasta.

EACH SERVING PROVIDES: $\frac{1}{4}$ Milk, $\frac{1}{2}$ Fat, $1\frac{1}{2}$ Vegetables, 2 Proteins, 2 Breads, 30 Optional Calories
PER SERVING: 355 Calories, 33 g Protein, 6 g Fat, 43 g Carbohydrate, 451 mg Sodium, 54 mg Cholesterol, 4 g Dietary Fiber

ROSEMARY CHICKEN WITH WILD RICE

MAKES 6 SERVINGS

6 ounces uncooked wild rice
1 tablespoon olive oil
1 pound, 3 ounces skinless boneless chicken breast, cubed
1½ cups diced carrots (½" dice)
1 tablespoon dried rosemary leaves
⅓ cup + 2 teaspoons reduced-calorie orange marmalade (8 calories per teaspoon)
¼ cup Dijon-style mustard
¼ teaspoon garlic powder
⅛ teaspoon freshly ground black pepper

1. In medium saucepan, bring 2½ cups water to a boil; stir in rice. Reduce heat to low; simmer, covered, about 45–50 minutes, or until rice is plump and tender. Set aside; keep warm.

2. Meanwhile, in large nonstick skillet, heat oil; add chicken and carrots. Cook over medium-high heat, stirring frequently, 3–4 minutes; stir in rosemary. Cook 3–4 minutes, until chicken is cooked through.

3. Add marmalade, mustard, garlic and pepper to chicken mixture; cook, stirring frequently, 3 minutes, until heated through. Add rice; toss to mix well.

EACH SERVING PROVIDES: ½ Fat, ½ Vegetable, 2½ Proteins, 1 Bread, 25 Optional Calories
PER SERVING: 270 Calories, 25 g Protein, 4 g Fat, 32 g Carbohydrate, 370 mg Sodium, 52 mg Cholesterol, 2 g Dietary Fiber

CHICKEN–BELL PEPPER CHILI

MAKES 4 SERVINGS

1 tablespoon + 1 teaspoon olive oil
1 medium red onion, chopped
1 medium red bell pepper, chopped
1 medium green bell pepper, chopped
1 medium yellow bell pepper, chopped
13 ounces ground chicken
1 tablespoon all-purpose flour
1 tablespoon chili powder
1 tablespoon ground cumin
1 teaspoon unsweetened cocoa powder
⅛ teaspoon ground red pepper
4½ cups canned crushed tomatoes
2 tablespoons balsamic vinegar
8 ounces cooked chick-peas

1. In large Dutch oven, heat oil; add onion and bell peppers. Cook over medium-high heat, stirring frequently, 5 minutes. Add chicken; cook, stirring frequently, 5–7 minutes, until no longer pink.

2. Sprinkle with flour, chili powder, cumin, cocoa powder and ground red pepper; cook, stirring quickly and constantly to combine, 1 minute. Add tomatoes and vinegar; bring to a boil. Reduce heat to low; simmer 30–40 minutes, stirring frequently, until thick. Stir in chick-peas; simmer 5 minutes, until heated through.

EACH SERVING PROVIDES: 1 Fat, 4 Vegetables, 2½ Proteins, 1 Bread, 10 Optional Calories
PER SERVING: 377 Calories, 25 g Protein, 16 g Fat, 37 g Carbohydrate, 545 mg Sodium, 76 mg Cholesterol, 6 g Dietary Fiber

CHICKEN-CHILI CASSEROLE

A marvelous way to use leftover chicken, this is an ideal crusty casserole to serve on a chilly night. Just add a salad and some fruit for an easy dinner.

MAKES 4 SERVINGS

6 ounces uncooked wide noodles
1 tablespoon + 1 teaspoon reduced-calorie tub margarine
1 tablespoon + 1½ teaspoons all-purpose flour
2 cups skim milk
1 tablespoon grated Parmesan cheese
8 ounces cubed cooked chicken
½ cup chopped red onion
2 tablespoons chopped canned green chilies
1 tablespoon Dijon-style mustard
1 tablespoon + 1½ teaspoons seasoned dried bread crumbs

1. In large pot of boiling water, cook noodles 8–10 minutes, until tender; drain.

2. Preheat oven to 375°F. Spray 2-quart casserole with nonstick cooking spray; set aside.

3. In medium saucepan, melt margarine over medium-high heat; sprinkle with flour. Cook, whisking quickly and constantly, for 2 minutes. Whisk in milk and cheese; cook, stirring constantly, 2–3 minutes, until thickened. Remove from heat.

4. Add noodles, chicken, onion, chilies and mustard to saucepan; toss to mix well. Spoon mixture into prepared casserole; sprinkle with bread crumbs. Bake 20–25 minutes, until browned and bubbly.

EACH SERVING PROVIDES: ½ Milk, ½ Fat, ¼ Vegetable, 2 Proteins, 2¼ Breads, 10 Optional Calories
PER SERVING: 371 Calories, 28 g Protein, 9 g Fat, 43 g Carbohydrate, 396 mg Sodium, 94 mg Cholesterol, 2 g Dietary Fiber

BARLEY-CHICKEN CASSEROLE

MAKES 6 SERVINGS

2 teaspoons vegetable oil
1 cup chopped onions
4½ ounces uncooked pearl barley
2 teaspoons chicken bouillon granules
2 teaspoons low-sodium chicken bouillon granules
13 ounces cubed cooked chicken breast
2 cups sliced mushrooms
2 ounces slivered almonds

1. Preheat oven to 350°F. In large ovenproof Dutch oven, heat oil; add onions and barley. Cook over medium heat, stirring frequently, 1–2 minutes, until onion is browned.

2. Add bouillon granules, low-sodium bouillon granules and 3 cups water to Dutch oven; stir to combine. Bake 45 minutes; remove from oven.

3. Add chicken, mushrooms and half of the almonds to chicken mixture; stir to combine. Bake 30 minutes.

4. To serve, sprinkle remaining almonds over chicken mixture.

EACH SERVING PROVIDES: 1 Fat, 1 Vegetable, 2½ Proteins, 1 Bread, 5 Optional Calories
PER SERVING: 272 Calories, 25 g Protein, 9 g Fat, 23 g Carbohydrate, 424 mg Sodium, 52 mg Cholesterol, 4 g Dietary Fiber

HERBED CHICKEN HASH

New York's famous "21" restaurant regulars often order their favorite food there, a rich chicken hash. Our version is easy to make and under 200 calories a serving.

MAKES 4 SERVINGS

2 slices white bread
1 tablespoon + 1½ teaspoons grated Parmesan cheese
⅛ teaspoon ground white pepper
1 tablespoon + 1 teaspoon reduced-calorie tub margarine
½ cup chopped red onion
½ cup chopped celery
10 ounces skinless boneless chicken breast, cut into ½" pieces
1 tablespoon all-purpose flour
1 teaspoon dried thyme leaves
½ teaspoon chives
¼ teaspoon salt
1 cup skim milk
1 medium green bell pepper, chopped
¼ teaspoon paprika

   1. In mini food processor or blender, combine bread, cheese and white pepper. Process until mixture is the consistency of coarse crumbs; set aside.

   2. Preheat oven to 350°F. Spray 1-quart casserole with nonstick cooking spray; set aside.

   3. In large nonstick skillet, melt margarine over medium-high heat; add onion and celery. Cook, stirring frequently, 4 minutes. Add chicken; sprinkle with flour, thyme, chives and salt; cook, stirring frequently, 5 minutes. Stir in milk; cook, stirring frequently, 2–3 minutes, until sauce thickens. Remove from heat; stir in bell pepper.

   4. Spoon chicken mixture into prepared casserole. Sprinkle with crumb mixture and paprika. Bake 30–35 minutes, until golden brown.

EACH SERVING PROVIDES: ¼ Milk, ½ Fat, 1 Vegetable, 2 Proteins, ½ Bread, 40 Optional Calories
PER SERVING: 185 Calories, 21 g Protein, 4 g Fat, 15 g Carbohydrate, 368 mg Sodium, 44 mg Cholesterol, 1 g Dietary Fiber

ORANGE COUSCOUS WITH CHICKEN

Couscous, the national dish of Morocco, gets a double dose of orange, complementing the grain and adding flavor to the cooked chicken; make this your leftover secret!

MAKES 6 SERVINGS

¾ cup orange juice
2 teaspoons low-sodium chicken bouillon granules
1 teaspoon chicken bouillon granules
6 ounces uncooked couscous
12 ounces shredded cooked chicken breast
1¾ cups drained canned mandarin orange sections
½ cup chopped fresh parsley

   1. In large Dutch oven, combine orange juice, ½ cup water, low-sodium bouillon granules and bouillon granules; bring to a boil. Remove from heat; stir in couscous. Cover; let stand 10 minutes.

   2. Add chicken, 1½ cups of the orange sections and the parsley to Dutch oven; stir to combine. Cook over low heat, stirring frequently, about 5 minutes, until heated through.

   3. To serve, in large serving bowl, arrange couscous mixture; garnish with the remaining ¼ cup orange sections.

EACH SERVING PROVIDES: ½ Fruit, 2 Proteins, 1 Bread, 25 Optional Calories
PER SERVING: 251 Calories, 23 g Protein, 2 g Fat, 34 g Carbohydrate, 239 mg Sodium, 48 mg Cholesterol, 0 g Dietary Fiber

CHICKEN-RICOTTA PASTA BAKE

MAKES 6 SERVINGS

6 ounces uncooked rotelle (spiral pasta)
8 sun-dried tomato halves (not packed in oil)
1 tablespoon olive oil
$1\frac{1}{2}$ cups coarsely chopped zucchini
1 medium green bell pepper, chopped
1 medium onion, thinly sliced and separated into rings
2 garlic cloves, minced
2 cups canned pasta-style tomatoes
1 cup chopped roasted red bell pepper
1 tablespoon balsamic vinegar
$1\frac{1}{2}$ cups nonfat ricotta cheese
1 tablespoon grated lemon zest
$\frac{1}{2}$ teaspoon dried basil leaves
4 ounces shredded cooked chicken
$4\frac{1}{2}$ ounces shredded part-skim mozzarella cheese

1. In large pot of boiling water, cook pasta 8–10 minutes, until tender. Drain and set aside.

2. Meanwhile, in small bowl, cover sun-dried tomatoes with boiling water; let stand 2 minutes. Drain and cut into strips.

3. In large nonstick skillet, heat oil; add zucchini, green bell pepper, onion and garlic. Cook over medium-high heat, stirring frequently, 4–5 minutes, until tender; add tomato strips, canned tomatoes, red bell pepper and vinegar. Reduce heat to low; simmer 10–15 minutes, until liquid is reduced and sauce is thickened; stir in pasta. Set aside.

4. Preheat oven to 350°F. Spray an 11 × 7" baking pan with nonstick cooking spray.

5. In medium bowl, combine ricotta cheese, lemon zest and basil. Arrange half of the pasta in prepared pan; spread with ricotta mixture and sprinkle with chicken. Top with remaining pasta mixture; sprinkle with mozzarella cheese. Bake 25–30 minutes, until heated through and bubbly.

EACH SERVING PROVIDES: $\frac{1}{2}$ Fat, $2\frac{3}{4}$ Vegetables, 2 Proteins, $1\frac{1}{4}$ Breads, 30 Optional Calories
PER SERVING: 324 Calories, 24 g Protein, 8 g Fat, 37 g Carbohydrate, 431 mg Sodium, 29 mg Cholesterol, 2 g Dietary Fiber

SHEPHERD'S PIE

MAKES 4 SERVINGS

1 tablespoon + 1 teaspoon reduced-calorie tub margarine
2 tablespoons all-purpose flour
1 cup low-sodium chicken broth
1 teaspoon reduced-sodium soy sauce
8 ounces cubed cooked turkey
2 cups blanched sliced carrots
1 cup chopped spinach leaves
1 cup chopped scallions
$\frac{1}{2}$ cup drained canned whole-kernel corn
$\frac{1}{2}$ cup evaporated skimmed milk
1 teaspoon dried thyme leaves
$\frac{1}{2}$ teaspoon ground marjoram
12 ounces potatoes, mashed
1 tablespoon grated Parmesan cheese
$\frac{1}{4}$ teaspoon paprika

1. To prepare gravy, in medium saucepan, melt margarine over medium-high heat; sprinkle in 1 tablespoon of the flour. Cook, stirring constantly, 2 minutes. Whisk in broth, $\frac{1}{4}$ cup water and soy sauce; bring to a boil. Reduce heat to low; simmer, stirring constantly, 3–4 minutes, until thickened. Set aside.

2. Preheat oven to 400°F. Spray a 2-quart casserole with nonstick cooking spray; set aside.

3. To prepare filling, in large bowl, combine turkey and remaining 1 tablespoon flour. Add carrots, spinach, scallions, corn, milk, thyme, marjoram and prepared gravy; toss to mix well. Spoon into prepared casserole.

4. Spread potatoes evenly over top of casserole; sprinkle with cheese and paprika. Bake 30–35 minutes, until bubbly and potatoes are golden.

EACH SERVING PROVIDES: $\frac{1}{4}$ Milk, $\frac{1}{2}$ Fat, 2 Vegetables, 2 Proteins, 1 Bread, 30 Optional Calories
PER SERVING: 297 Calories, 24 g Protein, 6 g Fat, 37 g Carbohydrate, 312 mg Sodium, 46 mg Cholesterol, 4 g Dietary Fiber

CHICKEN-TOMATO CHOWDER

Thick with vegetables, potatoes and beans, chowder is a great midweek supper for the whole family. If you have extra portions, take one along in a wide-mouth vacuum container for a hearty lunch.

MAKES 4 SERVINGS

1 tablespoon + 1 teaspoon olive oil
1 cup thinly sliced carrots
1 cup chopped scallions
1 cup chopped celery
2 garlic cloves, minced
2 cups canned crushed tomatoes
2 cups low-sodium chicken broth
10 ounces cubed pared potatoes
$\frac{1}{2}$ teaspoon ground marjoram
$\frac{1}{4}$ teaspoon ground oregano
$\frac{1}{4}$ teaspoon freshly ground black pepper
10 ounces skinless boneless chicken breast, cut into $\frac{1}{2}$" pieces
4 ounces cooked cannellini beans
2 tablespoons chopped fresh parsley

1. In medium saucepan, heat 2 teaspoons of the oil; add carrots, scallions, celery and garlic. Cook over medium-high heat, stirring frequently, 4–5 minutes, until tender. Stir in tomatoes and broth; bring to a boil. Stir in potatoes, marjoram, oregano and pepper. Reduce heat; simmer, covered, 30–40 minutes, until potatoes are tender.

2. Meanwhile, in medium nonstick skillet, heat the remaining 2 teaspoons of oil; add chicken. Cook, stirring frequently, 6–8 minutes, until cooked through. Stir into potato mixture.

3. Stir in beans and parsley; reduce heat to low. Simmer 5 minutes, until heated through.

EACH SERVING PROVIDES: 1 Fat, 2$\frac{1}{2}$ Vegetables, 2 Proteins, 1 Bread, 10 Optional Calories
PER SERVING: 277 Calories, 24 g Protein, 7 g Fat, 32 g Carbohydrate, 314 mg Sodium, 41 mg Cholesterol, 5 g Dietary Fiber

SAFFRON ARROZ CON POLLO

MAKES 4 SERVINGS

1 tablespoon + 1 teaspoon olive oil
1$\frac{1}{2}$ pounds whole chicken breast, skinned and split
1 teaspoon paprika
$\frac{1}{4}$ teaspoon salt
$\frac{1}{4}$ teaspoon freshly ground black pepper
1 medium green bell pepper, chopped
$\frac{1}{2}$ cup chopped celery
$\frac{1}{2}$ cup chopped red onion
2 garlic cloves, minced
2 cups canned stewed tomatoes
$\frac{1}{2}$ cup low-sodium chicken broth
4 ounces uncooked regular long-grain rice
1 tablespoon rinsed drained capers
$\frac{1}{2}$ teaspoon dried oregano leaves
$\frac{1}{4}$ teaspoon saffron
1 bay leaf
1 cup thawed frozen peas
1 cup chopped roasted red bell peppers

1. Preheat oven to 350°F. In large skillet, heat oil; add chicken. Sprinkle on both sides with paprika, salt and black pepper; cook over medium heat, 8–10 minutes, turning frequently, until browned. Transfer chicken to Dutch oven.

2. Add green bell pepper, celery, onion and garlic to skillet; cook over medium-high heat, stirring frequently, 4–5 minutes, until tender. Stir in tomatoes, broth and 2 tablespoons water; bring to a boil. Remove from heat; stir in rice, capers, oregano, saffron and bay leaf.

3. Spoon rice mixture over chicken in Dutch oven; cover and bake 25 minutes. Uncover and stir in peas and roasted bell peppers. Cover and bake 15 minutes longer. Remove bay leaf before serving.

EACH SERVING PROVIDES: 1 Fat, 2$\frac{1}{2}$ Vegetables, 3 Proteins, 1$\frac{1}{2}$ Breads, 3 Optional Calories
PER SERVING: 333 Calories, 26 g Protein, 6 g Fat, 43 g Carbohydrate, 635 mg Sodium, 49 mg Cholesterol, 6 g Dietary Fiber

CHICKEN WITH BROWN RICE AND SUN-DRIED TOMATOES

MAKES 4 SERVINGS

2 teaspoons olive oil
$1\frac{1}{2}$ pounds whole chicken breast, skinned and split
$\frac{1}{2}$ teaspoon ground oregano
$\frac{1}{4}$ teaspoon salt
$\frac{1}{4}$ teaspoon freshly ground black pepper
4 ounces uncooked brown rice
$\frac{1}{2}$ cup chopped celery
$\frac{1}{2}$ cup chopped scallions
4 garlic cloves, minced
1 cup mixed vegetable juice
10 sun-dried tomato halves (not packed in oil)
4 ounces cooked chick-peas

1. In large nonstick skillet, heat oil; add chicken. Sprinkle with oregano, salt and pepper. Cook over medium-high heat, turning frequently, 5–7 minutes, until browned on all sides. Transfer to plate.

2. Add rice, celery, scallions and garlic to skillet; stir to combine. Cook, stirring frequently, 2 minutes. Stir in juice, sun-dried tomatoes and 2 tablespoons of water; bring to a boil. Reduce heat to low; return chicken to skillet. Simmer, covered, 40–45 minutes, until liquid is absorbed. Uncover, and stir in chick-peas; cook 2 minutes, until heated through.

EACH SERVING PROVIDES: $\frac{1}{2}$ Fat, $2\frac{1}{4}$ Vegetables, 3 Proteins, $1\frac{1}{2}$ Breads
PER SERVING: 309 Calories, 26 g Protein, 5 g Fat, 40 g Carbohydrate, 439 mg Sodium, 49 mg Cholesterol, 4 g Dietary Fiber

TANDOORI-DIJON CHICKEN BREAST

MAKES 4 SERVINGS

$\frac{1}{3}$ cup + 2 teaspoons plain nonfat yogurt
1 tablespoon grated fresh ginger root
1 tablespoon red wine vinegar
1 tablespoon Dijon-style mustard
$\frac{1}{2}$ teaspoon ground cumin
$\frac{1}{4}$ teaspoon cinnamon
$\frac{1}{8}$ teaspoon ground red pepper
$1\frac{1}{2}$ pounds whole chicken breast, skinned and split

1. To prepare marinade, in gallon-size sealable plastic bag, combine yogurt, ginger, vinegar, mustard, cumin, cinnamon and red pepper; add chicken. Seal bag, squeezing out air; turn to coat chicken. Refrigerate at least 2 hours or overnight, turning bag occasionally. Drain and discard marinade.

2. Preheat broiler. Spray broiler rack with nonstick cooking spray. Arrange chicken on rack; broil, 6–8 inches from heat, 15–20 minutes, turning occasionally, until cooked through.

EACH SERVING PROVIDES: 3 Proteins, 10 Optional Calories
PER SERVING: 115 Calories, 19 g Protein, 3 g Fat, 3 g Carbohydrate, 171 mg Sodium, 49 mg Cholesterol, 0 g Dietary Fiber

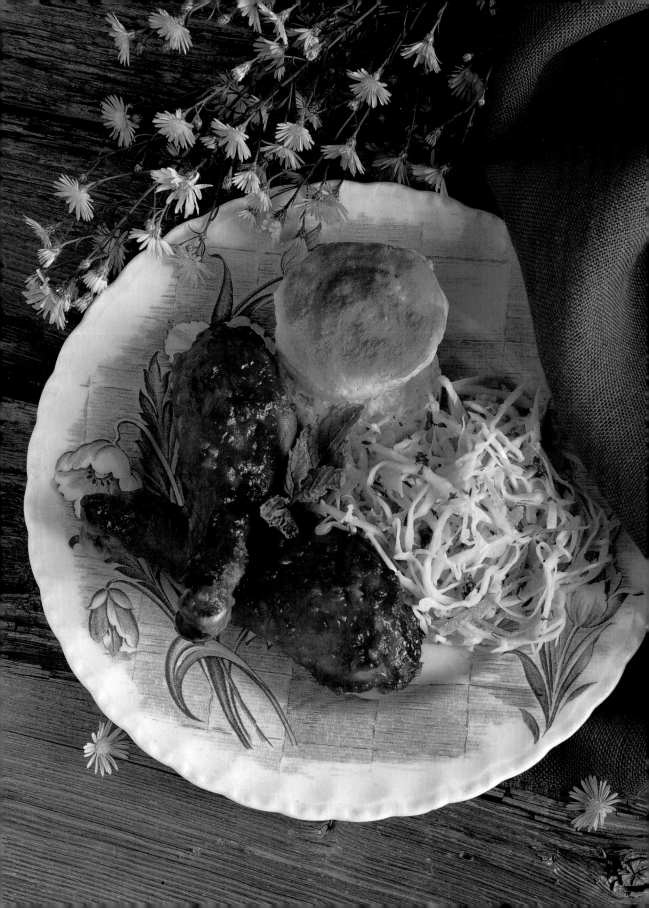

MOLASSES-BARBECUED CHICKEN LEGS

MAKES 4 SERVINGS

¼ cup spicy mixed vegetable juice
2 tablespoons chili sauce
1 tablespoon molasses
1 tablespoon drained horseradish
2 teaspoons red wine vinegar
1 teaspoon Dijon-style mustard
1 garlic clove, crushed
1 pound, 8 ounces chicken legs, skinned

1. Spray grill rack with nonstick cooking spray. Place grill rack 5" from coals. Prepare grill according to manufacturer's directions.

2. To prepare sauce, in small saucepan, combine juice, chili sauce, molasses, horseradish, vinegar, mustard and garlic; bring to a boil. Reduce heat to low; simmer 10 minutes, stirring frequently. Remove from heat; set aside.

3. Grill chicken 20–25 minutes, turning occasionally and brushing with sauce, until juices run clear when meat is pricked with a fork.

EACH SERVING PROVIDES: 3 Proteins, 20 Optional Calories
PER SERVING: 194 Calories, 23 g Protein, 8 g Fat, 7 g Carbohydrate, 282 mg Sodium, 80 mg Cholesterol, 0 g Dietary Fiber

ORANGE-CRUMBED BAKED CHICKEN THIGHS

MAKES 4 SERVINGS

2 tablespoons Dijon-style mustard
2 tablespoons orange juice
½ teaspoon reduced-sodium soy sauce
10 ounces skinless boneless chicken thighs
3 ounces flatbreads, made into crumbs
1 tablespoon grated orange zest
¼ teaspoon onion powder
¼ teaspoon freshly ground black pepper

1. Preheat oven to 350°F. Spray large baking sheet with nonstick cooking spray; set aside.

2. In medium bowl, combine mustard, orange juice and soy sauce. Brush chicken on both sides with mustard mixture; set aside.

3. On sheet of wax paper, combine flatbread crumbs, orange zest, onion powder and pepper. Dredge chicken, firmly pressing on crumb mixture, coating both sides.

4. On prepared baking sheet, arrange chicken; bake 15 minutes. Turn chicken; bake 15–20 minutes longer, until cooked through.

EACH SERVING PROVIDES: 2 Proteins, 1 Bread, 5 Optional Calories
PER SERVING: 179 Calories, 16 g Protein, 4 g Fat, 20 g Carbohydrate, 367 mg Sodium, 59 mg Cholesterol, 3 g Dietary Fiber

Molasses-Barbecued Chicken, Cole Slaw with Caraway-Mint Dressing (page 129)

DILLED CHICKEN DRUMSTICKS WITH RAISIN COUSCOUS

MAKES 4 SERVINGS

¾ cup plain nonfat yogurt
¼ cup chopped fresh dill
2 garlic cloves, crushed
¼ teaspoon paprika
¼ teaspoon salt
Pinch white pepper
1 pound, 8 ounces chicken drumsticks, skinned
2 teaspoons canola oil
1 cup thinly sliced carrots
1 cup chopped green bell pepper
2 teaspoons cornstarch
¼ cup low-sodium chicken broth
½ cup apple juice
⅓ cup + 2 teaspoons golden raisins
4 ounces uncooked whole-wheat couscous

1. To prepare marinade, in gallon-size sealable plastic bag, combine yogurt, dill, garlic, paprika, salt and white pepper; add chicken. Seal bag, squeezing out air; turn to coat chicken. Refrigerate at least 1 hour or overnight, turning bag occasionally.

2. Preheat oven to 350°F. In large nonstick skillet, heat oil; add carrots and bell pepper. Cook over medium-high heat, stirring frequently, 4–5 minutes, until tender.

3. In small bowl, dissolve cornstarch in broth; pour into skillet. Cook, stirring constantly, 1–2 minutes, until thickened.

4. With slotted spoon, remove chicken from marinade; arrange in an 8" baking pan. Drain marinade into vegetable mixture. Cook over medium heat, stirring constantly, until mixture comes to a boil. Remove from heat; pour over chicken. Cover and bake 15 minutes. Uncover and bake 15–20 minutes longer, until cooked through.

5. Meanwhile, in small saucepan, bring juice, ¼ cup water and raisins to a boil. Remove from heat; stir in couscous. Cover and let stand 5 minutes. Fluff with fork before serving.

EACH SERVING PROVIDES: ¼ Milk, ½ Fat, 1 Fruit, 1 Vegetable, 3 Proteins, 1 Bread, 5 Optional Calories
PER SERVING: 383 Calories, 31 g Protein, 8 g Fat, 46 g Carbohydrate, 269 mg Sodium, 80 mg Cholesterol, 2 g Dietary Fiber

Chicken Checklist

◆

You'll find this checklist comes in handy.

- *Check "sell by" date on package labels before buying.*
- *Refrigerate raw chicken immediately—don't leave it in the car while you run errands or on the countertop while you unpack groceries.*
- *While you can defrost chicken in the refrigerator, it will take about 24 hours to thaw a 4-pound chicken. To thaw more quickly, place chicken in a watertight plastic bag and place in cold water; change water frequently. A whole chicken will thaw in about 2 hours.*
- *Don't refreeze raw or cooked chicken that has thawed.*
- *Always marinate chicken in the refrigerator.*
- *When refrigerating a chicken with stuffing, remove the stuffing and refrigerate the chicken and the stuffing in separate containers.*

HONEY AND ANISE ROASTED CHICKEN THIGHS

MAKES 4 SERVINGS

½" piece pared fresh ginger root
2 garlic cloves, peeled
2 tablespoons honey
1 tablespoon grated orange zest
1 tablespoon reduced-sodium soy sauce
1 tablespoon balsamic vinegar
½ teaspoon anise seeds
¼ teaspoon ground cardamom
¼ teaspoon salt
1½ pounds chicken thighs, skinned

1. To prepare marinade, in mini food processor, combine ginger root and garlic; process until finely chopped. Add honey, orange zest, soy sauce, vinegar, anise, cardamom and salt; process marinade until combined.

2. Pour marinade into gallon-size sealable plastic bag; add chicken thighs. Seal bag, squeezing out air; turn to coat chicken. Refrigerate at least 1 hour, turning bag occasionally. Drain and discard marinade.

3. Preheat oven to 425°F. Spray broiler rack with nonstick cooking spray. Arrange chicken on rack; roast 20–30 minutes, turning once, until cooked through.

EACH SERVING PROVIDES: 3 Proteins, 30 Optional Calories
PER SERVING: 161 Calories, 15 g Protein, 6 g Fat, 10 g Carbohydrate, 336 mg Sodium, 54 mg Cholesterol, 0 g Dietary Fiber

CHICKEN WITH OLIVES AND DATES

Middle Eastern cooking often combines warm spices and fruit with poultry. Here, olives add another rich note.

MAKES 4 SERVINGS

1 tablespoon olive oil
2 garlic cloves, crushed
1 teaspoon ground ginger
1 teaspoon ground cumin
½ teaspoon paprika
¼ teaspoon turmeric
¼ teaspoon cinnamon
¼ teaspoon salt
15 ounces skinless boneless chicken drumsticks
¼ cup low-sodium chicken broth
6 dried apricot halves, chopped
2 coarsely chopped pitted dates
10 small Calamata olives, pitted and chopped
1 tablespoon grated lemon zest

1. To prepare marinade, in gallon-size sealable plastic bag, combine oil, garlic, ginger, cumin, paprika, turmeric, cinnamon and salt; add chicken. Seal bag, squeezing out air; turn to coat chicken. Refrigerate 1 hour, turning once. Drain and discard marinade.

2. Heat large nonstick skillet sprayed with nonstick cooking spray. Add chicken and broth; cover and cook over medium heat, 15 minutes. Uncover and turn chicken over; sprinkle with apricots, dates, olives, lemon zest and 1 tablespoon water. Cover and cook, checking occasionally, 15 minutes longer, until chicken is cooked through. If chicken begins to stick to bottom of skillet, add 1–2 tablespoons more water.

EACH SERVING PROVIDES: 1 Fat, ½ Fruit, 3 Proteins, 1 Optional Calorie
PER SERVING: 202 Calories, 23 g Protein, 8 g Fat, 9 g Carbohydrate, 296 mg Sodium, 82 mg Cholesterol, 1 g Dietary Fiber

CURRIED CHICKEN NUGGETS WITH SPINACH

In India, each household makes its own special curry blend as we have done here with cumin, turmeric, ginger and paprika. Adjust these seasonings to create your own custom-curry taste.

MAKES 4 SERVINGS

1 tablespoon + 1 teaspoon olive oil
2 teaspoons ground cumin
1 teaspoon turmeric
$\frac{1}{2}$ teaspoon ground ginger
$\frac{1}{8}$ teaspoon paprika
10 ounces skinless boneless chicken breast, cut into 1" pieces
4 cups coarsely chopped spinach leaves
2 tablespoons chopped green chilies
2 garlic cloves, minced
8 ounces cooked chick-peas
2 tablespoons chili sauce

1. In large nonstick skillet, heat oil; add cumin, turmeric, ginger and paprika. Cook over medium heat 1 minute; add chicken. Cook, stirring frequently, 6–8 minutes, until cooked through.

2. Add spinach, chilies and garlic to skillet; stir to combine. Cook 2–3 minutes, until spinach begins to wilt; stir in chick-peas and chili sauce. Reduce heat to low; simmer 2–3 minutes, until chick-peas are heated through.

EACH SERVING PROVIDES: 1 Fat, 2 Vegetables, 2 Proteins, 1 Bread, 10 Optional Calories
PER SERVING: 243 Calories, 24 g Protein, 7 g Fat, 22 g Carbohydrate, 211 mg Sodium, 41 mg Cholesterol, 3 g Dietary Fiber

CHICKEN AND ARTICHOKE PACKETS

Present these savory packets still in their foil wrappers and let each diner slit his or hers open. Remember to explain the need to be careful as steam escapes when you open the packets. For a more elegant presentation, use parchment paper instead of foil.
(See photo at right.)

MAKES 4 SERVINGS

Four 3-ounce skinless boneless chicken thighs
2 cups thawed frozen artichoke hearts
8 ounces cooked chick-peas
$\frac{1}{2}$ cup chopped fennel
$\frac{1}{2}$ cup shredded carrot
1 tablespoon grated Parmesan cheese
1 tablespoon chopped fresh thyme
$\frac{1}{4}$ teaspoon salt
$\frac{1}{4}$ cup Italian dressing

1. Preheat oven to 350°F. Cut four 12" squares of heavy-duty foil.

2. Arrange 1 chicken thigh in center of each piece of foil; top each with one-fourth of the artichoke hearts, chick-peas, fennel, carrot, cheese, thyme and salt. Drizzle each with 1 tablespoon dressing. Fold foil over chicken; securely seal ends to make packets.

3. On large baking sheet, arrange chicken packets; bake 20–30 minutes, until cooked through. To serve, carefully cut a cross in center of each packet to release steam.

EACH SERVING PROVIDES: 2 Fats, 1$\frac{1}{2}$ Vegetables, 2 Proteins, 1 Bread, 10 Optional Calories
PER SERVING: 310 Calories, 25 g Protein, 13 g Fat, 26 g Carbohydrate, 410 mg Sodium, 72 mg Cholesterol, 6 g Dietary Fiber

Chicken and Artichoke Packets

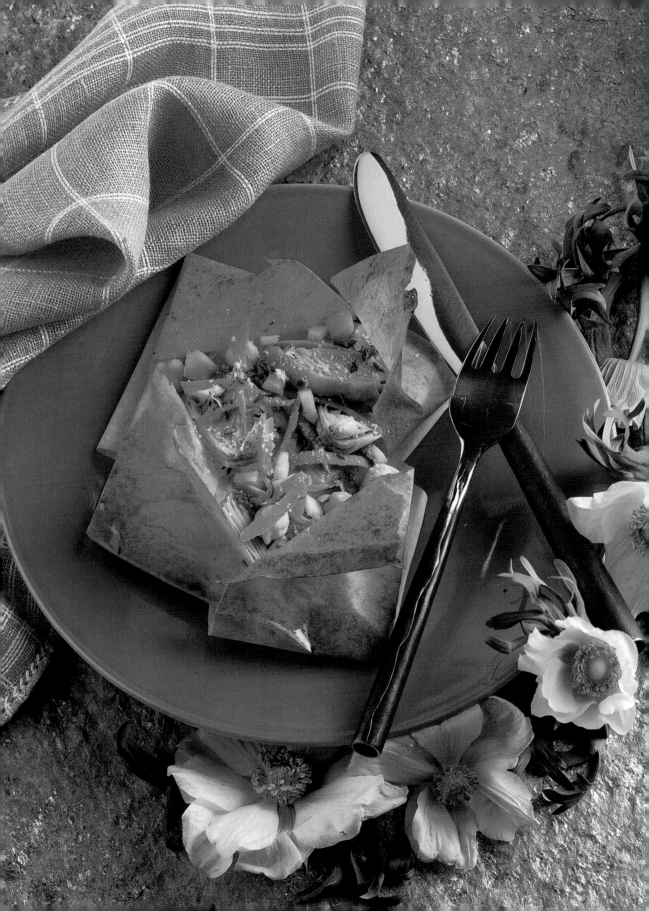

WARM CHICKEN SALAD WITH ROASTED RED PEPPER DRESSING

MAKES 4 SERVINGS

10 ounces skinless boneless chicken breast,
   pounded to $\frac{1}{4}$" thickness
3 garlic cloves, crushed
2 medium red bell peppers, sliced
1 medium yellow onion, sliced
2 teaspoons olive oil
$\frac{1}{4}$ cup chicken broth
1 teaspoon chopped fresh rosemary
1 tablespoon red wine vinegar
$\frac{1}{4}$ teaspoon freshly ground black pepper
$\frac{1}{8}$ teaspoon salt
3 cups torn red leaf lettuce
3 cups torn arugula leaves

1. On clean work surface, rub chicken with one-third of the garlic; transfer to small bowl with tight-fitting cover. Refrigerate, covered, at least 1 hour.

2. Preheat oven to 400°F. Spray medium nonstick skillet with nonstick cooking spray. Set aside.

3. To prepare dressing, in a 2-quart casserole, combine bell peppers, onion, the remaining garlic and the olive oil; roast 25 minutes. Stir in broth, $\frac{1}{4}$ cup water and the rosemary. Cover with foil; roast 20 minutes, until tender. Let cool slightly.

4. Transfer mixture to food processor or blender. Add vinegar and $\frac{1}{8}$ teaspoon of the pepper; purée until smooth.

5. In prepared skillet, cook chicken over medium-high heat 4–5 minutes, until golden; sprinkle with salt and remaining $\frac{1}{8}$ teaspoon pepper. Turn chicken; cook 4 minutes longer, until cooked through. Transfer to cutting board; let rest 5 minutes. Cut chicken into diagonal slices.

6. To serve, on serving platter combine lettuce and arugula; toss to mix well. Arrange sliced chicken on top; drizzle with dressing.

EACH SERVING PROVIDES: $\frac{1}{2}$ Fat, $4\frac{1}{2}$ Vegetables, 2 Proteins, 1 Optional Calorie
PER SERVING: 137 Calories, 18 g Protein, 4 g Fat, 8 g Carbohydrate, 193 mg Sodium, 41 mg Cholesterol, 2 g Dietary Fiber

---

Storing Chicken

◆

It's always a good idea to have chicken on hand, and chicken is so versatile that it's tempting to stock up. Use the chart below as a guide to refrigerating and storing chicken. Before freezing raw chicken, remove the store's plastic wrapper and rinse and dry. To freeze, wrap in foil, heavy-duty plastic wrap or plastic sandwich bags. Press air out of wrapper before sealing, and label with date.

Fresh Raw Chicken	*Refrigerator*	*Freezer*
Whole Chicken	*1–2 days*	*1 year*
Chicken Parts	*1–2 days*	*9 months*
Giblets	*1–2 days*	*3–4 months*
Ground Chicken	*1–2 days*	*3–4 months*
Cooked Chicken Leftovers	*Refrigerator*	*Freezer*
Whole Roasted Chicken	*3–4 days*	*4 months*
Cooked Chicken Dishes	*3–4 days*	*4 months*
Chicken Parts (plain)	*3–4 days*	*4 months*
Chicken Nuggets or Patties	*1–2 days*	*1–3 months*

CHICKEN DUMPLINGS

MAKES 4 SERVINGS

2 tablespoons chili sauce
1 tablespoon minced cilantro
1 tablespoon reduced-sodium teriyaki sauce
1 teaspoon rice-wine vinegar
$\frac{1}{2}$ teaspoon grated fresh ginger root
Pinch ground red pepper
8 ounces skinless boneless chicken breast, finely
   chopped*
$\frac{1}{2}$ cup finely shredded napa cabbage
1 tablespoon minced scallion
2 teaspoons reduced-sodium soy sauce
1 teaspoon cornstarch, dissolved in 2 teaspoons
   water
$\frac{1}{4}$ teaspoon powdered mustard
$\frac{1}{8}$ teaspoon freshly ground black pepper
20 wonton skins (3" squares)
1 tablespoon + 1 teaspoon sesame oil
1 cup low-sodium chicken broth
1 teaspoon all-purpose flour
1 tablespoon sesame seeds, toasted

1. To prepare sauce, in small bowl, combine chili sauce, cilantro, teriyaki sauce, vinegar, ginger and pepper; set aside.

2. To prepare filling, in medium bowl, combine chicken, cabbage, scallion, soy sauce, dissolved cornstarch, mustard and pepper.

3. Cover wontons with plastic wrap. Working with one wonton at a time, spoon 2 teaspoonfuls of filling into center of each wonton. Moisten edges of wontons with water; fold diagonally over filling to form a triangle. Press edges to seal, pressing out air. Repeat procedure using remaining wontons and filling.

4. In large nonstick skillet, heat oil until very hot; arrange dumplings in a circle in skillet. Cook over medium-high heat 5–7 minutes, until bottoms are golden.

5. Meanwhile, in small saucepan bring broth to a boil; remove from heat. Sprinkle with flour and stir constantly, until flour is dissolved. Pour broth mixture over dumplings in skillet; cook, partially covered, until liquid evaporates. Uncover and cook until bottoms are crisp. Carefully loosen dumplings with spatula. Sprinkle with seeds and serve with sauce.

*Chicken can also be ground in food processor.

EACH SERVING PROVIDES: 1 Fat, $\frac{1}{4}$ Vegetable, 1$\frac{1}{2}$ Proteins, 1 Bread, 35 Optional Calories
PER SERVING: 262 Calories, 19 g Protein, 7 g Fat, 29 g Carbohydrate, 570 mg Sodium, 36 mg Cholesterol, 0 g Dietary Fiber

◆

PROVENÇAL CHICKEN STRIPS

MAKES 4 SERVINGS

2 teaspoons olive oil
10 ounces skinless boneless chicken breast, cut into
   2" strips
1 cup chopped scallions
2 garlic cloves, minced
2 cups chopped plum tomatoes
2 tablespoons chopped fresh parsley
1 tablespoon rinsed drained capers
1 teaspoon red-wine vinegar
$\frac{1}{4}$ teaspoon crushed dried rosemary leaves
3 cups cooked wide noodles (hot)

1. In large nonstick skillet, heat oil; add chicken. Cook over medium-high heat, stirring constantly, 4 minutes. Add scallions and garlic; cook, stirring frequently, 2–4 minutes, until chicken is cooked through.

2. Add tomatoes, parsley, capers, vinegar and rosemary to skillet; stir to combine. Simmer, 5–10 minutes, until liquid evaporates. To serve, arrange noodles on serving platter; top with chicken mixture.

EACH SERVING PROVIDES: $\frac{1}{2}$ Fat, 1$\frac{1}{2}$ Vegetables, 2 Proteins, 1$\frac{1}{2}$ Breads
PER SERVING: 288 Calories, 23 g Protein, 5 g Fat, 36 g Carbohydrate, 123 mg Sodium, 81 mg Cholesterol, 5 g Dietary Fiber

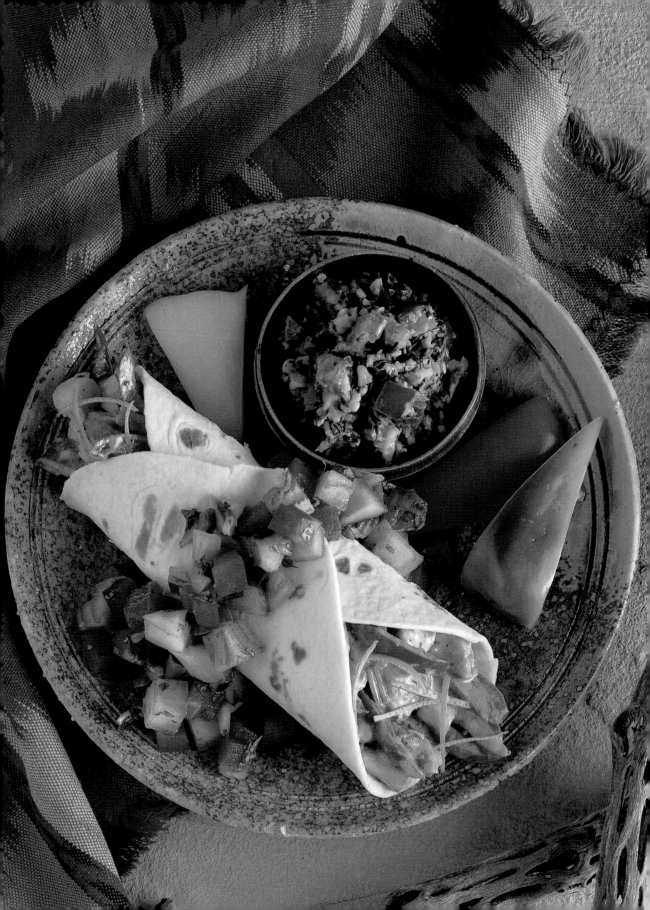

ORANGE-FLAVORED FAJITAS

MAKES 4 SERVINGS

4 flour tortillas (6" diameter)
$\frac{3}{4}$ cup plain nonfat yogurt
2 tablespoons orange juice
1 tablespoon grated orange zest
2 teaspoons canola oil
1 teaspoon ground cumin
$\frac{1}{4}$ teaspoon ground red pepper
10 ounces skinless boneless chicken breast, cut into strips
1 medium red bell pepper, cut into strips
1 cup chopped scallions ($\frac{1}{2}$" pieces)
2 garlic cloves, minced
$\frac{1}{4}$ cup salsa

1. Preheat oven to 350°F. Wrap tortillas in foil; bake 10 minutes, until soft. Set aside; keep warm in foil.

2. Meanwhile, in medium bowl, combine yogurt, juice and orange zest; set aside.

3. In large nonstick skillet, heat oil; add cumin and ground red pepper. Cook over medium-high heat, stirring frequently, 1 minute. Add chicken, bell pepper, scallions, and garlic; cook, stirring frequently, 6–8 minutes, until chicken is cooked through. Transfer chicken mixture to bowl with yogurt mixture; toss to mix well.

4. Unwrap 1 tortilla and spoon 1 tablespoon of salsa across tortilla; top with one-fourth of the chicken mixture. Roll up to enclose filling. Repeat procedure using remaining salsa and chicken mixture, making 3 more fajitas.

EACH SERVING PROVIDES: $\frac{1}{4}$ Milk, $\frac{1}{2}$ Fat, 1 Vegetable, 2 Proteins, 1 Bread, 5 Optional Calories
PER SERVING: 215 Calories, 21 g Protein, 5 g Fat, 21 g Carbohydrate, 270 mg Sodium, 42 mg Cholesterol, 2 g Dietary Fiber

CHICKEN "FRIED" RICE

MAKES 4 SERVINGS

8 ounces ground chicken
$\frac{1}{4}$ cup low-sodium chicken broth
1 tablespoon reduced-sodium teriyaki sauce
$\frac{1}{2}$ teaspoon ground coriander
$\frac{1}{4}$ teaspoon ground ginger
2 teaspoons peanut oil
2 large eggs, lightly beaten
1 cup chopped scallions
1 cup chopped green bell pepper
1 cup shredded carrots
$1\frac{1}{2}$ cups cooked brown rice
$\frac{1}{2}$ cup thawed frozen peas

1. Heat wok or large nonstick skillet sprayed with nonstick cooking spray over medium-high heat; add chicken. Cook, stirring frequently, 4–5 minutes, until browned. Transfer to medium bowl; add broth, teriyaki sauce, coriander and ginger. Stir and set aside.

2. Add 1 teaspoon of the oil to wok and heat; add eggs. Cook, stirring, until set but still moist. Transfer to small bowl.

3. Heat the remaining teaspoon of oil in same skillet; add scallions, pepper and carrots. Cook, stirring frequently, 3–4 minutes, until tender. Stir in rice and peas; cook until rice begins to brown. Add chicken mixture and cooked eggs; cook 5 minutes, until chicken is heated through.

EACH SERVING PROVIDES: $\frac{1}{2}$ Fat, $1\frac{1}{2}$ Vegetables, 2 Proteins, 1 Bread, 5 Optional Calories
PER SERVING: 272 Calories, 17 g Protein, 11 g Fat, 27 g Carbohydrate, 194 mg Sodium, 153 mg Cholesterol, 4 g Dietary Fiber

Orange-Flavored Fajitas

CHICKEN PITA PIZZAS

MAKES 4 SERVINGS

8 sun-dried tomato halves (not packed in oil)
4 small whole-wheat pita breads
$\frac{1}{4}$ cup low-sodium canned tomato sauce
6 ounces coarsely chopped cooked chicken
$\frac{1}{2}$ cup coarsely chopped arugula or watercress
20 small pitted black olives, thinly sliced
$1\frac{1}{2}$ ounces part-skim mozzarella cheese

1. Preheat oven to 425°F. Spray large baking sheet with nonstick cooking spray.

2. In small bowl, cover sun-dried tomatoes with boiling water; let stand 2 minutes. Drain and cut into thin strips; set aside.

3. On prepared baking sheet, arrange pitas; brush each with 1 tablespoon tomato sauce. Top each with one-fourth of the chicken, arugula, olives, tomato strips and cheese. Bake 10–12 minutes, until golden and cheese melts.

EACH SERVING PROVIDES: $\frac{1}{2}$ Fat, $1\frac{1}{2}$ Vegetables, 2 Proteins, 1 Bread
PER SERVING: 223 Calories, 19 g Protein, 8 g Fat, 22 g Carbohydrate, 372 mg Sodium, 44 mg Cholesterol, 4 g Dietary Fiber

DIJON CHICKEN STRIPS WITH CORN SALSA

MAKES 4 SERVINGS

Salsa:
1 cup drained canned whole-kernel corn
1 cup chopped green bell pepper
$\frac{1}{2}$ cup chopped tomato
$\frac{1}{2}$ cup chopped seeded cucumber
2 tablespoons chopped fresh cilantro
1 tablespoon chopped fresh parsley
1 tablespoon orange juice
1 tablespoon red wine vinegar
1 tablespoon canned chopped green chilies
$\frac{1}{2}$ teaspoon ground cumin
$\frac{1}{4}$ teaspoon salt
$\frac{1}{4}$ teaspoon chili powder
Chicken:
Four 3-ounce skinless boneless chicken breasts
2 tablespoons Dijon-style mustard
8 romaine lettuce leaves

1. To prepare salsa, in medium bowl, combine corn, bell pepper, tomato, cucumber, cilantro, parsley, juice, vinegar, chilies, cumin, salt and chili powder; set aside.

2. Heat indoor ridged grill sprayed with nonstick cooking spray until very hot. Or spray broiler rack with nonstick cooking spray. Preheat broiler.

3. Meanwhile, brush chicken on both sides with mustard; cut into 2" strips. For grill, arrange strips on grill; cook, 4–5 minutes, turning once, until cooked through. For broiler, arrange strips on rack and broil 4 inches from source of heat 4–5 minutes, turning once, until cooked through.

4. To serve, line 4 plates with 2 lettuce leaves each; top each with an equal amount of salsa. Arrange one-fourth of the chicken strips on each plate.

EACH SERVING PROVIDES: $1\frac{1}{2}$ Vegetables, 2 Proteins, $\frac{1}{2}$ Bread, 2 Optional Calories
PER SERVING: 164 Calories, 22 g Protein, 2 g Fat, 15 g Carbohydrate, 577 mg Sodium, 49 mg Cholesterol, 2 g Dietary Fiber

Dijon Chicken Strips with Corn Salsa

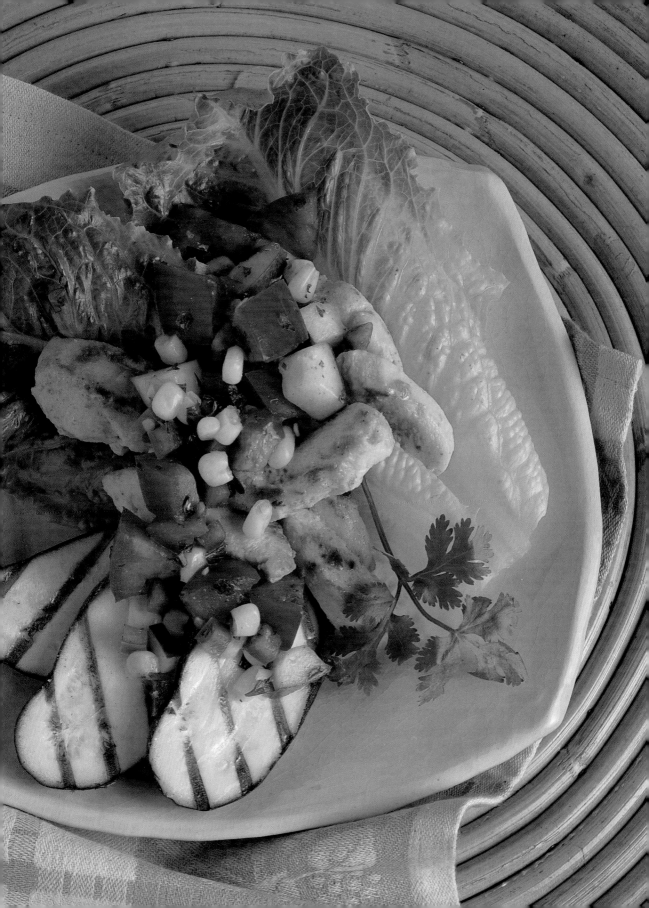

SAUTÉED CHICKEN WITH ARTICHOKE AND PEPPER SALAD

MAKES 4 SERVINGS

2 cups thawed frozen artichoke hearts, coarsely chopped
1 cup roasted red bell pepper
$\frac{1}{4}$ cup chopped fresh basil
2 tablespoons fresh lemon juice
1 tablespoon grated lemon zest
$\frac{1}{4}$ teaspoon salt
$\frac{1}{4}$ teaspoon freshly ground black pepper
3 tablespoons all-purpose flour
2 tablespoons uncooked yellow cornmeal
$\frac{1}{8}$ teaspoon white pepper
Four 3-ounce skinless boneless chicken breasts, thinly sliced
2 teaspoons olive oil

1. In medium bowl, combine artichokes, roasted bell pepper, basil, lemon juice, lemon zest, salt and pepper; set aside.

2. On sheet of wax paper, combine flour, cornmeal and white pepper. Dredge chicken in flour mixture, coating both sides.

3. In large nonstick skillet, heat oil until very hot; add chicken. Cook over medium-high heat, 3–4 minutes on each side, until cooked through.

4. To serve, arrange each chicken breast on plate with one-fourth of the salad.

EACH SERVING PROVIDES: $\frac{1}{2}$ Fat, 1$\frac{1}{2}$ Vegetables, 2 Proteins, $\frac{1}{2}$ Bread
PER SERVING: 199 Calories, 23 g Protein, 4 g Fat, 18 g Carbohydrate, 232 mg Sodium, 49 mg Cholesterol, 4 g Dietary Fiber

CLASSIC CHICKEN SALAD

In this light version of a salad classic, nonfat yogurt stands in for most of the mayonnaise. You'll never know the difference!

MAKES 4 SERVINGS

$\frac{3}{4}$ cup plain nonfat yogurt
2 tablespoons + 2 teaspoons reduced-calorie mayonnaise
1 tablespoon cider vinegar
2 teaspoons Dijon-style mustard
$\frac{1}{4}$ teaspoon celery seeds
$\frac{1}{4}$ teaspoon freshly ground black pepper
10 ounces cubed cooked chicken
2 cups blanched green beans
1 cup chopped celery
2 tablespoons grated onion

1. In small bowl, combine yogurt, mayonnaise, vinegar, mustard, celery seeds and pepper.

2. In medium bowl, combine chicken, beans, celery and onion. Add yogurt mixture; toss to mix well. Cover and refrigerate at least 1 hour before serving.

EACH SERVING PROVIDES: $\frac{1}{4}$ Milk, 1 Fat, 1$\frac{1}{2}$ Vegetables, 2$\frac{1}{2}$ Proteins
PER SERVING: 214 Calories, 24 g Protein, 8 g Fat, 10 g Carbohydrate, 252 mg Sodium, 67 mg Cholesterol, 2 g Dietary Fiber

ORIENTAL CHICKEN SALAD

MAKES 4 SERVINGS

¾ cup plain nonfat yogurt
1 tablespoon smooth peanut butter
1 tablespoon rice-wine vinegar
1 teaspoon sesame oil
1 garlic clove, crushed
¼ teaspoon ground coriander
8 ounces cubed cooked chicken
1½ cups cooked cellophane noodles
1 cup chopped scallions (1" pieces)
1 cup thinly sliced red bell pepper
¾ cup sliced water chestnuts
2 cups trimmed watercress or 2 cups mixed salad
    greens
1 tablespoon + 1 teaspoon toasted sesame seeds

1. In medium bowl, combine yogurt, peanut butter, vinegar, oil, garlic and coriander. Add chicken, cellophane noodles, scallions, bell pepper and water chestnuts; toss to mix well. Cover and refrigerate at least 1 hour.

2. To serve, arrange watercress evenly on 4 plates; top each with one-fourth of the chicken mixture. Sprinkle each with 1 teaspoon seeds.

EACH SERVING PROVIDES: ¼ Milk, ½ Fat, 2 Vegetables, 2¼ Proteins, 1 Bread, 15 Optional Calories
PER SERVING: 279 Calories, 22 g Protein, 9 g Fat, 28 g Carbohydrate, 118 mg Sodium, 51 mg Cholesterol, 2 g Dietary Fiber

CITRUS-GARLIC ROASTED HEN

MAKES 2 SERVINGS

1 tablespoon finely grated orange zest
1 tablespoon finely grated lemon zest
1 teaspoon dried thyme leaves
½ teaspoon onion powder
¼ teaspoon salt
¼ teaspoon freshly ground black pepper
One 1-pound game hen, split and skinned
2 teaspoons olive oil
1 medium green bell pepper, cut into strips
1 medium onion, thinly sliced and separated into
    rings
2 cups thawed frozen artichoke hearts
2 tablespoons low-sodium chicken broth
2 tablespoons fresh lemon juice
4 garlic cloves, cut into thin slices

1. Preheat oven to 375°F.

2. In small bowl, combine orange zest, lemon zest, thyme, onion powder, salt and pepper. Rub mixture on both sides of hen; set aside.

3. In large ovenproof skillet, heat oil; add bell pepper and onion. Cook over medium-high heat, stirring frequently, 4–5 minutes, until tender. Stir in artichokes, broth, juice and garlic; bring to a boil.

4. Remove skillet from heat; arrange hen on top of vegetable mixture. Bake, covered, 50–60 minutes, until juices run clear when meat is pricked with fork.

EACH SERVING PROVIDES: 1 Fat, 3½ Vegetables, 3 Proteins, 1 Optional Calorie
PER SERVING: 319 Calories, 31 g Protein, 12 g Fat, 25 g Carbohydrate, 431 mg Sodium, 76 mg Cholesterol, 8 g Dietary Fiber

TERIYAKI-ORANGE GAME HEN

MAKES 2 SERVINGS

2 tablespoons rice-wine vinegar
2 tablespoons reduced-sodium teriyaki sauce
1 tablespoon grated orange zest
1 tablespoon honey
1 tablespoon Dijon-style mustard
2 teaspoons sesame oil
One 1-pound Cornish hen, split

1. To prepare marinade, in gallon-size sealable plastic bag, combine vinegar, teriyaki sauce, orange zest, honey, mustard and oil; add hen. Seal bag, squeezing out air; turn to coat hen. Refrigerate at least 1 hour or overnight, turning bag occasionally.

2. Preheat broiler. Spray broiler rack with nonstick cooking spray. With slotted spoon, transfer hen to broiler rack. Drain marinade into small saucepan; bring to a boil. Remove from heat.

3. Broil hen, 6–8 inches from heat, 15–20 minutes, turning occasionally and basting with reserved marinade, until juices run clear when hen is pricked with a fork. Remove skin before serving.

EACH SERVING PROVIDES: 3 Proteins, 90 Optional Calories
PER SERVING: 267 Calories, 26 g Protein, 12 g Fat, 14 g Carbohydrate, 601 mg Sodium, 76 mg Cholesterol, 0 g Dietary Fiber

MUSHROOM-STUFFED TURKEY BREAST

Suitable for your best company, this beautiful roulade is filled with sautéed vegetables and carves into attractive pinwheel slices.

MAKES 12 SERVINGS

2 tablespoons stick margarine
1 cup chopped red onion
2 cups sliced mushrooms
1 cup shredded carrot
2 cups drained thawed frozen chopped spinach
2 tablespoons chopped fresh parsley
1 tablespoon grated Parmesan cheese
$\frac{1}{2}$ teaspoon dried basil leaves
1 slice reduced-calorie white bread, finely chopped
1 cup low-sodium chicken broth
1 tablespoon grated lemon zest
One 2-pound, 13-ounce skinless boneless turkey breast

1. In large nonstick skillet, melt margarine over medium-high heat; add onion. Cook, stirring frequently, 4 minutes. Add mushrooms and carrot; cook, stirring frequently, 4–5 minutes, until tender. Stir in spinach, parsley, cheese and basil; cook 2 minutes. Remove from heat; stir in bread, 2 tablespoons of the broth and the lemon zest. Set aside.

2. Preheat oven to 325°F. Spray a 13 × 9" baking pan with nonstick cooking spray.

3. Arrange turkey between two sheets of plastic wrap; with meat mallet or rolling pin, pound turkey to even thickness.

4. Remove top sheet of plastic wrap from turkey; spread mushroom mixture down center of turkey breast, leaving 2½" border on all sides. Starting with short side, roll turkey breast jelly-roll style to enclose filling. Secure roll at 2" intervals with poultry string; arrange seam-side down in prepared pan. Pour remaining ¾ cup + 2 tablespoons broth over turkey; cover with foil tent.

5. Bake 1 to 1½ hours, basting frequently with broth, until meat thermometer inserted in center of roll reaches 180°F. Transfer turkey to carving board; let stand 10 minutes before slicing.

EACH SERVING PROVIDES: ½ Fat, 1 Vegetable, 3 Proteins, 10 Optional Calories
PER SERVING: 162 Calories, 28 g Protein, 3 g Fat, 5 g Carbohydrate, 119 mg Sodium, 71 mg Cholesterol, 2 g Dietary Fiber

---

Easy Poaching

◆

Poaching is a delicious way to cook chicken. The liquid in which you poach the chicken can add wonderful flavor, and a poached chicken breast is lovely with a sauce, as in Creole Poached Chicken Breasts (page 142).

Poaching is also an easy way to cook chicken for recipes that require cooked chicken, such as Oriental Chicken Salad (page 169).

- *Place a boneless chicken breast in a deep skillet and add water just to cover. Add a dash of salt, pepper and onion powder.*
- *Place wax paper on top of chicken to hold in steam. Bring to a simmer and cook 4 to 8 minutes or until the thickest part of the meat becomes white and opaque. (You can reserve the liquid for soup stock.)*
- *Drain meat; cool slightly before refrigerating.*

POACHED BALSAMIC TURKEY ON SPINACH

MAKES 4 SERVINGS

½ cup apple juice
1 cinnamon stick
Four 3-ounce turkey cutlets
½ cup orange juice
¼ cup dark raisins
¼ cup balsamic vinegar
1 tablespoon grated orange zest
1 tablespoon chopped fresh mint
2 teaspoons olive oil
1 teaspoon firmly packed light brown sugar
¼ teaspoon freshly ground black pepper
4 cups spinach leaves

1. In large nonstick skillet, bring apple juice and cinnamon stick to a boil; add turkey. Reduce heat to low; simmer, partially covered, 7–9 minutes, until cooked through. With slotted spoon, transfer turkey to plate; reserve juice; discard cinnamon stick.

2. Add orange juice, raisins, vinegar, orange zest, mint, oil, brown sugar and pepper to skillet; bring to a boil. Reduce heat to low; simmer 4–5 minutes, until reduced by half.

3. To serve, line 4 plates with one-fourth of the spinach leaves; top each with a turkey cutlet. Spoon equal amount of sauce over each cutlet.

EACH SERVING PROVIDES: ½ Fat, 1 Fruit, 2 Vegetables, 2 Proteins, 5 Optional Calories
PER SERVING: 192 Calories, 23 g Protein, 3 g Fat, 18 g Carbohydrate, 91 mg Sodium, 53 mg Cholesterol, 2 g Dietary Fiber

TOASTED ALMOND TURKEY CUTLETS

MAKES 4 SERVINGS

Four 3-ounce turkey cutlets
1 tablespoon grated Parmesan cheese
$\frac{1}{4}$ teaspoon freshly ground black pepper
2 teaspoons olive oil
1 ounce sliced almonds
$\frac{1}{2}$ cup low-sodium chicken broth
2 tablespoons dry white wine
2 garlic cloves, crushed
2 tablespoons chopped fresh basil
1 teaspoon stick margarine
1 teaspoon lemon juice

1. On sheet of wax paper, sprinkle each cutlet on both sides with cheese and pepper. In large nonstick skillet, heat 1 teaspoon of the oil; add turkey. Cook over medium-high heat, 4–6 minutes on each side, until cooked through. Transfer to serving platter; keep warm.

2. In same skillet, heat the remaining teaspoon of oil; add almonds. Cook, stirring constantly, 1 minute, until golden. Transfer to small bowl.

3. To same skillet, add broth, wine, 2 tablespoons of water and the garlic; bring to a boil. Cook until reduced by half; remove from heat. Stir in toasted almonds, basil, margarine and juice.

4. To serve, top turkey with sauce.

EACH SERVING PROVIDES: 1$\frac{1}{4}$ Fats, 2$\frac{1}{4}$ Proteins, 15 Optional Calories
PER SERVING: 183 Calories, 23 g Protein, 8 g Fat, 3 g Carbohydrate, 85 mg Sodium, 54 mg Cholesterol, 0 g Dietary Fiber

TURKEY CUTLETS WITH CRANBERRY SAUCE

MAKES 4 SERVINGS

Four 3-ounce turkey cutlets
$\frac{1}{4}$ teaspoon salt
$\frac{1}{4}$ teaspoon freshly ground black pepper
2 teaspoons canola oil
$\frac{1}{2}$ cup chopped red onion
1 cup low-calorie cranberry juice cocktail
1 tablespoon firmly packed dark brown sugar
1 tablespoon red wine vinegar
1 teaspoon green peppercorns
$\frac{1}{2}$ teaspoon dried thyme leaves
$\frac{1}{3}$ cup + 2 teaspoons dried cranberries
1 tablespoon cornstarch, dissolved in 2 tablespoons water

1. On sheet of wax paper, sprinkle each cutlet on both sides with salt and pepper. In large nonstick skillet, heat oil; add turkey and onion. Cook over medium-high heat, stirring occasionally and turning turkey once, 5–7 minutes on each side, until cooked through. Transfer to serving platter; keep warm.

2. To same skillet, stir in juice, brown sugar, vinegar, peppercorns and thyme; bring to a boil. Stir in cranberries; reduce heat to low and simmer 5 minutes. Stir in dissolved cornstarch; bring to a boil. Cook 1 minute, stirring constantly, until thickened. To serve, spoon sauce over turkey.

EACH SERVING PROVIDES: $\frac{1}{2}$ Fat, 1 Fruit, $\frac{1}{4}$ Vegetable, 2 Proteins, 20 Optional Calories
PER SERVING: 189 Calories, 21 g Protein, 3 g Fat, 19 g Carbohydrate, 183 mg Sodium, 53 mg Cholesterol, 0 g Dietary Fiber

TURKEY AND RICE-WINE VINEGAR STIR-FRY

Stir-fried in fragrant sesame oil, these marinated turkey strips are a hearty meal when potatoes, rice and vegetables are served alongside.

MAKES 4 SERVINGS

1 cup orange juice
1 tablespoon grated fresh ginger root
10 ounces turkey cutlets, cut into strips
1 tablespoon + 1 teaspoon Oriental sesame oil
10 ounces baking potatoes, pared and cubed
2 medium carrots, thinly sliced
1 medium onion, thinly sliced and separated into rings
1/2 teaspoon fennel seeds
1/4 teaspoon red pepper flakes
2 1/2 cups green beans
1 cup cooked brown rice
1 tablespoon reduced-sodium soy sauce
1 tablespoon rice-wine vinegar
1 tablespoon sesame seeds, toasted

1. To prepare marinade, in gallon-size sealable plastic bag, combine juice and ginger; add turkey. Seal bag, squeezing out air; turn to coat turkey. Refrigerate at least 1 hour, turning bag occasionally. With slotted spoon, remove turkey from marinade, reserving marinade.

2. In large wok or nonstick skillet, heat oil; add turkey. Stir-fry 6–8 minutes, until cooked through. Transfer turkey to bowl. Add potatoes, carrots, onion rings, fennel seeds and pepper flakes to wok; stir-fry 8–10 minutes, until tender.

3. Meanwhile, drain reserved marinade into small saucepan; bring to a boil. Remove from heat.

4. Add beans, rice, soy sauce and vinegar to wok; stir-fry 4–5 minutes, until rice begins to brown. Add cooked turkey and marinade; stir-fry 4–6 minutes, until liquid is evaporated. Sprinkle with seeds.

EACH SERVING PROVIDES: 1 Fat, 1/2 Fruit, 2 1/2 Vegetables, 2 Proteins, 1 Bread, 10 Optional Calories
PER SERVING: 322 Calories, 23 g Protein, 7 g Fat, 43 g Carbohydrate, 216 mg Sodium, 44 mg Cholesterol, 5 g Dietary Fiber

TURKEY AND DRIED FRUIT PILAF

MAKES 4 SERVINGS

2 teaspoons olive oil
10 ounces thinly sliced turkey cutlets
1 cup chopped scallions
1 cup chopped celery
2 garlic cloves, minced
1 teaspoon cinnamon
1 teaspoon firmly packed dark brown sugar
1/4 teaspoon ground nutmeg
4 ounces uncooked regular long-grain rice
1 cup low-sodium chicken broth
1/4 cup dark raisins
12 dried apricot halves, coarsely chopped
1 tablespoon sesame seeds, toasted

1. Preheat oven to 350°F.

2. In large ovenproof skillet, heat oil; add turkey. Cook over medium-high heat 2–3 minutes on each side, until browned. Transfer to plate; set aside.

3. Add scallions, celery and garlic to skillet; cook, stirring frequently, 4–5 minutes, until tender. Reduce heat to medium-low. Stir in cinnamon, brown sugar and nutmeg; cook 1 minute. Stir in rice; cook 1 minute. Add broth; bring to a boil. Remove from heat; stir in cooked turkey.

4. Cover skillet with ovenproof lid; bake 40 minutes. Uncover; stir in raisins, apricots and sesame seeds. Cover and bake 10–15 minutes, until liquid is absorbed and rice is tender.

EACH SERVING PROVIDES: 1/2 Fat, 1 Fruit, 1 Vegetable, 2 Proteins, 1 Bread, 20 Optional Calories
PER SERVING: 297 Calories, 22 g Protein, 5 g Fat, 42 g Carbohydrate, 83 mg Sodium, 44 mg Cholesterol, 3 g Dietary Fiber

BROILED TURKEY CUTLETS WITH FETA-TOMATO SAUCE

MAKES 4 SERVINGS

4 sun-dried tomato halves (not packed in oil)
$1\frac{1}{2}$ ounces crumbled plain or peppercorn-flavored feta cheese
1 tablespoon minced scallion
2 garlic cloves, minced
$\frac{1}{2}$ teaspoon dried basil leaves
$\frac{1}{4}$ teaspoon dried oregano leaves
Four 3-ounce turkey cutlets

1. Preheat broiler. Spray broiler rack with nonstick cooking spray.

2. In small bowl, cover sun-dried tomatoes with boiling water; let stand 2 minutes. Drain and finely chop; return tomatoes to bowl.

3. Add cheese, scallion, garlic, basil and oregano to same bowl; stir to combine.

4. Broil turkey on rack, 4" from heat, 4 minutes; turn and top each cutlet with one-fourth of the cheese mixture. Broil 4–5 minutes longer, until cooked through and cheese begins to melt.

EACH SERVING PROVIDES: $\frac{1}{2}$ Vegetable, $2\frac{1}{2}$ Proteins
PER SERVING: 136 Calories, 23 g Protein, 3 g Fat, 3 g Carbohydrate, 164 mg Sodium, 62 mg Cholesterol, 1 g Dietary Fiber

MONTEREY JACK TURKEY BURGER

If you thought bacon-cheeseburgers were a thing of the past, think again. This delicious combo, served on a toasted bun, tastes great with ground turkey and turkey bacon.

MAKES 4 SERVINGS

10 ounces ground turkey
2 tablespoons minced scallion
1 tablespoon reduced-sodium soy sauce
1 tablespoon ketchup
$\frac{1}{4}$ teaspoon garlic powder
$\frac{1}{4}$ teaspoon freshly ground black pepper
$1\frac{1}{2}$ ounces shredded Monterey Jack cheese
4 strips turkey bacon
4 hamburger rolls (2 ounces each), split and toasted
1 medium tomato, cut into 4 slices

1. In large bowl, combine turkey, scallion, soy sauce, ketchup, garlic powder and pepper; mix well. Add cheese; stir to mix well. Shape turkey mixture into 4 equal patties.

2. Heat indoor ridged grill sprayed with nonstick cooking spray; add bacon. Cook 3–4 minutes on each side, until browned. Transfer to plate; set aside. Wipe grill clean; arrange burgers on grill; cook 6–8 minutes on each side, until cooked through.

3. To serve, layer rolls with burgers, bacon and tomato slices.

EACH SERVING PROVIDES: $\frac{1}{2}$ Vegetable, $2\frac{1}{2}$ Proteins, 2 Breads, 35 Optional Calories
PER SERVING: 352 Calories, 23 g Protein, 14 g Fat, 33 g Carbohydrate, 826 mg Sodium, 71 mg Cholesterol, 2 g Dietary Fiber

Monterey Jack Turkey Burger

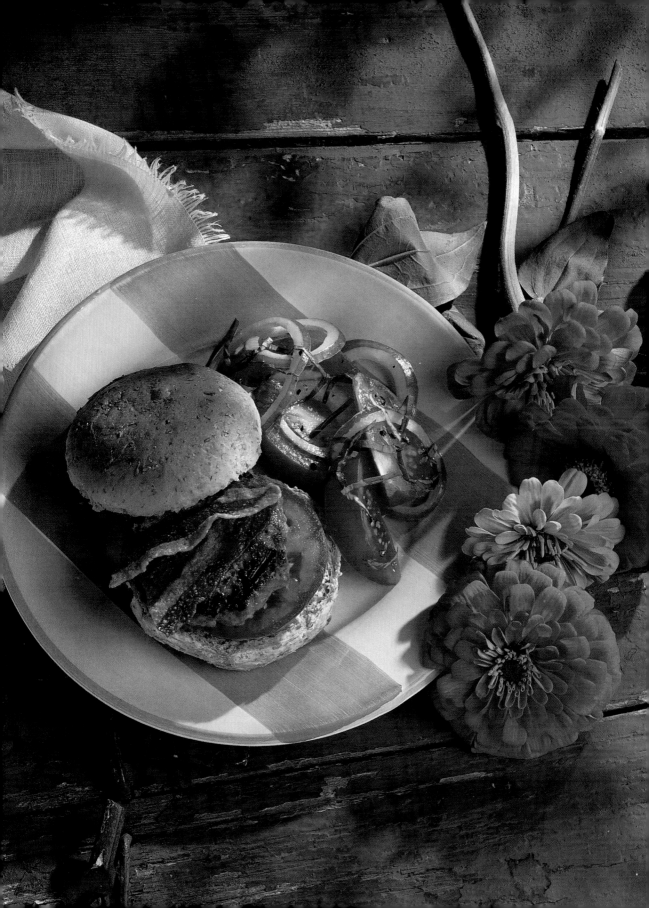

PARMESAN-TURKEY MEATLOAF

An American classic, the meatloaf gets a nutritional update when made with turkey, skim milk and egg white.

MAKES 8 SERVINGS

1 tablespoon + 1 teaspoon olive oil
1 medium onion, chopped
1 pound, 4 ounces ground turkey
4 slices whole-wheat bread, processed into fine crumbs
½ cup skim milk
1 large egg white, lightly beaten
3 tablespoons ketchup
2 tablespoons grated Parmesan cheese
½ teaspoon garlic powder
½ teaspoon ground basil
¼ teaspoon ground thyme
¼ teaspoon freshly ground black pepper

1. Preheat oven to 350°F. Spray an 8 × 5" loaf pan with nonstick cooking spray; set aside.

2. In small nonstick skillet, heat oil; add onion. Cook over medium-high heat, stirring frequently, 4–5 minutes, until tender.

3. In medium bowl, combine cooked onion, turkey, bread crumbs, milk, egg white, ketchup, cheese, garlic powder, basil, thyme and pepper; mix well.

4. Shape turkey mixture into a loaf and arrange in prepared pan. Bake 50–60 minutes, until browned and cooked through. Let stand 10 minutes; cut into slices.

EACH SERVING PROVIDES: ½ Fat, 2 Proteins, ½ Bread, 20 Optional Calories
PER SERVING: 181 Calories, 15 g Protein, 9 g Fat, 10 g Carbohydrate, 247 mg Sodium, 53 mg Cholesterol, 1 g Dietary Fiber

DILLED TURKEY MEATBALLS WITH VEGETABLE SAUCE

Our version of meatballs and sauce combines ground turkey with just the white of an egg and some bread crumbs; the sauce is rich with vegetables. Serve over your favorite pasta.

MAKES 4 SERVINGS

10 ounces ground turkey
1 large egg white, lightly beaten
3 tablespoons seasoned dried bread crumbs
2 tablespoons chopped fresh dill
1 tablespoon Dijon-style mustard
1 teaspoon salt-free lemon-herb seasoning
2 teaspoons olive oil
1 medium green bell pepper, chopped
1 medium red bell pepper, chopped
1 cup sliced zucchini
1 cup chopped fennel
2 garlic cloves, minced
3 cups canned stewed tomatoes
2 teaspoons grated lemon zest
½ teaspoon dried oregano leaves

1. In large bowl, combine turkey, egg white, bread crumbs, dill, mustard and seasoning; mix well. Shape into 12 equal meatballs.

2. In large nonstick skillet, heat oil; add meatballs. Cook over medium-high heat, turning frequently, 6–8 minutes, until browned on all sides. With slotted spoon, transfer meatballs to plate; set aside.

3. Add bell peppers, zucchini, fennel and garlic to skillet; cook, stirring frequently, 4–5 minutes, until tender. Stir in tomatoes, lemon zest and oregano. Reduce heat to low; simmer 5 minutes. Return meatballs to skillet; simmer, partially covered, 10 minutes, frequently spooning sauce over meatballs.

EACH SERVING PROVIDES: ½ Fat, 3½ Vegetables, 2 Proteins, ¼ Bread, 5 Optional Calories
PER SERVING: 229 Calories, 17 g Protein, 8 g Fat, 23 g Carbohydrate, 859 mg Sodium, 52 mg Cholesterol, 6 g Dietary Fiber

Dilled Turkey Meatballs with Vegetable Sauce

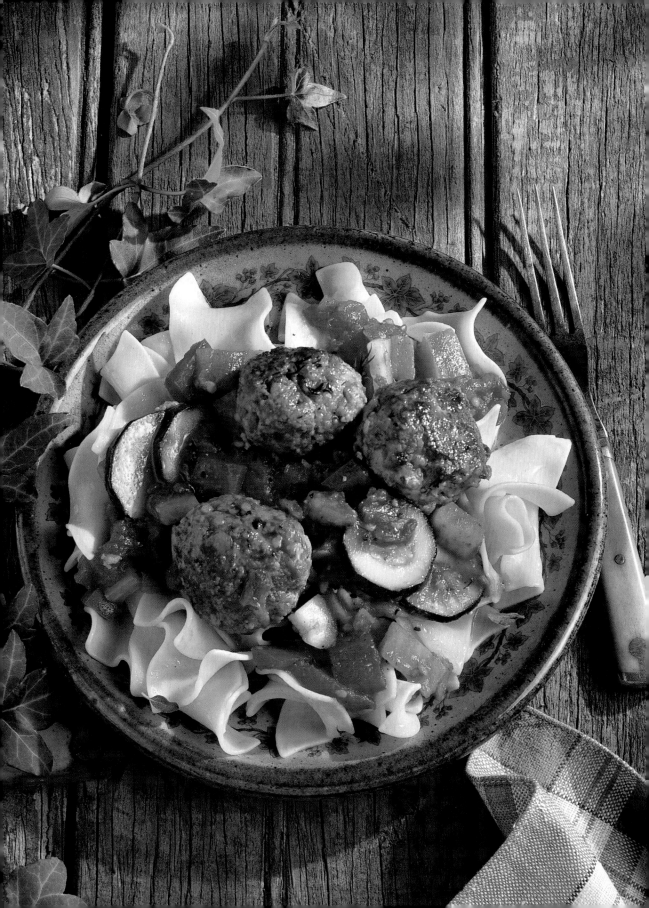

STUFFED ONIONS

MAKES 4 SERVINGS

4 large yellow onions (6 ounces each), peeled
5 ounces hot Italian turkey sausage (90% or more fat free), casings removed
2 garlic cloves, minced
½ cup seasoned dried bread crumbs
2 tablespoons orange juice
1 tablespoon chopped fresh sage
1 tablespoon chopped fresh parsley
2 teaspoons grated orange zest

1. With large stainless steel knife, cut off stem of each onion, flush with base so that onions will stand upright; cut ½" slice from top of each onion.

2. In medium saucepan with 1" of gently boiling water, arrange onions, stem-end down. Simmer, covered, 20 minutes, until tender. With slotted spoon, transfer onions to several layers of paper towels; drain. With melon scoop or sharp-edged teaspoon, hollow out the inside of each onion, leaving ½" walls and bottom; reserve shells and onion centers.

3. Preheat oven to 400°F. Finely chop onion centers; set aside.

4. Heat large nonstick skillet that has been sprayed with nonstick cooking spray; add one-half of the chopped onions, sausage and garlic. Discard or reserve remaining chopped onions for another use. Cook over medium heat, stirring frequently to break up sausage, 5–7 minutes, until lightly browned. Stir in bread crumbs, juice, sage, parsley and orange zest; remove from heat.

5. Spoon one-fourth of the sausage mixture into each onion shell; arrange stuffed onions in a 13 × 9" baking pan. Pour 1 cup of water in pan; bake 30 minutes, until lightly browned.

EACH SERVING PROVIDES: 1½ Vegetables, 1 Protein, ½ Bread, 20 Optional Calories
PER SERVING: 181 Calories, 10 g Protein, 5 g Fat, 26 g Carbohydrate, 595 mg Sodium, 29 mg Cholesterol, 2 g Dietary Fiber

ITALIAN-STYLE PEPPERS AND ONIONS

This 20-minute skillet supper combines everyone's favorite Italian flavors. Serve with an escarole salad and garlic bread for an authentic trattoria meal.

MAKES 4 SERVINGS

5 ounces hot Italian turkey sausage (90% or more fat free), cut into ¼" slices
1 medium red bell pepper, cut into ¼" strips
1 medium green bell pepper, cut into ¼" strips
1 medium yellow bell pepper, cut into ¼" strips
1 medium onion, cut into ¼" slices
¼ cup chicken broth
3 garlic cloves, minced
¼ teaspoon red pepper flakes
¼ teaspoon dried oregano leaves

1. Heat large nonstick skillet that has been sprayed with nonstick cooking spray; add sausage. Cook over medium heat, stirring frequently to break up sausage, 4–6 minutes, until no longer pink.

2. Add bell peppers, onion, broth, garlic, pepper flakes and oregano; cook, stirring frequently, 5 minutes, until most of the liquid has evaporated.

3. Reduce heat to low; simmer, covered, 3–4 minutes, until peppers are tender.

EACH SERVING PROVIDES: 1¾ Vegetables, 1 Protein, 1 Optional Calorie
PER SERVING: 92 Calories, 7 g Protein, 4 g Fat, 7 g Carbohydrate, 256 mg Sodium, 29 mg Cholesterol, 1 g Dietary Fiber

PENNE WITH PROSCIUTTO AND SAUSAGE

MAKES 4 SERVINGS

6 ounces uncooked penne pasta
2½ cups broccoli florets
8 ounces hot Italian turkey sausage (90% or more fat free), cut into ½" slices
1 tablespoon + 1 teaspoon olive oil
1 medium red bell pepper, cut into strips
1 medium yellow bell pepper, cut into strips
1 medium red onion, thinly sliced and separated into rings
1 cup thinly sliced mushrooms
2 ounces prosciutto, cut into thin strips
2 garlic cloves, minced
¼ teaspoon red pepper flakes
¼ cup chopped fresh basil
1 tablespoon grated Parmesan cheese

1. In large pot of boiling water, cook pasta 6 minutes; add broccoli. Cook, 2–4 minutes, until tender. Drain and transfer to serving bowl; keep warm.

2. Meanwhile, heat large nonstick skillet sprayed with nonstick cooking spray; add sausage. Cook over medium-high heat, stirring frequently, 6–8 minutes, until cooked through. Transfer to bowl with pasta; keep warm.

3. In same skillet, heat 2 teaspoons of the oil; add bell peppers and onion. Cook, stirring frequently, 4 minutes. Add mushrooms, prosciutto, garlic and pepper flakes; cook, stirring frequently, 3–4 minutes, until tender. Transfer to bowl with pasta.

4. Add the remaining 2 teaspoons oil, basil and cheese to pasta mixture; toss to mix well.

EACH SERVING PROVIDES: 1 Fat, 3 Vegetables, 2 Proteins, 2 Breads, 10 Optional Calories
PER SERVING: 368 Calories, 21 g Protein, 13 g Fat, 44 g Carbohydrate, 572 mg Sodium, 57 mg Cholesterol, 5 g Dietary Fiber

TURKEY SAUSAGE WITH CHICK-PEAS

MAKES 4 SERVINGS

2 teaspoons olive oil
10 ounces hot Italian turkey sausage (90% or more fat free), casings removed
1 medium green bell pepper, coarsely chopped
1 cup chopped celery
4 garlic cloves, minced
½ teaspoon ground thyme
½ teaspoon fennel seeds
1 cup low-sodium chicken broth
1 tablespoon cornstarch
1 tablespoon Worcestershire sauce
¾ cup spicy mixed vegetable juice
4 ounces uncooked couscous
8 ounces cooked chick-peas

1. In large nonstick skillet, heat oil; add sausage. Cook over medium-high heat, stirring frequently to break up sausage, 6–8 minutes, until browned. Add bell pepper, celery, garlic, thyme and fennel seeds; cook, stirring frequently, 4–5 minutes, until tender.

2. Meanwhile, in a 1-cup liquid measure, combine broth, cornstarch and Worcestershire sauce, stirring to dissolve cornstarch. In small saucepan, bring juice to a boil; remove from heat. Stir in couscous, cover, and let stand, about 5 minutes.

3. Stir broth mixture and chick-peas into sausage mixture; bring to a boil. Reduce heat to low; simmer 2–4 minutes, until sauce thickens.

4. To serve, fluff couscous with fork; divide evenly onto each of 4 plates. Top each with one-fourth of the sausage mixture.

EACH SERVING PROVIDES: ½ Fat, 1½ Vegetables, 2 Proteins, 2 Breads, 15 Optional Calories
PER SERVING: 358 Calories, 20 g Protein, 10 g Fat, 47 g Carbohydrate, 538 mg Sodium, 51 mg Cholesterol, 3 g Dietary Fiber

SAUSAGE AND CHEESE GRITS

Cheddar cheese and turkey sausage transform the bland taste of grits into a real treat, especially nice for a weekend brunch as a change from the usual egg dishes.

MAKES 6 SERVINGS

$4\frac{1}{2}$ ounces uncooked old-fashioned hominy grits
$4\frac{1}{2}$ ounces grated reduced-fat cheddar cheese
4 ounces cooked turkey sausage, crumbled
1 cup skim milk
2 eggs
1 teaspoon dried thyme leaves
$\frac{1}{2}$ teaspoon garlic powder

1. Preheat oven to 350°F. Spray an 11 × 7" baking dish with nonstick cooking spray.
2. In Dutch oven bring 3 cups water to a boil; stir in grits. Return to a boil; cook, stirring constantly, 4 minutes. Remove from heat.
3. Add 4 ounces of the cheese and the sausage to Dutch oven; stir until cheese melts. Set aside.
4. In small bowl, with whisk, combine milk, eggs, thyme and garlic powder; gradually whisk into grits mixture, mixing thoroughly. Transfer to prepared baking dish.
5. Bake 30–40 minutes or until all liquid is absorbed. Top with remaining $\frac{1}{2}$ ounce of cheese; bake about 5 minutes, until cheese is bubbly.

EACH SERVING PROVIDES: 2 Proteins, 1 Bread, 15 Optional Calories
PER SERVING: 219 Calories, 15 g Protein, 8 g Fat, 20 g Carbohydrate, 295 mg Sodium, 104 mg Cholesterol, 0 g Dietary Fiber

LAYERED MEXICAN CASSEROLE

MAKES 4 SERVINGS

2 teaspoons canola oil
5 ounces hot Italian turkey sausage (90% or more fat free), casings removed
1 medium red bell pepper, chopped
1 cup chopped scallions
1 teaspoon chili powder
$\frac{1}{2}$ teaspoon ground cumin
1 cup canned stewed tomatoes
8 ounces cooked black beans
2 cups nonfat cottage cheese
1 large egg white, lightly beaten
$\frac{1}{8}$ teaspoon white pepper
6 flour tortillas (6" diameter)
$1\frac{1}{2}$ ounces shredded reduced-fat Monterey Jack cheese

1. Preheat oven to 350°F. Spray a 2-quart casserole with nonstick cooking spray; set aside.
2. In large nonstick skillet, heat oil; add sausage, bell pepper and scallions. Cook over medium-high heat, stirring frequently to break up sausage, 6–8 minutes, until browned. Add chili powder and cumin; cook, stirring, 1 minute. Stir in tomatoes and beans. Reduce heat to low; simmer 5 minutes.
3. Meanwhile, in medium bowl, combine cottage cheese, egg white and white pepper.
4. Arrange 2 tortillas in bottom of prepared casserole; top with half of the turkey mixture, then half of the cottage cheese. Arrange 2 more tortillas on top of cottage cheese and repeat layers, ending with last 2 tortillas; sprinkle with cheese.
5. Bake 30–35 minutes, until heated through and cheese is melted. Let stand 10 minutes before serving.

EACH SERVING PROVIDES: $\frac{1}{2}$ Fat, $1\frac{1}{2}$ Vegetables, 2 Proteins, $2\frac{1}{2}$ Breads, 5 Optional Calories
PER SERVING: 404 Calories, 31 g Protein, 11 g Fat, 46 g Carbohydrate, 973 mg Sodium, 47 mg Cholesterol, 5 g Dietary Fiber

ORANGE-GLAZED SAUSAGE KABOBS

MAKES 4 SERVINGS

¼ cup orange spreadable fruit
¼ cup orange juice
1 tablespoon grated onion
1 garlic clove, crushed
Pinch ground red pepper
10 ounces hot Italian turkey sausage, cut into 1" pieces
2 cups chopped zucchini (1" pieces)
2 cups whole mushrooms
12 cherry tomatoes

1. Spray grill rack with nonstick cooking spray. Place grill rack 5" from coals. Prepare grill according to manufacturer's directions.

2. In small saucepan, combine spreadable fruit, juice, onion, garlic and red pepper; cook over medium heat, stirring constantly, 2–3 minutes, until spreadable fruit melts. Remove from heat; set aside.

3. Onto each of 4 metal or bamboo skewers, alternating ingredients, thread one-fourth of the sausage, zucchini, mushrooms and tomatoes.

4. Arrange kabobs on grill rack; grill 20–25 minutes, turning and brushing frequently with orange mixture, until sausage is cooked through.

EACH SERVING PROVIDES: 2½ Vegetables, 2 Proteins, 70 Optional Calories
PER SERVING: 194 Calories, 14 g Protein, 8 g Fat, 18 g Carbohydrate, 391 mg Sodium, 59 mg Cholesterol, 1 g Dietary Fiber

RAISIN AND SAGE BREAD STUFFING

MAKES 4 SERVINGS

2 tablespoons + 2 teaspoons reduced-calorie tub margarine
1 cup chopped celery
1 medium onion, chopped
½ cup chopped carrot
1 teaspoon ground sage
½ teaspoon ground thyme
¼ teaspoon crushed fennel seeds
¼ teaspoon ground marjoram
¼ teaspoon salt
¼ teaspoon freshly ground black pepper
8 slices 2-day-old reduced-calorie white bread, cut into cubes
½ cup golden raisins
2 tablespoons low-sodium chicken broth

1. Preheat oven to 350°F. Spray 2-quart casserole with nonstick cooking spray; set aside.

2. In large nonstick skillet, melt margarine over medium-high heat; add celery, onion and carrot. Cook, stirring frequently, 4–5 minutes, until tender. Stir in sage, thyme, fennel, marjoram, salt and pepper; cook 1 minute. Remove from heat; stir in bread cubes and raisins. Add broth; stir until bread is moistened.

3. Spoon stuffing into prepared casserole. Bake 30–35 minutes, until heated through and golden.

EACH SERVING PROVIDES: 1 Fat, 1 Fruit, 1 Vegetable, 1 Bread, 1 Optional Calorie
PER SERVING: 207 Calories, 5 g Protein, 6 g Fat, 40 g Carbohydrate, 453 mg Sodium, 0 mg Cholesterol, 7 g Dietary Fiber

GIBLET-SAGE DRESSING

MAKES 12 SERVINGS

15 ounces turkey giblets
1 tablespoon black peppercorns
1 bay leaf
$\frac{1}{4}$ cup reduced-calorie tub margarine, melted
2 cups thinly sliced mushrooms
1 cup chopped leeks, white part only
$\frac{1}{4}$ cup low-sodium chicken broth
1 teaspoon ground sage
12 slices 2-day-old whole-wheat bread, cut into cubes
1$\frac{1}{2}$ ounces toasted pecans, chopped
$\frac{1}{4}$ teaspoon celery seeds
$\frac{1}{4}$ teaspoon freshly ground black pepper

1. In large pot of boiling water, cook giblets, peppercorns and bay leaf, 20–30 minutes, until tender. Drain and discard peppercorns and bay leaf; let cool slightly. Finely chop giblets; set aside.

2. Preheat oven to 325°F. Spray 2-quart casserole with nonstick cooking spray.

3. In medium nonstick skillet, heat 1 tablespoon of the margarine over medium-high heat; add mushrooms and leeks. Cook, stirring frequently, 4–6 minutes, until tender. Stir in broth and sage. Reduce heat to low; simmer 2 minutes.

4. In large bowl, combine cooked giblets, mushroom mixture, bread cubes, the remaining 3 tablespoons margarine, pecans, celery seeds and pepper; mix until just combined.

5. Spoon dressing into prepared casserole. Bake 45–50 minutes, until golden.

EACH SERVING PROVIDES: 1 Fat, $\frac{1}{2}$ Vegetable, 1 Protein, 1 Bread
PER SERVING: 167 Calories, 10 g Protein, 7 g Fat, 16 g Carbohydrate, 220 mg Sodium, 100 mg Cholesterol, 2 g Dietary Fiber

SAUSAGE AND RICE DRESSING

MAKES 4 SERVINGS

1 tablespoon + 1 teaspoon reduced-calorie tub margarine
5 ounces turkey sausage, casings removed
1 cup chopped celery
$\frac{1}{2}$ cup chopped onion
$\frac{1}{2}$ cup chopped fennel
2 garlic cloves, minced
3 cups cooked brown rice
$\frac{1}{4}$ cup low-sodium chicken broth
2 tablespoons chopped fresh sage
1 tablespoon grated lemon zest
$\frac{1}{4}$ teaspoon freshly ground black pepper

1. Preheat oven to 325°F. Spray 2-quart casserole with nonstick cooking spray.

2. In large nonstick skillet, melt 2 teaspoons of the margarine over medium-high heat; add sausage. Cook, stirring frequently to break up sausage, 8–10 minutes, until browned. With slotted spoon, transfer sausage to plate.

3. Melt the remaining 2 teaspoons margarine in skillet; add celery, onion, fennel and garlic. Cook, stirring frequently, 4–5 minutes, until tender. Stir in cooked sausage, rice, broth, sage, lemon zest and pepper. Reduce heat to low; simmer 5 minutes, until liquid evaporates.

4. Transfer dressing to prepared casserole. Bake 45–50 minutes, until heated through and golden.

EACH SERVING PROVIDES: $\frac{1}{2}$ Fat, 1 Vegetable, 1 Protein, 1$\frac{1}{2}$ Breads, 1 Optional Calorie
PER SERVING: 260 Calories, 11 g Protein, 8 g Fat, 38 g Carbohydrate, 335 mg Sodium, 25 mg Cholesterol, 3 g Dietary Fiber

CORNBREAD-CRANBERRY DRESSING

A soon-to-be holiday tradition, try this with your turkey dinner. The dried cranberries add a tart hint to the slightly sweet cornbread.

MAKES 12 SERVINGS

3¾ ounces (½ cup + 2 tablespoons) uncooked yellow cornmeal
½ cup + 1 tablespoon all-purpose flour
¼ cup chopped scallions
2 tablespoons chopped fresh dill
1 tablespoon granulated sugar
½ teaspoon baking powder
½ teaspoon baking soda
¼ teaspoon salt
3 large egg whites
½ cup skim milk
2 tablespoons canola oil
1 cup apple juice
12 dried apricot halves, chopped
¼ cup dried cranberries
1 cinnamon stick
4 slices 2-day-old whole-wheat bread, cut into cubes

1. Preheat oven to 425°F. Spray 8" baking pan with nonstick cooking spray; set aside.

2. To prepare cornbread, in medium bowl, combine cornmeal, flour, scallions, dill, sugar, baking powder, baking soda and salt. In separate medium bowl, combine 2 of the egg whites, milk and oil; pour over cornmeal mixture. With wooden spoon, beat mixture 30 seconds.

3. Spoon batter into prepared pan. Bake 12–15 minutes, until edges are golden and toothpick inserted in center comes out clean. Cool in pan 10 minutes. Remove from pan; cool completely on rack.

4. Meanwhile, in small saucepan, combine apple juice, apricots, cranberries and cinnamon stick; bring to a boil. Reduce heat to low; simmer 5–10 minutes, until liquid is reduced by half. Discard cinnamon stick.

5. Preheat oven to 325°F. Spray 2-quart casserole with nonstick cooking spray; set aside.

6. In large bowl, crumble prepared cornbread. Add juice mixture, the remaining egg white, and bread cubes; mix until just combined. Spoon into prepared casserole. Bake 40–50 minutes, until golden.

EACH SERVING PROVIDES: ½ Fat, ½ Fruit, 1 Bread, 15 Optional Calories
PER SERVING: 137 Calories, 4 g Protein, 3 g Fat, 24 g Carbohydrate, 188 mg Sodium, 0 mg Cholesterol, 2 g Dietary Fiber

WILD RICE–MUSHROOM STUFFING

MAKES 4 SERVINGS

1 cup low-sodium chicken broth
4 ounces uncooked wild rice, rinsed
1 tablespoon + 1 teaspoon reduced-calorie tub margarine
2 cups thinly sliced shiitake mushrooms
1 medium red bell pepper, cut into strips
$\frac{1}{2}$ cup chopped celery
$\frac{1}{2}$ cup chopped shallots
1 teaspoon dried thyme leaves
$\frac{1}{4}$ teaspoon salt
$\frac{1}{4}$ teaspoon freshly ground black pepper
2 fluid ounces ($\frac{1}{4}$ cup) dry red wine
1 cup chopped spinach leaves

1. In small saucepan, combine broth and 1 cup water; bring to a boil. Stir in rice; reduce heat to low. Simmer, covered, 50–60 minutes, until rice is tender; set aside.

2. Preheat oven to 325°F. Spray 2-quart casserole with nonstick cooking spray.

3. Meanwhile, in large nonstick skillet, melt margarine over medium-high heat; add mushrooms, bell pepper, celery, shallots, thyme, salt and pepper. Cook, stirring frequently, 4 minutes, until tender; stir in wine. Reduce heat to low; simmer 2–3 minutes, until liquid evaporates. Remove from heat. Add spinach and cooked rice; stir to combine.

4. Spoon rice mixture into prepared casserole; bake 30–40 minutes, until heated through.

EACH SERVING PROVIDES: $\frac{1}{2}$ Fat, 2$\frac{1}{2}$ Vegetables, 1 Bread, 20 Optional Calories
PER SERVING: 174 Calories, 7 g Protein, 3 g Fat, 30 g Carbohydrate, 216 mg Sodium, 0 mg Cholesterol, 3 g Dietary Fiber

Steak with Two Peppers (page 187)

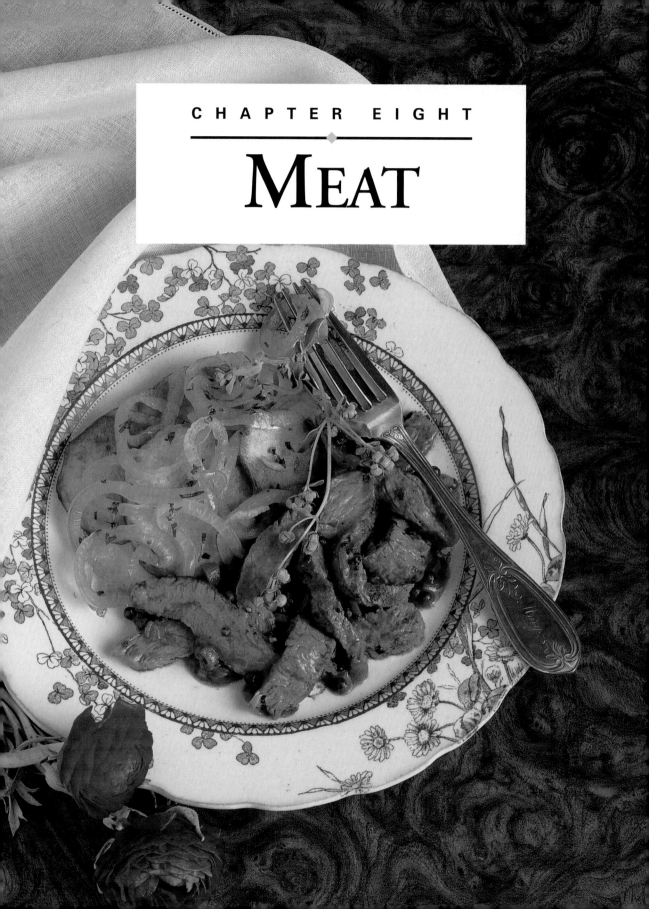

CHAPTER EIGHT

MEAT

LONDON BROIL

MAKES 4 SERVINGS

15 ounces top round or sirloin tip
4 fluid ounces (½ cup) dry red wine
1 garlic clove, finely chopped
Freshly ground black pepper to taste
1 sprig fresh rosemary, chopped, or 1 teaspoon
    dried leaves, crumbled
Salt to taste

1. Place steak in a gallon-size sealable plastic bag. Add wine, garlic and pepper. Lightly massage marinade into meat. Add rosemary sprig (if using dried, add with other ingredients). Seal bag, squeezing out air; turn to coat steak. Refrigerate overnight or up to 24 hours, turning bag occasionally.

2. Remove meat from refrigerator at least 30 minutes before broiling. Preheat broiler for at least 20 minutes. Lift meat from marinade, and discard marinade. Broil on rack 3" from heat approximately 4 minutes on each side, salting cooked side and turning only once.

3. Remove steak from broiler; allow it to rest for 2–3 minutes. Slice thinly across the grain and serve immediately.

EACH SERVING (3 ounces) PROVIDES: 3 Proteins, 25 Optional Calories
PER SERVING: 176 Calories, 27 g Protein, 4 g Fat, 1 g Carbohydrate, 54 mg Sodium, 71 mg Cholesterol, 0 g Dietary Fiber

BROILED T-BONE STEAK

This steak is also great on the grill. The perfect accompaniment? Grilled vegetables, such as eggplant, squash and onion.

MAKES 4 SERVINGS

One 1 pound, 2-ounce T-bone or rib steak (at least
    1–1½" thick), excess fat trimmed
1 tablespoon + 1 teaspoon extra virgin olive oil
2 teaspoons chopped fresh rosemary
2 teaspoons chopped fresh sage
Salt and freshly ground black pepper to taste

1. Preheat broiler. Spray rack with nonstick cooking spray.

2. In small bowl, mix oil, rosemary and sage. Rub steak with herb mixture.

3. Broil steak 3" from heat, 6 minutes for rare, turning once, or until cooked to desired doneness. Season with salt and pepper as soon as steak is done. Slice and serve.

EACH SERVING (3 ounces) PROVIDES: 1 Fat, 3 Proteins
PER SERVING: 223 Calories, 24 g Protein, 13 g Fat, 0 g Carbohydrate, 56 mg Sodium, 68 mg Cholesterol, 0 g Dietary Fiber

MARINATED FLANK STEAK

MAKES 4 SERVINGS

¼ cup reduced-sodium soy sauce

2 teaspoons honey

2 teaspoons grated fresh ginger root, or 1 teaspoon ground

2 teaspoons finely chopped fresh lemon grass, or grated lemon zest

2 garlic cloves, finely chopped

½ fluid ounce (1 tablespoon) dry sherry

Pinch crushed red pepper flakes

15 ounces flank steak

2 teaspoons olive oil

Salt and freshly ground black pepper to taste

1. To prepare marinade, in gallon-size sealable plastic bag, combine soy sauce, honey, ginger, lemon grass, garlic, sherry and red pepper flakes; add steak. Seal bag, squeezing out air; turn to coat steak. Refrigerate overnight or up to 24 hours, turning bag occasionally. Remove meat from refrigerator at least 30 minutes before broiling.

2. Preheat broiler. Drain and discard marinade; dry meat with paper towel. Rub very lightly with oil. Broil on a rack 3 inches from heat approximately 4 minutes each side, turning only once and salting cooked side only.

3. Season with pepper. Allow meat to rest about 2–3 minutes before carving into thin diagonal slices.

EACH SERVING (3 ounces) PROVIDES: 3 Proteins, 35 Optional Calories
PER SERVING: 226 Calories, 24 g Protein, 11 g Fat, 6 g Carbohydrate, 671 mg Sodium, 57 mg Cholesterol, 0 g Dietary Fiber

STEAK WITH TWO PEPPERS

MAKES 4 SERVINGS

1 tablespoon drained canned green peppercorns packed in brine

1 teaspoon cracked black pepper

15 ounces boneless top loin steak (excess fat trimmed), pounded slightly

2 teaspoons olive oil

Salt to taste

2 teaspoons stick margarine

1 tablespoon freshly chopped shallots or red onion

2 fluid ounces (¼ cup) dry red wine

1 teaspoon tomato paste

⅓ cup low-sodium beef broth

1. Using your fingers, press 2 teaspoons of the green peppercorns and the black pepper into the steak.

2. Place medium nonstick skillet over medium-high heat. When hot, add olive oil and sauté steak 1–2 minutes per side, salting the cooked side and turning only once. Remove meat and keep warm between two plates.

3. Heat 1 teaspoon of the margarine over medium heat; add shallots; sauté, stirring, until wilted, about 1 minute. Add wine; cook, stirring, until wine evaporates, about 2 minutes. Dissolve tomato paste in the beef broth and add with the remaining 1 teaspoon green peppercorns. Cook until liquid reduces slightly, about another 2–3 minutes; swirl in the remaining 1 teaspoon margarine. Quickly return steak and any accumulated juices to sauce and reheat about 30 seconds to 1 minute. Remove steak and slice. Pour sauce over steak and serve.

EACH SERVING (3 ounces) PROVIDES: 1 Fat, 3 Proteins, 15 Optional Calories
PER SERVING: 204 Calories, 23 g Protein, 10 g Fat, 1 g Carbohydrate, 153 mg Sodium, 63 mg Cholesterol, 0 g Dietary Fiber

Beef Roasting Timetable
General Procedures

1. Place meat (straight from refrigerator) on rack in open roasting pan.
2. Season either before or after cooking.
3. Insert meat thermometer into thickest part of roast, not touching bone.
4. Do not add water. Do not cover.
5. Roast in oven until meat thermometer registers 5° to 10°F below desired doneness. During the standing time the roast will continue to rise 5° to 10°F and reach the final meat thermometer reading. (Oven does not have to be preheated.)
6. Allow roast to stand 15 to 20 minutes before serving. Temperature will rise and roast will be easier to carve.

BEEF

Beef Cut	Approx. Weight in Pounds	Oven Temperature	Final Meat Thermometer Reading	Approx. Cooking Time* (min./lb.)
Beef Rib Roast	4 to 6	325°F	140°F (rare)	26 to 30
			160°F (medium)	34 to 38
	6 to 8	325°F	140°F (rare)	23 to 25
			160°F (medium)	27 to 30
	8 to 10	325°F	140°F (rare)	19 to 21
			160°F (medium)	23 to 25
Beef Rib Eye Roast	4 to 6	350°F	140°F (rare)	18 to 20
			160°F (medium)	20 to 22
	8 to 10	350°F	140°F (rare)	13 to 15
			160°F (medium)	16 to 18
Beef Tenderloin, Whole	4 to 6	425°F	140°F (rare)	45 to 60 (total time)
Beef Tenderloin, Half	2 to 3	425°F	140°F (rare)	35 to 40 (total time)
Beef Round Tip Roast	2½ to 4	325°F	140°F (rare)	30 to 35
			160°F (medium)	35 to 40
	4 to 6	325°F	140°F (rare)	25 to 30
			160°F (medium)	30 to 35
	8 to 10	325°F	140°F (rare)	18 to 22
			160°F (medium)	23 to 25
Beef Top Round Roast	2½ to 4	325°F	140°F (rare)	25 to 30
			160°F (medium)	30 to 35
	4 to 6	325°F	140°F (rare)	20 to 25
			160°F (medium)	25 to 30
	6 to 10	325°F	140°F (rare)	17 to 19
			160°F (medium)	22 to 24
Beef Top Loin Roast	4 to 6	325°F	140°F (rare)	17 to 21
			160°F (medium)	21 to 25
	6 to 8	325°F	140°F (rare)	14 to 17
			160°F (medium)	17 to 21

*Cooking times are based on meat taken directly from the refrigerator.
Chart courtesy of the National Live Stock and Meat Board.

PEPPERED ROAST TENDERLOIN

Leftovers can be used for cold beef salads, stir-fries or sandwiches.

MAKES 10 SERVINGS

2 pounds, 6 ounces tenderloin of beef
2 garlic cloves, cut lengthwise into slivers
1 tablespoon + 2 teaspoons olive oil
1 tablespoon cracked black peppercorns
1 teaspoon finely chopped fresh rosemary, or $\frac{1}{2}$ teaspoon dried leaves
1 teaspoon finely chopped fresh thyme, or $\frac{1}{2}$ teaspoon dried leaves
1 teaspoon finely chopped sage, or $\frac{1}{2}$ teaspoon dried leaves
Salt to taste

1. Preheat oven to 425°F. Make small incisions in the tenderloin with a small sharp knife; insert a sliver of garlic in each incision. Rub tenderloin with oil; combine the peppercorns, rosemary, thyme, sage and salt; pat the mixture on all sides of tenderloin.

2. Place tenderloin in a small, shallow roasting pan and roast for 10 minutes. Reduce heat to 350°F; roast another 15 minutes for rare, 20 minutes for medium. Allow roast to rest outside of oven for 10 minutes before slicing.

EACH SERVING (3 ounces) PROVIDES: $\frac{1}{2}$ Fat, 3 Proteins
PER SERVING: 210 Calories, 24 g Protein, 12 g Fat, 0 g Carbohydrate, 52 mg Sodium, 71 mg Cholesterol, 0 g Dietary Fiber

BEEF STEW

MAKES 4 SERVINGS

1 tablespoon + 1 teaspoon olive oil
1 tablespoon finely chopped onion
1 tablespoon finely chopped carrot
1 tablespoon finely chopped celery
15 ounces beef round, cut into $1\frac{1}{2}$" cubes
1 cup chopped canned plum tomatoes, with juice
4 fluid ounces ($\frac{1}{2}$ cup) dry red wine
1 teaspoon finely chopped fresh thyme or $\frac{1}{2}$ teaspoon dried leaves
1 bay leaf
Salt and freshly ground black pepper to taste
Eight $1\frac{1}{2}$-ounce onions, peeled, roots trimmed, with ends intact
2 medium carrots, pared and cut into 1" chunks
15 ounces pared potato cut into 1" cubes
1 cup hot water
1 cup thawed frozen peas
1 tablespoon finely chopped fresh flat-leaf parsley
1 tablespoon finely chopped fresh mint

1. In medium casserole or heavy saucepan, heat oil over medium heat. Sauté chopped onion, carrot and celery until onion is translucent, about 5–6 minutes. Add beef. Raise heat to medium-high and sauté, stirring, for 5 minutes. Add tomatoes, wine, thyme, bay leaf, salt and pepper. Bring to a boil and lower heat. Simmer gently, partially covered, 45 minutes, stirring occasionally.

2. Add onions, carrots, potato and hot water. Cover and cook another 40 minutes.

3. Add peas. Cook 4 minutes; add parsley and mint, and cook 1 more minute. Remove bay leaf before serving.

EACH SERVING ($1\frac{1}{4}$ cups) PROVIDES: 1 Fat, $2\frac{1}{2}$ Vegetables, 3 Proteins, $1\frac{1}{4}$ Breads, 25 Optional Calories
PER SERVING: 348 Calories, 29 g Protein, 10 g Fat, 31 g Carbohydrate, 226 mg Sodium, 62 mg Cholesterol, 2 g Dietary Fiber

POT ROAST WITH VEGETABLES

You'll relish this pot roast, which delivers great, old-fashioned taste, complete with modern instructions for sure-fire, low-fat gravy.

MAKES 8 SERVINGS

2 tablespoons + 2 teaspoons olive oil
1 pound, 14 ounces bottom or top round boneless roast
1 cup finely chopped onion
1/2 cup finely chopped carrot
1/2 cup finely chopped celery
2 garlic cloves, finely chopped
1 1/2 teaspoons finely chopped rosemary or 1/2 teaspoon dried leaves, crumbled
1 1/2 teaspoons finely chopped fresh sage
6 juniper berries, crushed (optional)
4 fluid ounces (1/2 cup) dry red wine
1 cup chopped canned plum tomatoes with juice
1 cup low-sodium beef broth
Salt and freshly ground black pepper to taste

What's the Beef?

◆

Recently, meat has had a bad reputation in the protein game, yet it's a reputation that's really undeserved. It's easy to incorporate beef into a healthy eating plan when you follow a few sensible guidelines:

- *Select the leanest cuts of beef—top round, top loin strip steak, top sirloin, eye round, tip and extra-lean (10 percent or less) ground beef.*
- *For pork, tenderloin, leg (fresh ham) and loin chops are good choices.*
- *Look for reduced-fat luncheon and processed meats.*
- *Trim all visible fat from beef, then roast, broil or bake on a rack to keep any untrimmed fat from being reabsorbed.*

---

1. In heavy casserole, heat oil. Add roast and brown on all sides over medium-high heat. Remove roast. Lower heat to medium and add onion, carrot, celery, garlic, rosemary, sage and juniper, if using. Sauté, stirring constantly, about 10 minutes, until vegetables are golden and fragrant.

2. Add wine, turning up the heat slightly and scraping the browned bits on the bottom of the pan; then return roast to casserole. Cook for 2 minutes. Add tomatoes and stir. Add broth, salt and pepper. Liquid should only cover about one-third of the meat. Cover and bring to a boil, leaving cover slightly askew. Lower heat and simmer gently, turning meat occasionally, until tender when tested with a fork, about 2 hours. Skim all fat from liquid before serving.*

*Note: For best fat removal: Make pot roast ahead of time. Remove meat and cool both gravy and meat to room temperature. Wrap meat in plastic and refrigerate meat and gravy separately. When cold, fat is easily removed from gravy with a large spoon or spatula. To serve: slice meat thinly across the grain and reheat it in the gravy over low heat until heated through. If a thicker gravy is desired, quickly reduce over high heat, keeping sliced meat warm.

EACH SERVING PROVIDES: 3/4 Vegetable, 3 Proteins, 55 Optional Calories
PER SERVING: 218 Calories, 24 g Protein, 10 g Fat, 5 g Carbohydrate, 121 mg Sodium, 62 mg Cholesterol, 1 g Dietary Fiber

SPICY MEATLOAF WITH HERBS

As always, leftover meatloaf makes a very satisfying sandwich. Try it in a Pita (page 68) topped with Dijon mustard.

MAKES 4 SERVINGS

2 teaspoons vegetable oil
1 cup mushrooms, finely chopped
$\frac{1}{2}$ cup finely chopped onion
$\frac{1}{4}$ cup finely chopped carrot
2 tablespoons finely chopped celery
2 tablespoons finely chopped green bell pepper
14 ounces extra-lean ground beef (10% or less fat)
$1\frac{1}{2}$ ounces quick-cooking oats
1 egg
2 tablespoons tomato paste
1 tablespoon Worcestershire sauce
2 teaspoons finely chopped garlic
1 teaspoon finely chopped fresh rosemary, or $\frac{1}{2}$ teaspoon dried crumbled leaves
1 teaspoon finely chopped fresh sage, or pinch dried leaves
1 teaspoon finely chopped fresh thyme, or $\frac{1}{2}$ teaspoon dried leaves
$\frac{1}{4}$ teaspoon hot pepper sauce
$\frac{1}{4}$ cup tomato purée or tomato sauce, diluted with $\frac{1}{4}$ cup water

1. Spray a shallow 9" square pan with non-stick cooking spray; set aside. In large nonstick skillet, heat oil; add mushrooms, onion, carrot, celery, and bell pepper. Cook, stirring frequently, until softened, about 5 minutes.

2. Preheat oven to 350°F. In large bowl, combine beef, oats, tomato paste, egg, Worcestershire sauce, garlic, rosemary, sage, thyme and pepper sauce. Form into an oblong loaf approximately 7 × 5 × 2" and place in prepared loaf pan.

3. Bake 1 hour, basting with tomato purée mixture after the first 30 minutes. Allow meatloaf to stand about 10 minutes before slicing.

EACH SERVING PROVIDES: $\frac{1}{2}$ Fat, $1\frac{1}{2}$ Vegetables, 3 Proteins, $\frac{1}{2}$ Bread
PER SERVING: 288 Calories, 25 g Protein, 15 g Fat, 15 g Carbohydrate, 271 mg Sodium, 115 mg Cholesterol, 2 g Dietary Fiber

SPINACH MEATBALLS

MAKES 4 SERVINGS

10 ounces extra-lean ground beef (10% or less fat)
$\frac{1}{2}$ cup finely chopped spinach or thawed frozen spinach, squeezed dry
$\frac{1}{2}$ cup + 2 tablespoons finely chopped onion
1 egg
$\frac{3}{4}$ ounce grated Parmesan cheese
1 garlic clove, finely chopped
$\frac{1}{8}$ teaspoon grated nutmeg
Salt and freshly ground black pepper to taste
4 cups low-sodium tomato purée
1 tablespoon finely chopped carrot
1 tablespoon finely chopped celery
Pinch crushed red pepper flakes
3 tablespoons very fine dried bread crumbs
1 tablespoon + 1 teaspoon olive oil

1. In medium bowl, combine ground beef, spinach, 2 tablespoons of the onion, the egg, Parmesan, garlic, nutmeg, salt and pepper. Form into 16 meatballs; refrigerate for at least 30 minutes.

2. In 3-quart saucepan combine tomato purée, the remaining $\frac{1}{2}$ cup onion, the carrot, celery and red pepper flakes. Bring to a boil over high heat; reduce heat to low; simmer, partially covered, 30–40 minutes, stirring occasionally.

3. Place bread crumbs in a shallow bowl. In a 10-inch nonstick skillet over medium-high heat, heat oil; when oil is very hot, roll each meatball lightly in the bread crumbs and place gently in the pan. Sauté, turning occasionally, until meatballs are browned on all sides.

4. As meatballs are browned, add them to sauce. Simmer together over low heat 15–20 minutes, gently stirring occasionally.

EACH SERVING (4 meatballs) PROVIDES: 1 Fat, $4\frac{3}{4}$ Vegetables, $2\frac{1}{2}$ Proteins, $\frac{1}{4}$ Bread
PER SERVING: 340 Calories, 23 g Protein, 15 g Fat, 32 g Carbohydrate, 268 mg Sodium, 101 mg Cholesterol, 7 g Dietary Fiber

BEEF AND BEAN CHILI

MAKES 4 SERVINGS

1 tablespoon + 1 teaspoon olive oil
1 cup chopped onions
1/2 cup chopped carrot
1/4 cup chopped celery
1/4 cup chopped green bell pepper
2 teaspoons finely chopped garlic
1 teaspoon finely chopped seeded jalapeño pepper
  (or to taste)
10 ounces extra-lean ground beef (10% or less fat)
1 tablespoon chili powder
2 teaspoons ground cumin
1 teaspoon dried oregano leaves
1/2 teaspoon ground coriander
2 cups chopped canned plum tomatoes with juice
16 ounces rinsed drained cooked pinto or kidney
  beans
1/2 teaspoon salt
Pinch pepper
1/4 cup chopped fresh cilantro
1/4 cup nonfat sour cream
1/4 cup chopped red onion
Chopped fresh cilantro

1. In large saucepan, heat oil; add onions, carrot, celery, bell pepper, garlic and jalapeño. Cook over medium heat, stirring occasionally, until onion is translucent, about 15 minutes.

2. Add beef, breaking it up with a wooden spoon; sauté until no longer pink, about 2–3 minutes. Add chili powder, cumin, oregano and coriander; cook and stir 1 minute.

3. Add tomatoes, beans, salt and pepper; reduce heat to low and simmer gently, partially covered, 20 minutes, stirring occasionally. Stir in cilantro before serving. Top each serving with 1 tablespoon each of sour cream, red onion and some cilantro.

EACH SERVING (1 cup) PROVIDES: 1 Fat, 2 Vegetables, 2 Proteins, 2 Breads, 10 Optional Calories
PER SERVING: 388 Calories, 27 g Protein, 13 g Fat, 43 g Carbohydrate, 566 mg Sodium, 44 mg Cholesterol, 7 g Dietary Fiber

SLOPPY JOES

Sloppy Joes are great on hamburger buns, but you can also serve them without the buns.

MAKES 4 SERVINGS

1 tablespoon + 1 teaspoon olive oil
1 cup finely chopped onions
1/3 cup finely chopped celery
1/3 cup finely chopped carrot
1/3 cup finely chopped green bell pepper
1/2 teaspoon dried oregano leaves
1/2 teaspoon dried thyme leaves
15 ounces extra-lean ground beef (10% or less fat)
1 cup chopped canned plum tomatoes with juice
2 tablespoons tomato paste
1 tablespoon Worcestershire sauce
2 teaspoons red-wine vinegar
1/4 teaspoon hot pepper sauce
Salt and freshly ground black pepper to taste
Four 2-ounce rolls or hamburger buns
4 unsweetened medium pickles, optional

1. In a medium saucepan, heat oil; add onions, celery, carrot and bell pepper. Sauté, stirring occasionally, until onions are translucent, about 10–12 minutes. Add oregano, thyme and beef, breaking up beef with a wooden spoon. Sauté until beef is no longer pink, about 3–4 minutes.

2. Combine tomatoes, water and tomato paste, and add to beef mixture. Cook for 1 minute. Add Worcestershire sauce, vinegar, red pepper sauce, salt and pepper; bring to a boil, lower heat and simmer for 10 minutes, stirring occasionally. Serve on rolls with pickles, if using.

EACH SERVING (3/4 cup) PROVIDES: 1 Fat, 1 3/4 Vegetables, 3 Proteins, 2 Breads
PER SERVING: 431 Calories, 28 g Protein, 18 g Fat, 39 g Carbohydrate, 619 mg Sodium, 66 mg Cholesterol, 3 g Dietary Fiber

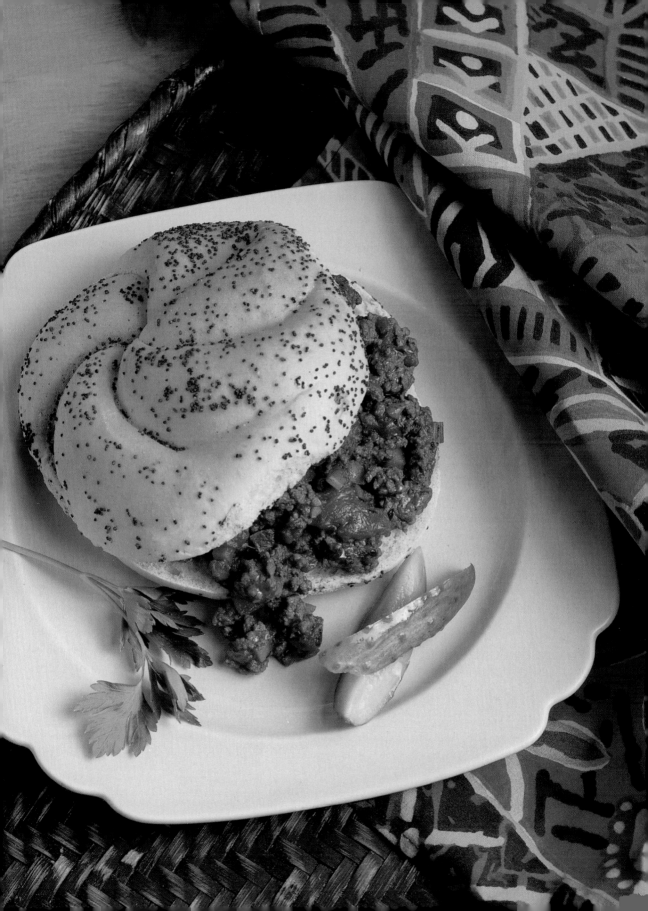

MUSHROOM HAMBURGERS

These hamburgers are great with sautéed onions. Slice the onions, then sauté in a nonstick pan with a little beef bouillon, until tender.

MAKES 4 SERVINGS

2 teaspoons olive oil
$\frac{1}{2}$ cup finely chopped red or yellow bell pepper
$\frac{1}{4}$ cup finely chopped onion
2 tablespoons finely chopped carrot
2 tablespoons finely chopped celery
2 garlic cloves, finely chopped
2 cups finely chopped mushrooms
10 ounces extra-lean ground beef (10% or less fat)
1 tablespoon steak sauce
Salt and freshly ground black pepper to taste

1. In a 10-inch nonstick skillet, heat oil; add bell pepper, onion, carrot, celery and garlic. Sauté, stirring, until onion is translucent, about 8–10 minutes. Add mushrooms; raise heat to high and sauté, stirring, until mushrooms brown and liquid evaporates, about 8 minutes. Allow mixture to come to room temperature. Preheat broiler.

2. Combine mushroom mixture with ground beef, steak sauce, salt and pepper. Form into 4 hamburgers. Spray broiler rack with nonstick cooking spray. Broil burgers on rack 3–4" from heat, 3–4 minutes on each side for medium-rare.

EACH SERVING PROVIDES: $\frac{1}{2}$ Fat, 1$\frac{1}{2}$ Vegetables, 2 Proteins, 5 Optional Calories
PER SERVING: 164 Calories, 15 g Protein, 10 g Fat, 5 g Carbohydrate, 127 mg Sodium, 44 mg Cholesterol, 1 g Dietary Fiber

CUBAN-STYLE BEEF CASSEROLE

MAKES 4 SERVINGS

1 tablespoon + 1 teaspoon olive oil
1 cup chopped onions
$\frac{1}{2}$ cup chopped red bell pepper
2 garlic cloves, finely chopped
15 ounces extra-lean ground beef (10% or less fat)
1$\frac{1}{2}$ cups chopped canned plum tomatoes with juice
$\frac{1}{2}$ cup low-sodium beef broth
2 tablespoons raisins
2 teaspoons seeded finely chopped jalapeño pepper
Grated zest of 1 orange or lemon
$\frac{1}{8}$ teaspoon ground cloves
$\frac{1}{8}$ teaspoon cinnamon
$\frac{1}{8}$ teaspoon freshly grated nutmeg
1 tablespoon chopped rinsed drained capers
4 cups cooked regular long-grain rice

1. Preheat oven to 400°F. In an ovenproof (2$\frac{1}{2}$-quart) medium casserole, heat oil over medium-high heat. Add onions, bell pepper and garlic; sauté, stirring frequently, until onion is golden, about 12–15 minutes.

2. Add ground beef; sauté, stirring, just until it loses its red color, about 1–2 minutes. Add tomatoes, broth, raisins, jalapeño pepper, zest, cloves, cinnamon and nutmeg. Raise heat to high and bring to a boil.

3. Place casserole in preheated oven for 15 minutes. Stir in capers; return to oven for 5–10 minutes, until mixture thickens; add a few tablespoons of water if mixture appears too dry. Serve over rice.

EACH SERVING ($\frac{3}{4}$ cup) PROVIDES: 1 Fat, $\frac{1}{4}$ Fruit, 1$\frac{1}{2}$ Vegetables, 3 Proteins, 2 Breads, 3 Optional Calories
PER SERVING: 542 Calories, 29 g Protein, 16 g Fat, 70 g Carbohydrate, 285 mg Sodium, 66 mg Cholesterol, 3 g Dietary Fiber

Baked Beef and Pasta

Makes 4 Servings

1 tablespoon + 1 teaspoon olive oil
1 cup finely chopped onions
$\frac{1}{2}$ cup finely chopped carrot
$\frac{1}{2}$ cup finely chopped celery
2 teaspoons finely chopped garlic
2 teaspoons finely chopped fresh thyme (or 1 teaspoon dried leaves)
8 ounces extra-lean ground beef (10% or less fat)
4 fluid ounces ($\frac{1}{2}$ cup) dry red wine
2 cups chopped canned plum tomatoes with juice
1 cup cooked tiny green peas, or thawed frozen peas
$4\frac{1}{2}$ ounces small cut pasta (tubetti, ditilini or elbows) cooked until very tender and drained
$1\frac{1}{2}$ ounces grated pecorino-romano or imported provolone cheese
2 tablespoons chopped fresh mint or basil

1. Preheat oven to 350°F. Spray a 2–2$\frac{1}{2}$-quart ovenproof casserole with nonstick cooking spray. In a medium nonstick skillet, heat oil; add onions, carrot, celery, garlic and thyme; sauté, stirring, until onion is translucent, about 8–10 minutes.

2. Add beef, breaking it up with a wooden spoon, and sauté until no longer pink, about 3–4 minutes. Add wine; turn up heat to high; cook 2 minutes. Stir in tomatoes and peas and lower heat to medium; cook, stirring occasionally, for 20 minutes.

3. Toss pasta, cheese and mint into beef mixture and place in prepared casserole. Bake 20 minutes.

EACH SERVING (1$\frac{1}{4}$ cups) PROVIDES: 1 Fat, 2 Vegetables, 2 Proteins, 2 Breads, 25 Optional Calories
PER SERVING: 400 Calories, 23 g Protein, 14 g Fat, 41 g Carbohydrate, 451 mg Sodium, 46 mg Cholesterol, 5 g Dietary Fiber

Eggplant and Beef Casserole

Makes 4 Servings

2 medium eggplants, ends trimmed and thinly sliced lengthwise ($\frac{1}{4}$-inch slices)
1 tablespoon + 1 teaspoon olive oil
1 cup finely chopped onions
10 ounces extra-lean ground beef (10% or less fat)
$1\frac{1}{2}$ cups chopped canned plum tomatoes with juice
1 tablespoon chopped fresh mint or basil
1 tablespoon chopped fresh flat-leaf parsley
1 teaspoon dried oregano leaves
Salt and freshly ground black pepper to taste
2 ounces (2 tablespoons) regular long-grain rice, boiled 2 minutes and drained
$1\frac{1}{2}$ ounces grated Parmesan cheese

1. Lightly salt eggplant and let stand for $\frac{1}{2}$ hour.

2. Preheat broiler 15 minutes. Wipe eggplant slices with paper towels to remove excess moisture and salt. Spray both sides of eggplant lightly with nonstick cooking spray, and place on rack about 4 inches from heat. Broil on each side for about 3–4 minutes or until slices are soft and turn golden. Set aside. Lower oven temperature to 350°F.

3. In a 10-inch nonstick skillet, heat oil; add onions. Sauté until onions are translucent, about 5–6 minutes. Add beef; sauté until it loses its red color and browns slightly, about 4 minutes.

4. Add tomatoes, mint, parsley, oregano, salt and pepper; lower heat very slightly and simmer until mixture thickens somewhat, about 10 minutes. Mix in rice.

5. Spray a 3-quart ovenproof casserole lightly with nonstick cooking spray. In the casserole, place a layer of eggplant, then a layer of meat sauce. Continue layering, ending with meat sauce. Sprinkle with cheese and bake about 35 minutes, until hot and bubbly.

EACH SERVING (1$\frac{1}{2}$ cups) PROVIDES: 1 Fat, 4$\frac{1}{4}$ Vegetables, 2$\frac{1}{2}$ Proteins, $\frac{1}{2}$ Bread
PER SERVING: 362 Calories, 24 g Protein, 15 g Fat, 35 g Carbohydrate, 408 mg Sodium, 52 mg Cholesterol, 5 g Dietary Fiber

STUFFED PEPPERS

MAKES 4 SERVINGS

10 ounces extra-lean ground beef (10% or less fat)
$\frac{1}{2}$ cup finely chopped onion
$\frac{1}{4}$ cup cooked tiny green peas or thawed frozen peas
2 ounces regular long-grain rice, boiled 7 minutes and drained
1$\frac{1}{2}$ ounces grated Parmesan cheese
2 tablespoons tomato paste
3 garlic cloves, finely chopped
1 teaspoon finely chopped fresh thyme, or $\frac{1}{2}$ teaspoon dried leaves
1 teaspoon finely chopped fresh mint or basil
$\frac{1}{2}$ teaspoon finely chopped fresh sage
$\frac{1}{2}$ teaspoon finely chopped fresh rosemary, or $\frac{1}{4}$ teaspoon dried and crumbled leaves
4 medium green, red or yellow bell peppers, tops cut off, cored and ribs removed
$\frac{1}{2}$ cup tomato purée or tomato sauce

1. Preheat oven to 350°F. Combine all ingredients except peppers and tomato purée. Loosely stuff peppers with mixture; stand them upright in a baking dish or casserole just large enough to hold them. Pour tomato purée over peppers; add enough water that liquid comes about one-fourth up the sides of the peppers. Cover baking pan.

2. Bake, basting occasionally with the liquid in the pan, 45 minutes. Uncover pan, and continue baking until the peppers are tender and filling is completely cooked, about 20 minutes. Remove from oven, cover and allow to rest for 5 minutes before serving.

EACH SERVING PROVIDES: 3 Vegetables, 2$\frac{1}{2}$ Proteins, $\frac{1}{2}$ Bread, 10 Optional Calories
PER SERVING: 286 Calories, 22 g Protein, 11 g Fat, 26 g Carbohydrate, 458 mg Sodium, 52 mg Cholesterol, 3 g Dietary Fiber

TACOS

MAKES 4 SERVINGS

2 ripe medium tomatoes, cut into small pieces
1 tablespoon + 1 teaspoon olive oil
$\frac{1}{2}$ cup finely chopped onion
2 garlic cloves, finely chopped
1 teaspoon finely chopped jalapeño pepper (or to taste)
2 teaspoons ground cumin
1 teaspoon dried oregano leaves
1 teaspoon paprika
15 ounces extra-lean ground beef (10% or less fat)
1 cup chopped canned plum tomatoes with juice
Salt and freshly ground black pepper to taste
$\frac{1}{2}$ cup finely chopped fresh cilantro leaves
$\frac{1}{2}$ cup finely chopped red onion
2 tablespoons fresh lime juice
Eight $\frac{1}{2}$-ounce taco shells
2 cups shredded iceberg or romaine lettuce
$\frac{1}{4}$ cup nonfat sour cream

1. Place fresh tomatoes in strainer or colander. Drain for 20–30 minutes.

2. In medium saucepan, heat oil; add onion, garlic and jalapeño pepper. Sauté, stirring occasionally, until garlic is golden, about 6–8 minutes. Add cumin, oregano and paprika; sauté, stirring, for 1 minute. Add beef and sauté, breaking up beef, until it loses its red color, about 3 minutes. Add canned tomatoes, salt and pepper; lower heat and simmer until thickened, about 10 minutes.

3. To prepare salsa, combine fresh tomatoes, cilantro, red onion and juice. Season with salt and pepper to taste.

4. To assemble: Divide beef mixture evenly ($\frac{1}{4}$ cup each) among 8 taco shells; top with lettuce, then salsa, and finally 1$\frac{1}{2}$ teaspoons of sour cream.

EACH SERVING (2 tacos) PROVIDES: 1 Fat, 3 Vegetables, 3 Proteins, 1 Bread, 10 Optional Calories
PER SERVING: 430 Calories, 27 g Protein, 22 g Fat, 34 g Carbohydrate, 408 mg Sodium, 66 mg Cholesterol, 5 g Dietary Fiber

TACO SALAD

MAKES 4 SERVINGS

$\frac{1}{2}$ cup plain nonfat yogurt
$\frac{1}{4}$ cup chopped fresh cilantro leaves
$\frac{1}{4}$ cup nonfat sour cream
1 garlic clove, crushed
$\frac{1}{8}$ teaspoon salt
2 teaspoons olive oil
$\frac{3}{4}$ cup chopped onions
2 garlic cloves, minced
$\frac{1}{2}$ cup chopped carrot
$\frac{1}{2}$ cup diced celery
$\frac{1}{4}$ cup chopped red bell pepper
$\frac{1}{4}$ cup chopped green bell pepper
1 tablespoon + 1 teaspoon chili powder
1 teaspoon ground cumin
1 teaspoon dried oregano leaves, crumbled
$\frac{1}{4}$ teaspoon ground red pepper
$\frac{1}{4}$ teaspoon freshly ground black pepper
1 bay leaf
8 ounces cooked ground beef
2 cups canned plum tomatoes with juice
$\frac{1}{2}$ cup tomato paste
4 cups shredded iceberg lettuce
$\frac{1}{2}$ cup shredded carrot
4 corn tortillas (6" diameter), lightly toasted, each
   cut into 4 triangles
3 ounces low-fat shredded cheddar cheese

1. To prepare dressing, in small bowl, combine yogurt, cilantro, sour cream, crushed garlic and salt; let stand 30 minutes.

2. In large nonstick skillet, heat oil; add $\frac{1}{2}$ cup of the onions and the minced garlic. Sauté over medium-high heat until onion is translucent; add chopped carrot, celery, red bell pepper, green bell pepper, chili powder, cumin, oregano, ground red pepper, black pepper and bay leaf. Cook, stirring constantly, 2 minutes. Add beef; cook, stirring to break up meat. Stir in tomatoes, reserved liquid, 1 cup water and the tomato paste; bring to a boil. Reduce heat to low; simmer, covered, 20 minutes. Uncover; continue to cook, stirring occasionally, 15 minutes, until dry.

3. Meanwhile, in large bowl, combine lettuce, shredded carrot and one-fourth of the cilantro dressing; toss to coat.

4. To serve, arrange lettuce mixture evenly on 4 plates; mound one-fourth of the meat mixture in center of each. Surround each mound with 4 tortilla triangles; sprinkle each with one-fourth of the cheese and 1 tablespoon of the remaining onion. Pour one-fourth of the remaining dressing over each salad.

EACH SERVING PROVIDES: $\frac{1}{2}$ Fat, $5\frac{1}{2}$ Vegetables, 3 Proteins, 1 Bread, 25 Optional Calories
PER SERVING: 429 Calories, 29 g Protein, 19 g Fat, 38 g Carbohydrate, 845 mg Sodium, 65 mg Cholesterol, 7 g Dietary Fiber

BEEF KABOBS WITH MOROCCAN SPICES

For these kabobs, 10-inch wooden skewers work well. Soak the skewers in water for about half an hour before cooking, to keep them from catching fire.

MAKES 4 SERVINGS

1 medium onion, cubed

Grated zest of 1 lemon

2 tablespoons fresh lemon juice

1 tablespoon + 1 teaspoon olive oil

2 garlic cloves

1 teaspoon ground cumin

1 teaspoon chopped fresh thyme or $\frac{1}{2}$ teaspoon dried leaves

1 teaspoon chopped fresh mint

$\frac{1}{2}$ teaspoon paprika

Dash ground red pepper

15 ounces boneless beef tenderloin, cut into 1-inch cubes

1 bay leaf

1 medium onion, cut into 8 wedges and blanched

1 medium seeded and cored red bell pepper, cut into 8 squares, blanched

8 medium mushroom caps, blanched

Chopped fresh flat-leaf parsley to garnish

1. To prepare marinade, in food processor or blender, place cubed onion, zest, juice, oil, garlic, cumin, thyme, mint, paprika and ground red pepper. Purée until blended. In a gallon-size sealable plastic bag, combine beef cubes, bay leaf and marinade. Seal bag, squeezing out air; turn to coat beef. Refrigerate 1 hour or overnight, turning bag occasionally. Allow meat to remain at room temperature 30 minutes before cooking. Drain marinade into small saucepan and bring to a boil; reserve.

2. While meat marinates, soak four 10" bamboo skewers in water for 1 hour.

3. Preheat broiler or grill 20 minutes. Thread vegetables and meat onto skewers, beginning and ending with onion wedges. Set skewers on rack, keeping rack about 2–3 inches from heat. Broil about 3 minutes per side, basting with the marinade when turning.

4. Heat remaining marinade and bring to a boil. Boil for 1 minute. Serve marinade with kabobs.

EACH SERVING (1 kabob) PROVIDES: 1¼ Vegetables, 3 Proteins, 40 Optional Calories
PER SERVING: 243 Calories, 23 g Protein, 13 g Fat, 7 g Carbohydrate, 61 mg Sodium, 66 mg Cholesterol, 1 g Dietary Fiber

---

Super Stir-Fries

◆

Stir-fries are a terrific way to use meat—they showcase meat as part of a delicious meal that includes fresh vegetables and just the smallest bit of oil. Serve over pasta or rice, and you have a complete meal. Try Spicy Pork Stir-Fry (page 213) or Beef Stir-Fry with Mixed Vegetables (page 199) and you'll be hooked! It's simple to create your own stir-fries, combining meat and vegetables in a wok or heavy skillet. Have all your ingredients ready before you start, as stir-fries cook in a flash. Below you'll find suggestions of beef (pick one) and vegetables (pick a few!) to combine.

Beef	*Vegetables*
Sirloin Tip	*Mushrooms*
Strip Steak	*Broccoli*
Bottom Round	*Bok Choy*
Tenderloin	*Cabbage*
Top Round Steak	*Spinach*
Round Tip Steak	*Pea Pods*

Beef and Asparagus Stir-Fry

Sherry adds a lovely flavor to this stir-fry, but if it's unavailable, you can substitute a bit more soy sauce. Reduce Optional Calories to 5 per serving.

Makes 4 Servings

1 fluid ounce (2 tablespoons) dry sherry
1 tablespoon finely chopped fresh ginger root
Zest from 1 orange, julienned
2 garlic cloves, finely chopped
1 tablespoon dark sesame oil
2 teaspoons dark soy sauce
10 ounces boneless beef tenderloin, cut into thin strips
1 teaspoon cornstarch
2 teaspoons vegetable oil
24 asparagus spears, trimmed and cut diagonally into 2-inch pieces
$\frac{1}{4}$ cup thinly sliced scallions
1 teaspoon sesame seeds

    1. To prepare marinade, in a gallon-size sealable plastic bag, combine sherry, ginger, zest, garlic, sesame oil and soy sauce; add beef. Seal bag, squeezing out air; turn to coat beef. Refrigerate 1 hour, turning bag occasionally.

    2. Strain marinade into measuring cup. Add enough water to make $\frac{1}{3}$ cup liquid. Add cornstarch and stir to dissolve.

    3. Heat a nonstick wok or large nonstick skillet over high heat. Add vegetable oil and beef; stir-fry until beef loses its red color, about 1 minute. Remove beef with slotted spoon and reserve. Reduce heat slightly and add asparagus; stir-fry 2–3 minutes. Return beef and reserved marinade to wok; raise heat to high and stir-fry until sauce thickens, about 2 minutes. To serve, sprinkle with scallions and sesame seeds.

EACH SERVING (1$\frac{1}{4}$ cups) PROVIDES: 1$\frac{1}{4}$ Fats, 1$\frac{1}{4}$ Vegetables, 2 Proteins, 15 Optional Calories
PER SERVING: 209 Calories, 18 g Protein, 12 g Fat, 6 g Carbohydrate, 214 mg Sodium, 44 mg Cholesterol, 1 g Dietary Fiber

Beef Stir-Fry with Mixed Vegetables

Makes 4 Servings

1 tablespoon vegetable oil
10 ounces boneless beef tenderloin, cut into thin strips
1 cup broccoli stems, peeled and cut into bite-size pieces*
1 medium carrot, pared and diagonally sliced
1 medium onion, cut into 8 wedges
$\frac{1}{2}$ medium red bell pepper, seeded and cut into 8 pieces
$\frac{1}{2}$ medium yellow bell pepper, seeded and cut into 8 pieces
8 medium shiitake mushroom caps, halved
1 cup snow peas, ends trimmed
1$\frac{1}{2}$ tablespoons soy sauce
1 tablespoon finely chopped fresh ginger root
2 garlic cloves, finely chopped
1 teaspoon dark sesame oil
Pinch red pepper flakes
1 teaspoon sesame seeds

    1. Heat nonstick wok or large nonstick skillet over high heat. Add oil and beef; stir-fry until meat loses its red color, about 1 minute. Remove with slotted spoon; reserve.

    2. Stir in broccoli and carrot; cover and steam 1 minute. Uncover and stir in onion, bell pepper and mushrooms. Stir-fry another 3 minutes. Add snow peas, soy sauce, ginger, garlic, sesame oil, red pepper flakes and reserved beef. Stir continuously for another minute. Sprinkle sesame seeds on top and serve.

*Reserve florets for another use.

EACH SERVING (1$\frac{3}{4}$ cups) PROVIDES: 1 Fat, 2$\frac{1}{2}$ Vegetables, 2 Proteins, 5 Optional Calories
PER SERVING: 214 Calories, 18 g Protein, 11 g Fat, 12 g Carbohydrate, 443 mg Sodium, 44 mg Cholesterol, 3 g Dietary Fiber

Spicy Beef and Broccoli Stir-Fry

Makes 4 Servings

1 fluid ounce (2 tablespoons) dry sherry
2 tablespoons soy sauce
1 tablespoon finely chopped fresh ginger root
1 tablespoon finely chopped garlic
1 teaspoon dark sesame oil
$\frac{1}{4}$ teaspoon red pepper flakes or to taste
10 ounces boneless beef tenderloin, cut into thin
   strips
1 teaspoon cornstarch
1 tablespoon vegetable oil
4 cups broccoli stems, peeled and cut into bite-size
   pieces*
$\frac{1}{4}$ cup thinly sliced scallions

1. To prepare marinade, in a gallon-size seal-able plastic bag, combine sherry, soy sauce, ginger, garlic, sesame oil and red pepper flakes; add beef. Seal bag, squeezing out air, turn to coat beef. Refrigerate 1 hour, turning bag occasionally.

2. Strain marinade into small saucepan and bring to a boil. Cool slightly; add enough water to make $\frac{1}{3}$ cup liquid. Add cornstarch and stir to dissolve.

3. Heat a nonstick wok or large nonstick skillet over high heat. Add oil and beef; stir-fry until beef loses its red color, about 1 minute. Remove with slotted spoon; lower heat slightly. Add broccoli; stir-fry 3 minutes. Cover and steam 1 minute. Return beef and reserved marinade to wok; increase heat to high and stir-fry until sauce thickens, about 2–3 minutes. Sprinkle with scallions.

*Reserve florets for another use.

EACH SERVING (1$\frac{1}{4}$ cups) PROVIDES: 1 Fat, 2$\frac{1}{4}$ Vegetables, 2 Proteins, 10 Optional Calories
PER SERVING: 204 Calories, 18 g Protein, 10 g Fat, 8 g Carbohydrate, 579 mg Sodium, 44 mg Cholesterol, 3 g Dietary Fiber

Roast Beef Salad with Arugula

Makes 4 Servings

1 medium red onion, halved lengthwise and sliced
   ($\frac{1}{4}$" slices)
1 tablespoon balsamic vinegar
2 teaspoons Dijon mustard
Salt and freshly ground black pepper to taste
1 tablespoon + 1 teaspoon extra virgin olive oil
10 sun-dried tomato halves (not packed in oil),
   soaked in boiling water for 2 minutes, then
   drained, dried and finely diced
8 cups arugula, thick stems removed
1 cup thinly sliced mushrooms
8 ounces cooked roast beef, cut into 8 julienned
   slices
Cracked black pepper to taste
1 lemon, cut into 4 wedges

1. Soak red onion in ice water for 1 hour; drain and pat dry.

2. To prepare dressing, in small bowl, whisk vinegar, mustard, salt and pepper together. Whisk in oil, a little at a time. Add sun-dried tomatoes and beat in 1 tablespoon water.

3. In medium bowl, toss arugula with 1 tablespoon dressing. Place on 4 plates. Toss onion and mushrooms with another tablespoon of dressing and divide among 4 plates. Toss roast beef with remaining dressing and place on top of salads. Sprinkle with cracked black pepper and serve with lemon wedges.

EACH SERVING PROVIDES: 1 Fat, 6 Vegetables, 2 Proteins
PER SERVING: 195 Calories, 20 g Protein, 9 g Fat, 12 g Carbohydrate, 152 mg Sodium, 46 mg Cholesterol, 4 g Dietary Fiber

Roast Beef Salad with Arugula

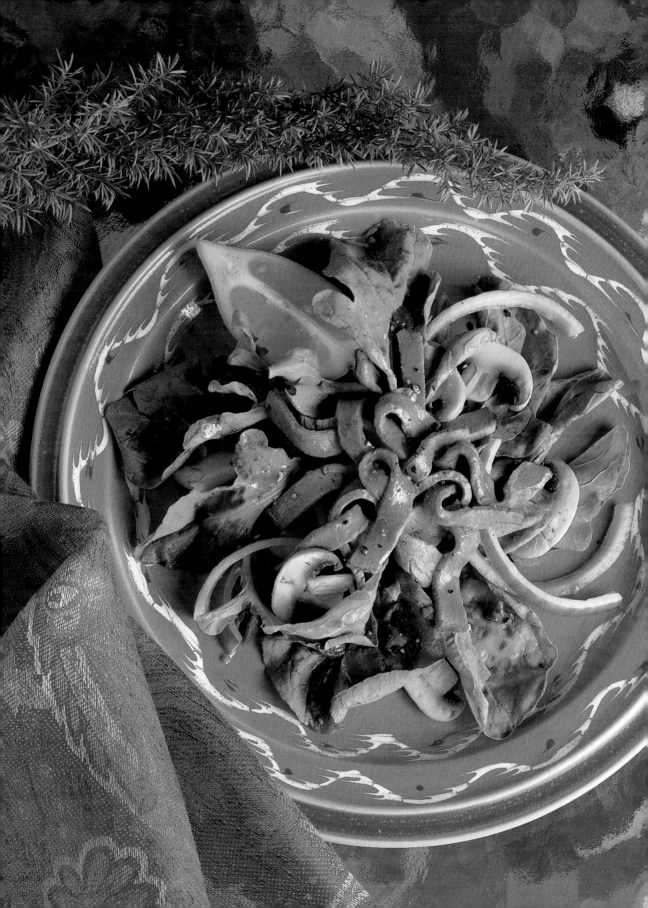

ASIAN ROAST BEEF SALAD

MAKES 4 SERVINGS

1 medium sweet onion, cut into $\frac{1}{4}$" rings
1 tablespoon fresh lime juice
2 teaspoons dark sesame oil
2 teaspoons vegetable oil
1 teaspoon oyster or fish sauce
1 teaspoon soy sauce
8 ounces cold roast beef, cut into $\frac{1}{2}$" julienne slices
1 medium cucumber, pared, halved lengthwise, seeded and thinly sliced
1 stalk fresh lemon grass, tender yellow part thinly sliced into rings, or 2 teaspoons of grated lemon zest
1 small jalapeño pepper, seeded and finely chopped
8 cups salad greens (such as romaine, baby kale or mustard, arugula, Boston and Bibb)
$\frac{1}{4}$ cup chopped fresh mint
$\frac{1}{4}$ cup chopped scallions
1 medium red bell pepper, seeded and diced
8 red radishes, trimmed and thinly sliced
Freshly ground black pepper to taste

1. Soak onion rings in ice water for 30 minutes; drain and pat dry.

2. To prepare dressing, whisk together lime juice, sesame oil, vegetable oil, oyster sauce and soy sauce. Toss roast beef, onion, cucumber, lemon grass and jalapeño with about half of the dressing.

3. Toss greens, mint and scallions with remaining dressing; divide equally among 4 plates. Top each with one-fourth of the roast beef mixture. Top with bell pepper, radish slices and black pepper.

EACH SERVING PROVIDES: 1 Fat, 5$\frac{1}{2}$ Vegetables, 2 Proteins, 3 Optional Calories
PER SERVING: 205 Calories, 20 g Protein, 9 g Fat, 12 g Carbohydrate, 212 mg Sodium, 46 mg Cholesterol, 4 g Dietary Fiber

SPICY STEAK SALAD

MAKES 4 SERVINGS

1 tablespoon + 1 teaspoon finely chopped fresh ginger root
1 tablespoon finely chopped garlic
2$\frac{1}{2}$ teaspoons dark sesame oil
2 teaspoons fresh lemon juice
1 tablespoon finely chopped fresh cilantro
$\frac{1}{2}$ teaspoon freshly ground black pepper
Pinch ground red pepper
15 ounces flank steak
1 medium red onion, thinly sliced
7 cups romaine lettuce, torn into bite-size pieces
$\frac{1}{2}$ cup coarsely chopped fresh cilantro
4 medium scallions, thinly sliced
1$\frac{1}{2}$ teaspoons olive oil
1 tablespoon steak sauce
1 tablespoon lemon juice
2 ripe medium tomatoes, each cut into 8 wedges

1. To prepare marinade, in small bowl, combine 1 tablespoon of the ginger, the garlic, 1 teaspoon of the sesame oil, the fresh lemon juice, cilantro, black pepper and ground red pepper. Rub flank steak with marinade ingredients; place in a resealable plastic bag. Seal bag, squeezing out air. Refrigerate overnight or 24 hours. Allow to stand at room temperature 30 minutes before broiling.

2. Soak onion slices in ice water 30 minutes; drain and pat dry.

3. Preheat broiler. Remove meat from marinade; dry with paper towel. Broil on a rack 3 inches from heat approximately 4 minutes per side, turning only once.

4. Allow steak to cool to room temperature; thinly slice across the grain into diagonal slices. Save juices.

5. Combine lettuce, onion, cilantro, scallions and the remaining 1 teaspoon ginger in a large mixing bowl. Whisk together olive oil, the remaining 1$\frac{1}{2}$ teaspoons sesame oil, the steak sauce, lemon juice and reserved juices. Toss lettuce mixture with half the dressing; divide evenly among 4 plates. Toss steak with remaining dressing; divide evenly, placing on top of lettuce. Add tomato wedges to each plate.

EACH SERVING PROVIDES: ¾ Fat, 5 Vegetables, 3 Proteins, 25 Optional Calories
PER SERVING: 267 Calories, 26 g Protein, 14 g Fat, 10 g Carbohydrate, 160 mg Sodium, 57 mg Cholesterol, 3 g Dietary Fiber

◆

MOROCCAN-STYLE ROAST LEG OF LAMB

Leftover lamb freezes well. After defrosting, it can be served in sandwiches or used in a stir-fry such as Lamb and Pepper Stir-Fry, or in Curried Lamb and Spinach (both page 207).

MAKES 8 SERVINGS

1 tablespoon + 1 teaspoon olive oil
2 teaspoons fresh lemon juice
2 teaspoons paprika
½ teaspoon ground cumin
1 tablespoon finely chopped fresh mint leaves
1½ teaspoons finely chopped garlic
Pinch ground red pepper
Salt and freshly ground black pepper to taste
2 pounds, 4 ounces half leg of lamb (preferably butt end)

1. Preheat oven to 375°F. In small bowl, thoroughly mix together oil, juice, paprika, cumin, mint, garlic, ground red pepper, salt and pepper. Rub mixture all over lamb.

2. Place in a shallow roasting pan; roast until meat is tender, about 2½ hours (internal temperature 160°F). Allow roast to stand at room temperature 10 minutes before carving.

EACH SERVING (3 ounces) PROVIDES: ½ Fat, 3 Proteins
PER SERVING: 186 Calories, 24 g Protein, 9 g Fat, 1 g Carbohydrate, 58 mg Sodium, 76 mg Cholesterol, 0 g Dietary Fiber

LAMB CHOPS WITH TOMATO-DILL SALSA

MAKES 4 SERVINGS

1 medium onion, cubed
3 tablespoons fresh lemon juice
2 garlic cloves
1 tablespoon + 1 teaspoon olive oil
1 teaspoon dried oregano leaves
½ teaspoon freshly ground black pepper
½ teaspoon ground coriander
½ teaspoon paprika
Salt to taste
Four 5-ounce loin lamb chops, with bone, about 1–1¼" thick
¾ cup diced ripe tomato
2 tablespoons finely chopped red onion
2 tablespoons finely chopped fresh dill
1 teaspoon paprika
Finely ground black pepper to taste

1. To prepare marinade, in blender or food processor, place onion, juice, garlic, 2 teaspoons of the olive oil, the oregano, pepper, coriander, paprika and salt. Purée until blended. Place lamb chops in a gallon-size sealable plastic bag; add marinade, turning bag to coat lamb. Refrigerate 3 hours or overnight, turning bag occasionally. Remove from refrigerator 1 hour before broiling.

2. To prepare salsa, combine tomato, onion, dill, the remaining 2 teaspoons of the olive oil, the paprika and pepper. Toss and keep at room temperature.

3. Preheat broiler. Place chops on rack; broil 3–4 inches from heat 4–5 minutes per side for medium-rare chops, turning only once. (Add 1–2 extra minutes per side for medium or well done chops.) Top each chop with one-fourth of the salsa.

EACH SERVING PROVIDES: ½ Fat, ¾ Vegetable, 3 Proteins, 20 Optional Calories
PER SERVING: 251 Calories, 26 g Protein, 13 g Fat, 6 g Carbohydrate, 77 mg Sodium, 81 mg Cholesterol, 1 g Dietary Fiber

Lamb Roasting Timetable
General Procedures

1. Place roast (straight from refrigerator) on rack in open roasting pan.
2. Season either before or after cooking.
3. Insert meat thermometer into thickest part of roast, not touching bone.
4. Do not add water. Do not cover.
5. Roast in oven until meat thermometer registers 5° to 10°F below desired doneness. During the standing time the roast will continue to rise 5° to 10°F and reach the final meat thermometer reading. (Oven does not have to be preheated.)
6. Allow roast to stand 15 to 20 minutes before serving. Temperature will rise and roast will be easier to carve.

LAMB

Lamb Cut	Approx. Weight in Pounds	Oven Temperature	Final Meat Thermometer Reading	Approx. Cooking Time* (min./lb.)
Lamb Leg	5 to 7	325°F	140°F (rare)	20 to 25
			160°F (medium)	25 to 30
			170°F (well)	30 to 35
	7 to 9	325°F	140°F (rare)	15 to 20
			160°F (medium)	20 to 25
			170°F (well)	25 to 30
Lamb Leg, Boneless	4 to 7	325°F	140°F (rare)	25 to 30
			160°F (medium)	30 to 35
			170°F (well)	35 to 40
Lamb Leg, Shank Half	3 to 4	325°F	140°F (rare)	30 to 35
			160°F (medium)	40 to 45
			170°F (well)	45 to 50
Lamb Leg, Sirloin Half	3 to 4	325°F	140°F (rare)	25 to 30
			160°F (medium)	35 to 40
			170°F (well)	45 to 50
Lamb Shoulder, Boneless	$3\frac{1}{2}$ to 5	325°F	140°F (rare)	30 to 35
			160°F (medium)	35 to 40
			170°F (well)	40 to 45
Lamb Rib Roast	$1\frac{1}{2}$ to 2	375°F	140°F (rare)	30 to 35
			160°F (medium)	35 to 40
			170°F (well)	40 to 45
	2 to 3	375°F	140°F (rare)	25 to 30
			160°F (medium)	30 to 35
			170°F (well)	35 to 40

*Cooking times are based on meat taken directly from the refrigerator.
Chart courtesy of the National Live Stock and Meat Board.

LAMB CHOPS WITH YOGURT-MINT SAUCE

Fresh mint and cucumber give this sauce a cooling tang. If fresh mint is unavailable, don't substitute dried mint. Instead, try Lamb Chops with Tomato-Dill Salsa (page 203).

MAKES 4 SERVINGS

Four 5-ounce loin lamb chops, about 1" thick (with bone)
¾ cup plain nonfat yogurt
½ cup chopped cucumber, pared and seeded
¼ cup fresh mint
¼ cup chopped scallions
1 garlic clove, chopped
Salt, crushed red pepper and black pepper to taste
Paprika to garnish (optional)
Chopped chives to garnish (optional)

1. Preheat broiler. Remove lamb chops from refrigerator 1 hour before cooking.

2. In a blender or food processor, purée yogurt, cucumber, mint, scallions and garlic. Season to taste with salt and crushed red pepper. Let stand at room temperature.

3. Meanwhile, season lamb with salt and black pepper. Place on broiler rack and broil 3–4 inches from heat, 4–5 minutes per side for medium-rare. (Add 1–2 minutes extra per side for medium or well-done chops.) Top each chop with one-fourth of the yogurt-mint sauce (about ¼ cup); sprinkle lightly with paprika and chopped chives, if desired.

EACH SERVING PROVIDES: ¼ Milk, ½ Vegetable, 3 Proteins
PER SERVING: 214 Calories, 28 g Protein, 8 g Fat, 5 g Carbohydrate, 106 mg Sodium, 82 mg Cholesterol, 0 g Dietary Fiber

SAVORY LAMB STEW

MAKES 4 SERVINGS

1 tablespoon + 1 teaspoon olive oil
½ cup finely chopped onion
¼ cup finely chopped carrot
¼ cup finely chopped celery
2 garlic cloves, finely chopped
15 ounces boneless lamb leg, cut into 1½" cubes
4 fluid ounces (½ cup) dry white wine
1 cup drained canned chopped plum tomatoes
1 cup hot water
2 teaspoons finely chopped fresh rosemary or 1 teaspoon dried leaves
2 teaspoons finely chopped fresh sage or 1 teaspoon dried leaves
2 teaspoons finely chopped fresh thyme or 1 teaspoon dried leaves
½ teaspoon grated lemon zest
Salt and freshly ground black pepper to taste
10 ounces all-purpose potatoes, cubed
2 cups cut green beans
1 tablespoon minced fresh parsley

1. Preheat oven to 350°F. In medium ovenproof flameproof casserole, heat oil over medium heat. Add onion, carrot, celery and garlic; sauté, stirring frequently, until onion is translucent, about 8 minutes. Add lamb; sauté, stirring frequently, until no longer pink, about 3 minutes. Add wine and cook for 2 minutes; add tomatoes, ½ cup of the hot water, rosemary, sage, thyme, zest, salt and pepper. Bring to a boil and place cover partially over casserole. Bake 40 minutes, stirring occasionally.

2. Add potatoes, green beans and the remaining ½ cup hot water; cover tightly and bake until tender, about 20 minutes more. If sauce seems thin, remove lamb, keep warm; reduce sauce over medium-high heat until thickened. Return lamb to sauce and stir. To serve, sprinkle with parsley.

EACH SERVING PROVIDES: 1 Fat, 2 Vegetables, 3 Proteins, ½ Bread, 25 Optional Calories
PER SERVING: 298 Calories, 25 g Protein, 10 g Fat, 23 g Carbohydrate, 183 mg Sodium, 68 mg Cholesterol, 3 g Dietary Fiber

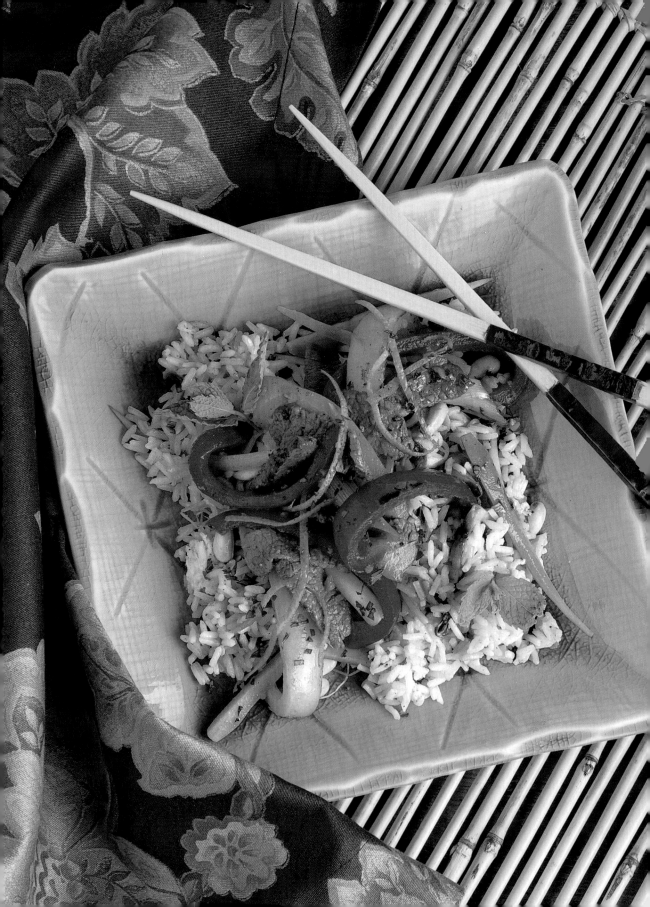

LAMB AND PEPPER STIR-FRY

MAKES 4 SERVINGS

1 tablespoon + 1 teaspoon vegetable oil
15 ounces boneless lamb (from the loin), cut into thin strips
1 tablespoon + 1½ teaspoons soy sauce
2 teaspoons honey
1 medium red bell pepper, cored, seeded and cut into ½" strips
1 medium yellow bell pepper, cored, seeded and cut into ½" strips
8 medium scallions, cut into 2" pieces
2 teaspoons finely chopped garlic
2 teaspoons finely chopped fresh ginger root
Zest from 1 orange, julienned
¼ teaspoon crushed red pepper flakes (or to taste)
2 tablespoons low-sodium chicken broth
Coarsely ground black pepper to taste
1 tablespoon chopped fresh mint to garnish (optional)

1. Heat a nonstick wok or large skillet over high heat. Add oil, then lamb, and stir-fry until lamb loses its red color, about 1–2 minutes. Remove with slotted spoon and reserve.

2. In measuring cup, combine soy sauce and honey; reserve.

3. Add bell peppers to wok; stir-fry until peppers soften slightly, about 4 minutes. Add scallions, garlic, ginger, zest, red pepper flakes and soy sauce mixture. Stir-fry 30 seconds more. Return lamb to wok. Add broth and black pepper; stir-fry another 30 seconds to reheat lamb and blend flavors. To serve, sprinkle mint over stir-fry, if desired.

EACH SERVING PROVIDES: 1 Fat, 1¼ Vegetables, 3 Proteins, 10 Optional Calories
PER SERVING: 244 Calories, 24 g Protein, 11 g Fat, 12 g Carbohydrate, 304 mg Sodium, 70 mg Cholesterol, 2 g Dietary Fiber

CURRIED LAMB AND SPINACH

MAKES 4 SERVINGS

1 tablespoon + 1 teaspoon vegetable oil
15 ounces boneless lamb (cut from the leg), cut into 1-inch cubes
½ cup finely chopped onion
1 tablespoon finely chopped garlic
1 tablespoon finely chopped fresh ginger root
½ cup drained canned chopped plum tomatoes
3 tablespoons chopped fresh cilantro
2 teaspoons turmeric
2 teaspoons ground cumin
2 teaspoons ground coriander
Pinch ground cloves
Pinch cinnamon
10 ounces thawed frozen spinach, or 2 cups fresh steamed, squeezed dry and chopped
½ cup low-sodium chicken broth mixed with ½ cup water
3 tablespoons fresh lemon juice
Salt, freshly ground black pepper and ground red pepper to taste
4 cups cooked regular long-grain rice

1. In 10" nonstick skillet, heat oil over medium-high heat. Add lamb; sauté, stirring, until browned, about 2 minutes. Add onion, garlic and ginger; sauté, stirring, 1 minute. Stir in tomatoes; cook another 2 minutes.

2. Lower heat to medium; add cilantro, tumeric, cumin, coriander, cloves and cinnamon; sauté, stirring frequently, 2 minutes. Add spinach, chicken broth, juice, salt, pepper and ground red pepper; stir. Bring to a boil. Cover and lower heat, simmering until meat is tender, about 10–20 minutes. Uncover; raise heat to high 1–2 minutes to reduce excess liquid, stirring frequently. Serve over rice.

EACH SERVING (1 cup) PROVIDES: 1 Fat, 1½ Vegetables, 3 Proteins, 2 Breads, 3 Optional Calories
PER SERVING: 491 Calories, 31 g Protein, 11 g Fat, 67 g Carbohydrate, 182 mg Sodium, 68 mg Cholesterol, 3 g Dietary Fiber

SHISH KABOB

MAKES 4 SERVINGS

$\frac{1}{2}$ cup chopped onion
2 tablespoons fresh lemon juice
1 tablespoon finely chopped garlic
1 tablespoon finely chopped fresh dill
1 tablespoon dried oregano leaves
1 tablespoon paprika
$\frac{1}{2}$ teaspoon freshly ground black pepper
15 ounces boneless lamb (from the leg), cut into
    $1\frac{1}{2}$" cubes
1 medium onion, cut into 8 wedges
1 medium red bell pepper, seeded, cored and cut
    into 8 wedges

1. To prepare marinade, in a blender or food processor, purée onion, juice, garlic, dill, oregano, paprika and pepper. Put lamb into a sealable plastic bag; add marinade. Seal bag, squeezing out air; turn bag to coat lamb. Refrigerate at least 3 hours or overnight, turning bag occasionally.

2. Remove lamb from refrigerator 1 hour before cooking. Soak four 10" bamboo skewers in water to cover for 1 hour, to avoid burning under the broiler.

3. Blanch onion wedges and bell pepper in boiling water for 2–3 minutes.

4. Preheat broiler. Alternately thread the lamb, onion and pepper onto the skewers. Place on broiler rack and broil 3–4 inches from heat 3–4 minutes per side for medium-rare. (Add 1–2 extra minutes per side for medium or well-done kabobs.)

EACH SERVING PROVIDES: 1 Vegetable, 3 Proteins
PER SERVING: 200 Calories, 25 g Protein, 7 g Fat, 8 g Carbohydrate, 61 mg Sodium, 76 mg Cholesterol, 1 g Dietary Fiber

TUSCAN-STYLE PORK ROAST

Try to slice only the amount to be served. Save the remainder unsliced. Leftovers can be refrigerated for 2 to 3 days (well wrapped). They make excellent sandwiches at room temperature. They can also be frozen. To serve, defrost and gently reheat in a microwave oven.

MAKES 8 SERVINGS

2 pounds, 4 ounces loin of pork (on the bone)
3 garlic cloves, cut into thin lengthwise slivers
1 tablespoon + 1 teaspoon olive oil
1 tablespoon finely chopped fresh rosemary
$\frac{1}{2}$ teaspoon freshly ground black pepper
$\frac{1}{2}$ teaspoon salt
4 fluid ounces ($\frac{1}{2}$ cup) dry white wine

1. Preheat oven to 350°F. Using a sharp paring knife, make small slits in the roast; insert slivers of garlic in slits. Rub roast with oil, rosemary, pepper and salt.

2. Place roast, bone-side down, in shallow roasting pan. Pour wine into pan; roast, basting occasionally with wine and pan juices, until cooked through and browned, about $1\frac{1}{2}$ hours (internal temperature 155°–160°F). Allow roast to rest 10 minutes before slicing.

EACH SERVING (3 ounces) PROVIDES: $\frac{1}{2}$ Fat, 3 Proteins, 15 Optional Calories
PER SERVING: 210 Calories, 24 g Protein, 10 g Fat, 1 g Carbohydrate, 182 mg Sodium, 69 mg Cholesterol, 0 g Dietary Fiber

HONEY-MUSTARD PORK CHOPS

If you like, you can liquefy the honey in a microwave. Place in a small, microwavable bowl and microwave on 25% power for 30 seconds.

MAKES 4 SERVINGS

1 tablespoon + 1 teaspoon honey
¼ cup Dijon mustard
1 teaspoon cider vinegar or wine vinegar
Salt and freshly ground black pepper to taste
Four 5-ounce loin pork chops, 1" thick (with bone)

1. To prepare marinade, in small saucepan heat honey over low heat until it liquefies. Add mustard, vinegar, salt and pepper; blend completely and cool to room temperature.

2. Place pork chops in a gallon-size sealable plastic bag. Pour marinade over chops. Seal bag, squeezing out air; turn bag to coat chops. Refrigerate overnight, turning bag occasionally.

3. Preheat broiler. Remove chops from refrigerator 30 minutes before broiling. Drain and discard marinade.

4. Broil on rack, close to heat source, until done, about 6–7 minutes per side.

EACH SERVING (3 ounces) PROVIDES: 3 Proteins, 20 Optional Calories
PER SERVING: 218 Calories, 24 g Protein, 9 g Fat, 8 g Carbohydrate, 505 mg Sodium, 67 mg Cholesterol, 0 g Dietary Fiber

BRAISED PORK CHOPS WITH ONION SALSA

MAKES 4 SERVINGS

1 medium red onion, peeled and sliced
1 medium tomato
Four 5-ounce loin pork chops (with bone)
Salt and freshly ground black pepper to taste
½ cup finely chopped fresh cilantro
1 tablespoon fresh lime juice
Grated zest of 1 orange
1 tablespoon orange juice
1 teaspoon finely chopped fresh ginger root
Pinch crushed red pepper flakes (or ground red pepper)
1 tablespoon + 1 teaspoon olive oil
¼ cup + 3 tablespoons apple juice or cider

1. Soak onion in cold water 30 minutes. Drain and chop finely. Chop tomato; drain in wire mesh strainer or colander 30 minutes.

2. Season chops with salt and pepper. To prepare onion salsa, in large bowl, combine onion, tomato, cilantro, lime juice, orange zest, orange juice, ginger and red pepper flakes. Reserve.

3. In a 10" nonstick skillet, heat oil over high heat. When hot, add chops and brown quickly on both sides, about 1–1½ minutes each side. Add apple juice, cover and lower heat to medium-low. Braise 15–20 minutes, until chops are tender and fully cooked, turning chops several times. Remove chops; turn up heat to reduce liquid. Pour sauce over chops; top with onion salsa.

EACH SERVING PROVIDES: 1 Fat, ¼ Fruit, ¾ Vegetable, 3 Proteins
PER SERVING: 239 Calories, 25 g Protein, 11 g Fat, 9 g Carbohydrate, 67 mg Sodium, 67 mg Cholesterol, 1 g Dietary Fiber

PORK CHOPS WITH PINEAPPLE-APPLE CHUTNEY

MAKES 4 SERVINGS

1 pound, 2 ounces pared and cored fresh
  pineapple, cut into small pieces
1 small Granny Smith apple, pared, cored and
  chopped finely
½ cup golden raisins, chopped
½ cup finely chopped red bell pepper
⅓ cup finely chopped red onion
¼ cup cider vinegar
2 tablespoons finely chopped fresh ginger root
1 tablespoon + 1 teaspoon orange marmalade
1 small jalapeño pepper, seeded and finely chopped
1 teaspoon finely chopped garlic
1 teaspoon yellow mustard seeds (optional)
¼ teaspoon cinnamon
Pinch ground cloves
Salt and freshly ground black pepper to taste
1 tablespoon + 1 teaspoon olive oil or vegetable oil
Four 5-ounce loin pork chops (with bone)

1. To prepare chutney, in a heavy medium saucepan, combine all ingredients except oil and pork chops; place over medium-low heat. Bring to simmer; if mixture is dry, add water, 1–2 tablespoons at a time, to keep mixture moist. Cook until mixture thickens and flavors blend, about 40–45 minutes. Preheat oven to 300°F.

2. In heavy 10-inch ovenproof skillet, heat oil over medium-high heat. When hot, add chops and sauté 1–1½ minutes each side, until browned. Place skillet in oven and cook another 10–15 minutes, turning occasionally. Serve with pineapple-apple chutney.

EACH SERVING PROVIDES: 1 Fat, 2 Fruits, ½ Vegetable, 3 Proteins, 15 Optional Calories
PER SERVING: 338 Calories, 26 g Protein, 13 g Fat, 31 g Carbohydrate, 63 mg Sodium, 67 mg Cholesterol, 2 g Dietary Fiber

PORK CHOPS WITH ARUGULA-TOMATO SALSA

MAKES 4 SERVINGS

1 tablespoon finely chopped fresh rosemary
1 tablespoon finely chopped fresh sage
1 tablespoon + 1 teaspoon extra virgin olive oil
½ teaspoon finely chopped fresh thyme or ¼
  teaspoon dried leaves
4 juniper berries, crushed (optional)
1 bay leaf, crumbled
Salt and freshly ground black pepper to taste
Four 5-ounce loin pork chops (with bone), about
  1" thick
2 cups arugula, thick stems removed and leaves
  torn into small pieces
1 diced seeded medium tomato
1 garlic clove, finely chopped
Fresh lemon juice to taste

1. To prepare marinade, combine rosemary, sage, 2 teaspoons of the oil, the thyme, juniper berries, if using, bay leaf, salt and pepper; rub on pork chops. Place in a gallon-size sealable plastic bag and seal, squeezing out air. Refrigerate 3 hours or overnight.

2. Bring chops to room temperature 1 hour before broiling. Preheat broiler 15–20 minutes before cooking.

3. To prepare salsa, in medium bowl, combine arugula, tomato, garlic, the remaining 2 teaspoons of oil, the juice, and additional salt and pepper.

4. Broil pork chops on rack, close to heat, 6–7 minutes per side. Top with arugula salsa.

EACH SERVING PROVIDES: ½ Fat, 1½ Vegetables, 3 Proteins, 20 Optional Calories
PER SERVING: 226 Calories, 27 g Protein, 12 g Fat, 3 g Carbohydrate, 62 mg Sodium, 70 mg Cholesterol, 1 g Dietary Fiber

Pork Chops with Arugula-Tomato Salsa

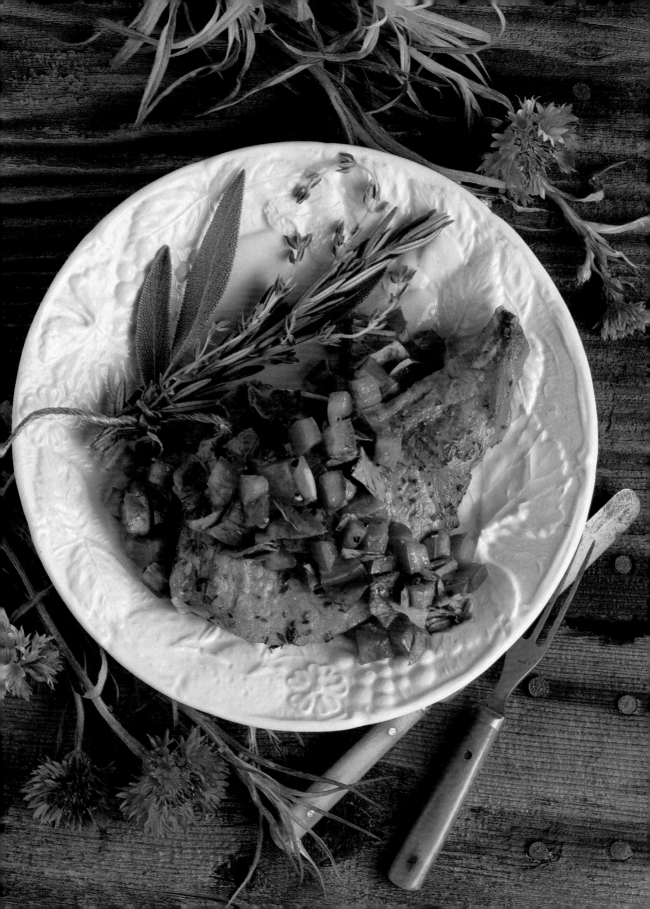

ITALIAN SAUSAGE WITH PEPPERS

You can control the heat of this hearty dish by using hot or sweet sausages, or a combination of the two.

MAKES 4 SERVINGS

2 teaspoons olive oil
1 Bermuda onion, halved lengthwise and thinly sliced into rings
1 medium red bell pepper, cored, seeded and thinly sliced
1 medium yellow bell pepper, cored, seeded and thinly sliced
1 medium green bell pepper, cored, seeded and thinly sliced
2 cups thinly sliced fresh fennel
2 garlic cloves, thinly sliced
1 cup chopped canned tomatoes with juice
Salt and freshly ground black pepper to taste
8 ounces cooked Italian pork sausages (hot, sweet or a combination)
6 ounces uncooked penne or other dried tubular pasta
$\frac{1}{4}$ cup chopped fresh basil
2 tablespoons chopped fresh flat-leafed parsley

1. In large nonstick skillet, heat oil over medium heat; add onion, bell peppers and fennel; sauté, stirring, until vegetables turn golden, about 8–10 minutes. Add garlic and stir; sauté another minute.

2. Add tomatoes, salt and pepper; stir. Lower heat and simmer, stirring occasionally, 15 minutes.

3. Add sausages to pan and stir. Cover and cook gently 20 minutes, stirring occasionally, until flavors blend. If mixture becomes too dry, add 1–2 tablespoons of water to keep mixture moist.

4. Meanwhile, in large pot of boiling water, cook the pasta; drain.

5. Add basil, parsley and pasta to sausage mixture and toss. Cook over medium-low heat for another minute and serve.

EACH SERVING PROVIDES: $\frac{1}{2}$ Fat, $3\frac{3}{4}$ Vegetables, 2 Proteins, 2 Breads
PER SERVING: 417 Calories, 19 g Protein, 18 g Fat, 44 g Carbohydrate, 683 mg Sodium, 44 mg Cholesterol, 4 g Dietary Fiber

Grilling Guide

◆

Steaks on the grill are a universal favorite, whether cooked in the great outdoors or on a handy indoor grill. All steaks take well to marinades, and you can use ours (see pages 350–352) or a favorite of your own. Just follow these guidelines for irresistible sizzle.

- *Trim excess fat before cooking to prevent flare-ups. Score edges of steaks before grilling to prevent curling. Use long-handled tongs to turn; piercing with a fork allows juices to escape.*
- *For cooking tender cuts such as club, rib-eye, T-bone, porterhouse and sirloin steaks, about $1\frac{1}{4}$" thick, sear over direct high heat on one side. Turn with tongs and continue to grill, reducing heat by raising the cooking rack.*

Time Table
Rare: 3–5 minutes first side, 8 minutes second side
Medium: 3–5 minutes first side, 10 minutes second side
Well Done: 3–5 minutes first side, 12 minutes second side

SPICY PORK STIR-FRY

MAKES 4 SERVINGS

1 tablespoon vegetable oil
15 ounces pork tenderloin, cut into thin slices $\frac{1}{8}$"
  to $\frac{1}{4}$" thick
1 medium red bell pepper, cored, seeded and cut
  into $\frac{1}{2}$" strips
8 medium scallions, cut into 2" pieces
2 cups drained canned pineapple chunks
1 medium tomato, cut into 8 wedges
1 medium jalapeño pepper, seeded and finely
  chopped
2 teaspoons finely chopped fresh ginger root
1 teaspoon finely chopped garlic
1 tablespoon + 1 teaspoon soy sauce
1 teaspoon dark sesame oil
$\frac{1}{4}$ cup chopped fresh cilantro

1. Heat nonstick wok or large skillet over high heat. Add vegetable oil, then pork slices. Stir-fry until pork is no longer pink, about 1–2 minutes. Remove with slotted spoon and reserve.

2. Add bell pepper; stir-fry 2–3 minutes, until edges blister slightly. Add scallions; stir-fry 30 seconds; add pineapple; stir-fry another 30 seconds. Add remaining ingredients except cilantro, return pork to wok and stir-fry 1–2 minutes more. Serve sprinkled with chopped cilantro.

EACH SERVING PROVIDES: 1 Fat, 1 Fruit, 1½ Vegetables, 3 Proteins
PER SERVING: 231 Calories, 24 g Protein, 9 g Fat, 15 g Carbohydrate, 403 mg Sodium, 69 mg Cholesterol, 2 g Dietary Fiber

ORANGE-GLAZED HAM AND PINEAPPLE

MAKES 4 SERVINGS

One 12-ounce ready-to-eat boneless ham steak
4 whole cloves
4 slices drained canned pineapple, quartered, with
  $\frac{1}{4}$ cup juice
$\frac{1}{2}$ cup orange juice
$\frac{1}{3}$ cup pineapple juice
2 tablespoons + 2 teaspoons orange marmalade
$\frac{1}{4}$ teaspoon cinnamon

1. Preheat oven to 400°F. Make several cuts along edge of ham; place in shallow ovenproof pan; stud with cloves. Place quartered pineapple slices around ham.

2. To make glaze, in small saucepan, combine orange juice, pineapple juice, reserved canned pineapple juice, marmalade and cinnamon. Bring to a boil over high heat; boil until slightly thickened, about 5–6 minutes. Pour glaze over ham. Bake 15 minutes, basting occasionally with glaze. Glaze should be thickened. If there is excess liquid, remove ham from pan; keep warm. Return pineapple and glaze to upper oven rack for several minutes, until glaze is thick.

3. Cut ham into 4 servings; top with pineapple and glaze.

EACH SERVING (3 ounces) PROVIDES: 1 Fruit, 3 Proteins, 30 Optional Calories
PER SERVING: 196 Calories, 17 g Protein, 4 g Fat, 23 g Carbohydrate, 1224 mg Sodium, 40 mg Cholesterol, 1 g Dietary Fiber

Ham Roasting Timetable
General Procedures

1. Place ham (straight from refrigerator) on rack in shallow roasting pan.
2. Insert a meat thermometer into thickest part of ham, not touching bone.
3. Cook ham according to specific directions shown below. If covering with aluminum foil, leave thermometer dial exposed.
4. Cook in 325°F oven until thermometer registers 135°F. (It is necessary to preheat oven for hams weighing less than 2 pounds.)
5. Remove cover and apply glaze during last 15 to 20 minutes of cooking time, if desired.
6. Allow ham to stand about 10 minutes or until thermometer registers 140°F. Ham will be easier to carve.

HAM

Fully-Cooked Smoked Cut	Approx. Weight in Pounds	Approx. Cooking Time (min./lb.)
Boneless Ham	1½ to 2	29 to 33
Cook in covered pan	3 to 4	19 to 23
with 1/2 cup water	6 to 8	16 to 20
	9 to 11	12 to 16
Bone-In Ham	6 to 8	13 to 17
Cook in covered pan	14 to 16	11 to 14
with no water		
Canned Ham	1½ to 2	23 to 25
Cook uncovered with	3	21 to 23
can juices	5	17 to 20
	8	15 to 18
	10	11 to 15

Chart courtesy of the National Live Stock and Meat Board.

HAM ROLLS WITH ASPARAGUS

These tasty ham rolls are topped with a delicious and creamy guilt-free mornay sauce.

MAKES 4 SERVINGS

24 medium asparagus spears (about 1¼ pounds), cut into 6" pieces
1 tablespoon + 1 teaspoon stick margarine
1 tablespoon + 1 teaspoon all-purpose flour
2 cups low-fat (1%) milk
Pinch salt
Freshly ground black pepper to taste
⅛ teaspoon grated nutmeg
⅛ teaspoon dried thyme leaves
1½ ounces grated Parmesan cheese
6 ounces boiled ham, cut into 8 slices
2 tablespoons finely chopped fresh flat-leaf parsley

1. Preheat oven to 350°F. In a shallow, wide non-aluminum pot, bring water to a boil. Add asparagus and cook until asparagus turns bright green, about 3–5 minutes. Remove from pot and immediately place asparagus in ice water to stop cooking; drain well when cool.

2. To prepare mornay sauce, in a heavy medium saucepan, melt margarine, whisk in flour; cook, whisking constantly, 1 minute. Gradually whisk in milk, salt, pepper, nutmeg and thyme. Bring to a boil, whisking constantly; lower heat and cook 1 minute. Remove from heat; whisk in Parmesan.

3. Lightly spray shallow baking dish, just large enough to contain asparagus, with nonstick cooking spray. Place 3 asparagus spears at the edge of each slice of ham and roll up. Place seam-side down in baking dish; whisk mornay sauce, then pour over rolls. Bake until sauce is bubbling and rolls are heated through, about 10 minutes. Sprinkle with parsley.

EACH SERVING PROVIDES: ½ Milk, 1 Fat, 1 Vegetable, 2 Proteins, 10 Optional Calories
PER SERVING: 225 Calories, 20 g Protein, 11 g Fat, 12 g Carbohydrate, 850 mg Sodium, 36 mg Cholesterol, 1 g Dietary Fiber

Storing Meat

◆

How long is it safe to store meat in your refrigerator or freezer? Use the chart below to ensure that your meat is stored properly.

Meat	Refrigerator	Freezer
Beef Cuts	3–4 days	6–12 months
Veal Cuts	1–2 days	6–9 months
Pork Cuts	2–3 days	6 months
Lamb Cuts	3–5 days	6–9 months
Ground Beef, Veal and Lamb	1–2 days	3–4 months
Ground Pork	1–2 days	1–3 months

Greek Kabobs with Turbot (page 248)

CHAPTER NINE

SEAFOOD

BARBECUED BLUEFISH WITH GRILLED VEGETABLES

Try the broiler variation for those times when you aren't able to fire up the grill. Marinate vegetables as in step one.

MAKES 4 SERVINGS

$\frac{1}{2}$ cup shredded fresh basil
$\frac{1}{4}$ cup fresh lemon juice
1 tablespoon + 1 teaspoon olive oil
1 tablespoon minced garlic
1 tablespoon honey
Salt and freshly ground black pepper to taste
2 cups unpeeled eggplant slices, $\frac{1}{8}$" thick
1 medium green bell pepper, cored, seeded and cut into 6 pieces
1 medium red bell pepper, cored, seeded and cut into 6 pieces
1 medium yellow bell pepper, cored, seeded and cut into 6 pieces
2 medium zucchini, cut into $\frac{1}{8}$" lengthwise slices
Four 5-ounce bluefish fillets

1. To prepare marinade, in gallon-size sealable plastic bag, combine basil, juice, oil, garlic, honey, salt and pepper; add eggplant, bell peppers and zucchini. Seal bag, squeezing out air; turn to coat vegetables. Refrigerate at least 2 hours.

2. Spray grill rack with nonstick cooking spray. Place grill rack 5" from coals. Prepare grill according to manufacturer's directions.

3. Drain marinade into small saucepan; bring to a boil and simmer 3 minutes. Place bluefish and vegetables on grill rack; brush with reserved marinade.

4. Grill fish and vegetables, turning once and brushing with any remaining marinade, 12–15 minutes, until fish flakes when tested with a fork and vegetables are tender-crisp.

EACH SERVING (1 bluefish fillet and $\frac{1}{4}$ of the vegetables) PROVIDES: $3\frac{1}{2}$ Vegetables, 2 Proteins, 55 Optional Calories
PER SERVING: 288 Calories, 31 g Protein, 11 g Fat, 17 g Carbohydrate, 92 mg Sodium, 84 mg Cholesterol, 2 g Dietary Fiber

BROILED BLUEFISH WITH GRILLED VEGETABLES

1. Spray broiler rack with nonstick cooking spray. Place vegetables on rack and broil 5–6 inches from heat 12–15 minutes.

2. Remove and keep warm. Place fish on broiler rack and broil 5–6 inches from heat 12–15 minutes, or until fish flakes easily when tested with fork.

◆

COD WITH PARSLEY SAUCE

MAKES 4 SERVINGS

1 cup low-fat (1%) milk
Four 5-ounce cod fillets
1 tablespoon + 1 teaspoon reduced-calorie tub margarine
3 tablespoons all-purpose flour
$\frac{1}{4}$ cup low-sodium chicken broth
2 tablespoons minced fresh parsley
$\frac{1}{2}$ teaspoon salt
$\frac{1}{4}$ teaspoon freshly ground black pepper
4 sprigs fresh parsley to garnish (optional)

1. In medium-size skillet, heat milk. Add cod fillets; cover and poach, 4–5 minutes, until fish is cooked and flakes easily when tested with a fork. Using a slotted spoon, transfer to a serving platter; keep warm. Reserve milk.

2. In medium-size saucepan, melt margarine; add flour. Cook over low heat 2 minutes, until bubbly. Remove from heat; whisk in hot milk and chicken broth; add minced parsley, salt and pepper. Return to low heat and cook, stirring constantly, 3 minutes, until sauce thickens. Pour over fish; garnish with parsley sprigs, if desired.

EACH SERVING (1 cod fillet and $\frac{1}{4}$ of the sauce) PROVIDES: $\frac{1}{4}$ Milk, $\frac{1}{2}$ Fat, 2 Proteins, $\frac{1}{4}$ Bread, 1 Optional Calorie
PER SERVING: 183 Calories, 28 g Protein, 4 g Fat, 8 g Carbohydrate, 421 mg Sodium, 63 mg Cholesterol, 0 g Dietary Fiber

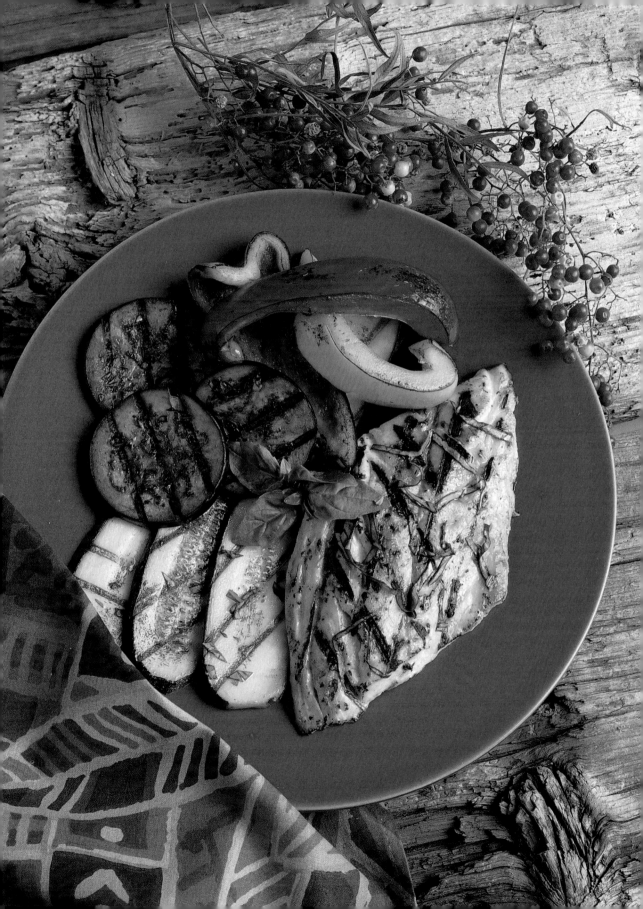

OVEN-FRIED CATFISH

MAKES 4 SERVINGS

1 pound, 4 ounces red-skinned potatoes, scrubbed
1 large egg
$\frac{1}{4}$ cup cornmeal
2 teaspoons dried parsley flakes
$\frac{1}{2}$ teaspoon salt
$\frac{1}{4}$ teaspoon freshly ground black pepper
Four 5-ounce catfish fillets
4 lemon wedges
2 cups fresh watercress, washed and large stalks
   removed

1. Preheat oven to 400°F. Spray 2 baking sheets with nonstick cooking spray.

2. Cut the potatoes into 2 × $\frac{1}{2}$" matchstick pieces; rinse under cold water and pat dry with paper towels. Spread potato sticks out on prepared baking sheet. Spray with nonstick cooking spray. Bake for 30 minutes until golden brown and crispy. Season with salt and pepper to taste.

3. Meanwhile, prepare catfish: In shallow bowl, lightly beat egg. On sheet of wax paper, combine cornmeal, parsley, salt and pepper. Dip catfish fillets in egg, then in cornmeal mixture, pressing gently to coat. Place on baking sheet; spray lightly with cooking spray.

4. Bake 10–15 minutes, until golden brown and fish flakes when tested with a fork. Serve with lemon wedges and potato sticks. Garnish with watercress.

EACH SERVING (1 fillet plus potatoes) PROVIDES: 1 Vegetable, 2$\frac{1}{4}$ Proteins, 1$\frac{1}{2}$ Breads
PER SERVING: 353 Calories, 27 g Protein, 12 g Fat, 34 g Carbohydrate, 355 mg Sodium, 100 mg Cholesterol, 3 g Dietary Fiber

NEW ENGLAND COD CASSEROLE

MAKES 4 SERVINGS

Four 5-ounce cod fillets
2 tablespoons + 2 teaspoons reduced-calorie tub
   margarine
1 tablespoon all-purpose flour
$\frac{2}{3}$ cup low-fat (1%) milk
1 cup canned cream-style corn
1 cup finely chopped scallions
$\frac{1}{2}$ teaspoon garlic salt
$\frac{1}{4}$ teaspoon dried basil leaves
$\frac{1}{4}$ teaspoon dried oregano leaves
$\frac{1}{4}$ teaspoon freshly ground black pepper
$\frac{1}{8}$ teaspoon paprika

1. Preheat oven to 400°F. Spray an 8" or 9" square shallow ovenproof dish with nonstick cooking spray. Arrange cod fillets on bottom. Bake 20–25 minutes, until fish is cooked and flakes easily when tested with a fork.

2. In medium-size saucepan, over medium heat, whisk margarine and flour; gradually whisk in milk, whisking until thickened. Stir in corn, scallions, garlic salt, basil, oregano, pepper and paprika. Bring to a boil. Remove from heat; cover and keep warm.

3. Remove fish to serving platter. Spoon warm sauce over fish.

EACH SERVING (1 cod fillet and $\frac{1}{4}$ of the sauce) PROVIDES: 1 Fat, $\frac{1}{2}$ Vegetable, 2 Proteins, $\frac{1}{2}$ Bread, 25 Optional Calories
PER SERVING: 231 Calories, 28 g Protein, 6 g Fat, 17 g Carbohydrate, 536 mg Sodium, 63 mg Cholesterol, 1 g Dietary Fiber

Oven-Fried Catfish

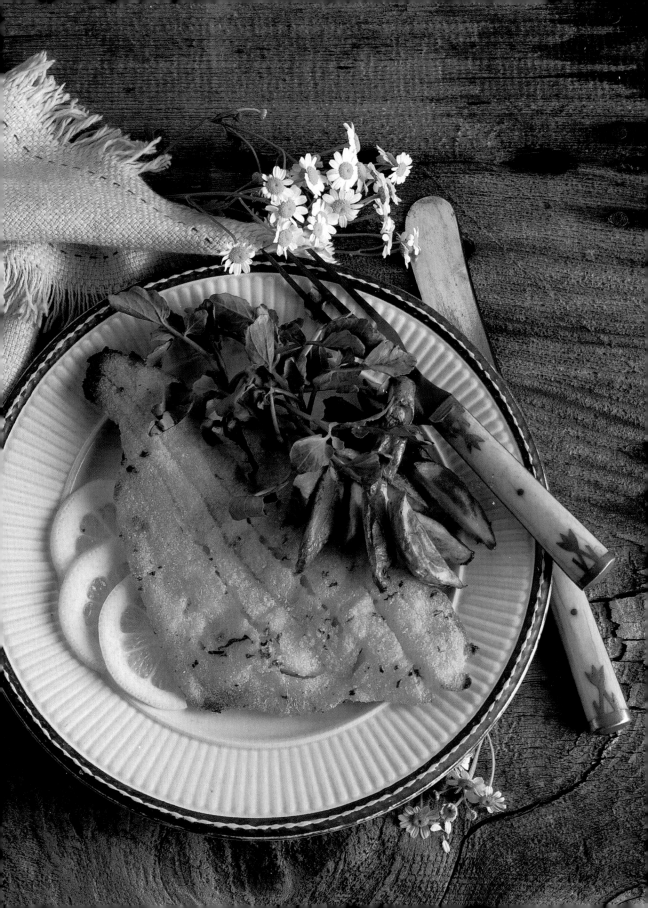

COD WITH SPAGHETTI

MAKES 4 SERVINGS

6 ounces uncooked spaghetti
1 tablespoon + 1 teaspoon olive oil
2 tablespoons minced garlic
1 pound, 4 ounces cod fillet, sliced into $\frac{1}{2}$" strips
2 cups chopped seeded tomatoes
1 cup shredded fresh basil
$\frac{1}{2}$ cup tomato purée
1 teaspoon salt
$\frac{1}{2}$ teaspoon freshly ground black pepper

1. In large pot of boiling water, cook spaghetti 8–10 minutes, until tender. Drain and place in serving bowl; keep warm.

2. In large skillet, heat oil. Add garlic, then cod. Cook 2–3 minutes, until fish is cooked and flakes when tested with a fork. Stir in tomatoes, basil, tomato purée, salt and pepper. Continue to cook just until heated through.

3. Pour into serving bowl with spaghetti. Toss to combine thoroughly.

EACH SERVING PROVIDES: 1 Fat, 1½ Vegetables, 2 Proteins, 2 Breads
PER SERVING: 365 Calories, 33 g Protein, 7 g Fat, 44 g Carbohydrate, 765 mg Sodium, 61 mg Cholesterol, 3 g Dietary Fiber

MEXICAN SALAD IN A TORTILLA

This pretty salad is served in a fresh twist in the tortilla—individual cups that are also crunchy treats.

MAKES 4 SERVINGS

Four 6" flour tortillas
12 ounces cooked codfish
2 cups chopped seeded peeled tomatoes
$\frac{1}{2}$ cup diced red onion
$\frac{1}{2}$ cup green bell pepper, cored, seeded and sliced
$\frac{1}{2}$ cup yellow bell pepper, cored, seeded and sliced
$\frac{1}{2}$ cup finely chopped cilantro
$\frac{1}{2}$ cup finely chopped scallions
2 tablespoons finely chopped jalapeño pepper
2 cups iceberg lettuce, shredded
$\frac{1}{4}$ cup fresh lime juice
2 tablespoons olive oil
$\frac{1}{4}$ teaspoon salt
4 lime wedges to garnish (optional)
4 sprigs fresh cilantro to garnish (optional)

1. Preheat oven to 350°F. Spray tortillas with nonstick cooking spray on both sides and place over upside-down ovenproof 6" baking dishes. To help hold shape, spray foil with nonstick cooking spray. Place foil, sprayed side down, on top of each baking dish and mold to cup. Place on baking sheet. Bake 5 minutes, until crisp. Remove from oven; cool.

2. In large bowl, combine codfish, tomatoes, red onion, bell peppers, cilantro, scallions and jalapeño pepper.

3. Place tortilla cups, flat-side down, on serving platter. Fill each with $\frac{1}{2}$ cup shredded lettuce and one-fourth of cod mixture.

4. In small bowl, whisk lime juice, oil and salt; drizzle over salads. Garnish with fresh lime and cilantro.

EACH SERVING (2 cups salad and 1 tortilla) PROVIDES: 1½ Fats, 3 Vegetables, 1½ Proteins, 1 Bread
PER SERVING: 267 Calories, 23 g Protein, 10 g Fat, 23 g Carbohydrate, 313 mg Sodium, 47 mg Cholesterol, 3 g Dietary Fiber

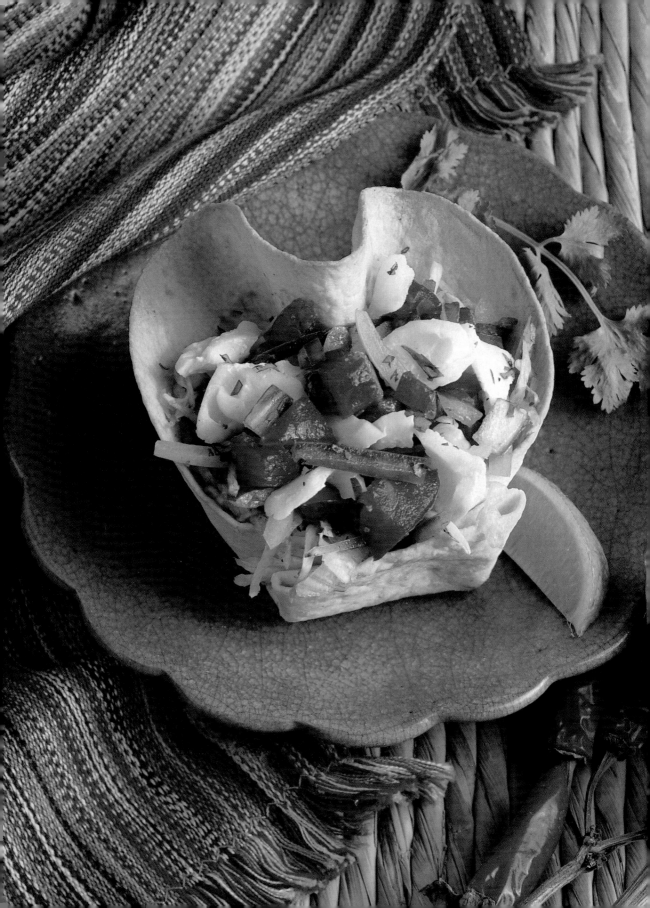

OVEN-FRIED FLOUNDER WITH TARTAR SAUCE

Enjoy guilt-free tartar sauce with our lightened version of the classic. Here, its creamy texture adds extra flavor to the lemon-spiced flounder.

MAKES 4 SERVINGS

$^3/_4$ cup nonfat plain yogurt
2 tablespoons minced dill pickle
2 tablespoons minced scallions
2 tablespoons minced parsley
1 tablespoon + 1 teaspoon reduced-calorie mayonnaise
1 tablespoon lemon juice
2 teaspoons pickle relish
2 teaspoons minced drained capers
1 teaspoon low-sodium Worcestershire sauce
$^1/_4$ teaspoon freshly ground black pepper
$^1/_8$ teaspoon ground red pepper
$^3/_4$ cup seasoned dried bread crumbs
2 ounces finely chopped mixed nuts, toasted
1 tablespoon dried thyme leaves
$1^1/_2$ teaspoons finely grated lemon zest
$^1/_2$ cup skim buttermilk
Four 5-ounce skinned and boned flounder fillets
4 lemon wedges to garnish (optional)

1. To prepare tartar sauce, in small bowl, mix together yogurt, pickle, scallions, parsley, mayonnaise, juice, pickle relish, capers, Worcestershire sauce, black pepper and ground red pepper. Cover with plastic wrap and refrigerate at least 1 hour.

2. Preheat oven to 400°F. Spray baking sheet with nonstick cooking spray.

3. On large plate, mix together bread crumbs, nuts, thyme and lemon zest; spread out on plate. Pour buttermilk into shallow bowl. Dip each fillet in buttermilk, then in bread crumb mixture, pressing gently to coat.

4. Place fillets on prepared baking sheet and spray with nonstick cooking spray. Bake for 10 minutes or until fish is cooked through and fish flakes when tested with a fork. Garnish with lemon wedges and serve with tartar sauce.

EACH SERVING (1 fillet and $^1/_3$ cup tartar sauce) PROVIDES: $^1/_4$ Milk, $1^1/_2$ Fats, $2^1/_2$ Proteins, 1 Bread, 15 Optional Calories
PER SERVING: 230 Calories, 9 g Protein, 10 g Fat, 27 g Carbohydrate, 853 mg Sodium, 4 mg Cholesterol, 0 g Dietary Fiber

◆

POACHED HALIBUT IN MUSHROOM BROTH

If wild mushrooms aren't available, substitute 1 cup of white button mushrooms, for a total of 2 cups.

MAKES 4 SERVINGS

3 ounces orzo
2 cups low-sodium chicken broth
1 cup mixed wild mushrooms (porcini, shiitake, cremini or oyster), sliced
1 cup white button mushrooms, sliced
4 fluid ounces ($^1/_2$ cup) dry white wine
2 tablespoons reduced-sodium soy sauce
$^1/_4$ teaspoon freshly ground black pepper
One 15-ounce skinned and boned halibut steak
2 tablespoons chopped chives to garnish (optional)

1. In large saucepan of boiling water, cook the orzo 8–10 minutes, until tender. Drain; keep hot.

2. In large skillet, place broth, wild mushrooms, white mushrooms, wine, soy sauce and pepper; bring to a boil. Reduce heat; simmer 5 minutes.

3. Stir in orzo; place halibut steak on top. Simmer, covered, 6–8 minutes, until fish is cooked through and flakes easily when tested with a fork.

4. Using slotted spatula, transfer halibut steak to cutting board; cut into 4 equal pieces. Transfer orzo-mushroom mixture to serving platter. Arrange halibut on top; garnish with chives, if desired.

EACH SERVING (1 piece of halibut and $^1/_4$ of the orzo mixture) PROVIDES: 1 Vegetable, $1^1/_2$ Proteins, 1 Bread, 35 Optional Calories
PER SERVING: 243 Calories, 27 g Protein, 4 g Fat, 19 g Carbohydrate, 283 mg Sodium, 34 mg Cholesterol, 1 g Dietary Fiber

MACKEREL POACHED WITH APPLES

Apples and mint add a sweet, satisfying flavor to the mackerel. Salmon can be successfully substituted for the mackerel.

MAKES 4 SERVINGS

1 vegetable bouillon cube
$\frac{1}{2}$ cup apple juice
3 small unpared McIntosh apples
1 cup finely chopped onions
$\frac{1}{2}$ cup chopped fresh mint
1 teaspoon salt
$\frac{1}{2}$ teaspoon freshly ground black pepper
Four 3-ounce mackerel fillets
8 lemon slices
4 sprigs fresh mint to garnish (optional)

1. To prepare poaching liquid, in large skillet, bring $1\frac{1}{2}$ cups water to a boil. Add bouillon cube, stirring until dissolved. Stir in apple juice; reduce heat to simmer.

2. Core one of the apples; slice crosswise into 8 slices. Add to simmering liquid and poach, just until tender, 2–3 minutes. Using slotted spoon, transfer apple slices to plate and keep warm.

3. Pare and chop the remaining 2 apples; add to simmering liquid. Stir in onions; simmer, covered, 5 minutes, until tender.

4. Stir in chopped mint, salt and pepper; place mackerel fillets in poaching liquid. Arrange lemon slices and reserved poached apple slices over the top of fillets. Continue poaching, covered, 5–8 minutes longer, until fish is cooked through and flakes when tested with a fork. Garnish with mint sprigs, if desired.

EACH SERVING (1 fillet and $\frac{1}{4}$ of the apple) PROVIDES: 1 Fruit, $\frac{1}{2}$ Vegetable, 2 Proteins, 3 Optional Calories
PER SERVING: 259 Calories, 17 g Protein, 12 g Fat, 22 g Carbohydrate, 860 mg Sodium, 60 mg Cholesterol, 2 g Dietary Fiber

CARIBBEAN MAHI MAHI

If mahi mahi is unavailable, try substituting orange roughy or flounder in this island-inspired dish.

MAKES 4 SERVINGS

1 medium banana, peeled and sliced $\frac{1}{2}$" thick
1 pound, 4 ounces mahi mahi fillets, cut into 2" pieces
$\frac{1}{2}$ cup mango slices
1 cup low-sodium chicken broth
$\frac{2}{3}$ cup pineapple juice
2 fluid ounces ($\frac{1}{4}$ cup) coconut milk
1 teaspoon salt
$\frac{1}{2}$ teaspoon freshly ground black pepper
4 cups cooked regular long-grain rice
1 cup fresh watercress to garnish (optional)

1. Spray large nonstick skillet with nonstick cooking spray. Cook banana 2–3 minutes, until golden brown on both sides. Add mahi mahi to skillet; cook 3–4 minutes, just until fish flakes easily when tested with a fork.

2. Stir in mango, broth, pineapple juice, coconut milk, salt and pepper; heat through.

3. Line a serving platter with the rice. Place $\frac{1}{2}$ cup watercress at each end if desired and spoon fish mixture in center.

EACH SERVING (2 cups) PROVIDES: $1\frac{1}{4}$ Fruits, $\frac{1}{2}$ Vegetable, 2 Proteins, 2 Breads, 45 Optional Calories
PER SERVING: 482 Calories, 33 g Protein, 5 g Fat, 73 g Carbohydrate, 695 mg Sodium, 104 mg Cholesterol, 1 g Dietary Fiber

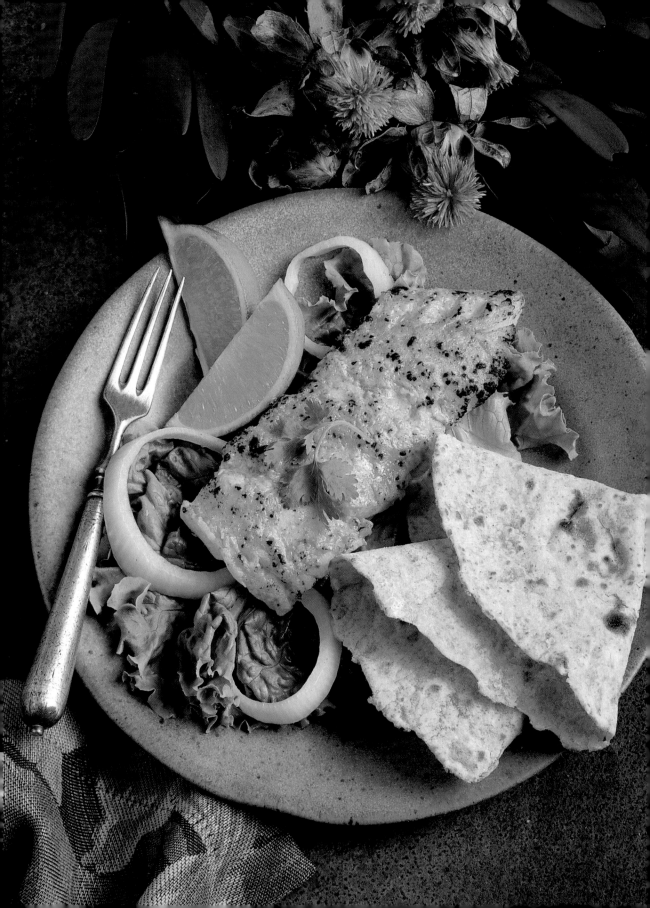

TANDOORI HADDOCK

MAKES 4 SERVINGS

This is very nice served with Pita (page 68).

1½ cups nonfat plain yogurt
½ cup chopped onion
2 tablespoons garam masala or curry powder
2 tablespoons fresh lemon juice
1 tablespoon minced seeded green chili pepper
1 tablespoon finely chopped fresh ginger root
1 large garlic clove
1 teaspoon salt
1 teaspoon turmeric
Four 4-ounce haddock fillets
2 cups shredded iceberg or other lettuce
½ cup onion slices, separated into rings
4 lime wedges to garnish (optional)
Fresh cilantro to garnish (optional)

1. To prepare marinade, in blender or food processor, combine yogurt, onion, garam masala, juice, chili pepper, ginger, garlic, salt and turmeric; purée until smooth. Pour into a gallon-size sealable plastic bag; add haddock fillets. Seal bag, squeezing out air; turn to coat fillets. Refrigerate 6–8 hours, turning bag occasionally.

2. Preheat broiler. Drain marinade into a small bowl. Place fillets in a shallow ovenproof dish. Spoon ¼ of the marinade over each fillet. Broil 4–6 minutes, until fillets are cooked and fish flakes easily when tested with a fork.

3. Line serving platter with shredded lettuce and onion rings; arrange fillets on top. Garnish with lime wedges and fresh cilantro, if desired.

EACH SERVING PROVIDES: ½ Milk, 1½ Vegetables, 1½ Proteins
PER SERVING: 209 Calories, 33 g Protein, 2 g Fat, 15 g Carbohydrate, 717 mg Sodium, 82 mg Cholesterol, 2 g Dietary Fiber

THAI MONKFISH WITH COCONUT SAUCE

MAKES 4 SERVINGS

One 15-ounce monkfish fillet, cut into 12 slices
1 tablespoon + 1 teaspoon chunky peanut butter
¼ cup low-fat (1%) milk stirred with ½ teaspoon coconut extract
1 tablespoon grated fresh ginger root
2 teaspoons minced seeded chili pepper
2 tablespoons chopped fresh cilantro
2 tablespoons fresh lime juice
1 teaspoon minced garlic
¾ teaspoon salt
¼ teaspoon freshly ground black pepper
4 lime slices
4 fresh cilantro sprigs to garnish (optional)
2 cups cooked regular long-grain white or basmati rice

1. Spray grill rack with nonstick cooking spray. Place grill rack 5" from coals. Prepare grill according to manufacturer's instructions.

2. Cut four 24" squares of double-thickness heavy-duty foil. Lay out on flat surface.

3. Arrange 3 slices monkfish in center of each foil square; dot each with 1 teaspoon of the peanut butter. Sprinkle evenly with milk mixture, ginger, chili pepper, cilantro, juice, garlic, salt and pepper; top each with a lime slice.

4. Fold bottom right-hand corner of foil over to meet top left-hand corner, forming a large triangular packet. Close the packet tightly by making overlapping folds along the two opened sides.

5. Place foil packets on grill; cook 30 minutes. Carefully transfer packets to serving plates; cut open in center, avoiding the steam. Garnish with cilantro sprigs, if desired. Serve each with ½ cup rice.

EACH SERVING (1 fillet and ½ cup rice) PROVIDES: 1 Fat, 1½ Proteins, 1 Bread, 5 Optional Calories
PER SERVING: 259 Calories, 20 g Protein, 5 g Fat, 32 g Carbohydrate, 467 mg Sodium, 27 mg Cholesterol, 1 g Dietary Fiber

SALMON EN PAPILLOTE

MAKES 4 SERVINGS

2 cups julienned carrots
2 cups julienned celery
2 cups julienned leeks
1½ tablespoons julienned pared fresh ginger root
Four 3-ounce salmon fillets
1 vegetable bouillon cube
½ cup boiling water
2 fluid ounces (¼ cup) dry white wine
½ teaspoon salt
½ teaspoon freshly ground black pepper
1 tablespoon + 1 teaspoon reduced-calorie tub
   margarine
4 sprigs fresh dill to garnish (optional)
4 fresh lemon slices to garnish (optional)

1. Preheat oven to 425°F. Spray 2 baking sheets with nonstick cooking spray. In medium saucepan, bring 1 inch of water to a boil; add carrots, celery, leeks and ginger. Reduce heat; cover and steam 1–2 minutes, until slightly wilted, but still crunchy.

2. Cut out four 12" squares of baking parchment paper; fold each 2 times into a 6" square. Unfold and lay out flat on a clean surface.

3. Place one-eighth of the vegetables in the top left-hand square of each paper.

4. Top each vegetable mound with a salmon fillet, then one-fourth more of the remaining vegetable mixture.

5. In small heatproof bowl, dissolve the vegetable bouillon cube in the ½ cup boiling water; spoon 2 tablespoons liquid over each of the fish-vegetable stacks. Sprinkle each with 1 tablespoon wine and season with salt and pepper. Place 1 teaspoon margarine on top of the vegetables.

6. Fold the bottom right-hand corner of each paper over to meet the top left-hand corner, forming 4 triangular packets. Close each packet tightly, overlapping folds along the 2 opened sides, making semicircular packets.

7. Place on baking sheets and bake for 5 minutes. Place each parcel on a serving plate. Standing back to avoid the steam, cut each packet open slightly in the center. Garnish each serving with 1 dill sprig and 1 lemon slice, if desired.

EACH SERVING (1 fillet and ¾ cup vegetables) PROVIDES: ½ Fat, 3 Vegetables, 2 Proteins, 15 Optional Calories
PER SERVING: 220 Calories, 19 g Protein, 8 g Fat, 16 g Carbohydrate, 660 mg Sodium, 47 mg Cholesterol, 3 g Dietary Fiber

On the Grill

Fast, easy and delicious, fish and shellfish are ideal choices for grilling. Here are a few pointers for perfect results.

- *Seafood cooks best over moderately hot fire; if you're grilling a whole fish, bank coals on either side of grill and place fish in the center.*
- *Fish steaks, fillets, kabobs and shellfish should be cooked over direct heat. For fragile fish, use a hinged basket or a mesh rack, or place fish on a sheet of perforated aluminum foil. Grills, baskets or foil should be sprayed with nonstick spray.*
- *Whole fish steaks should be turned halfway through cooking time; fillets under one inch do not need to be turned.*
- *To estimate time, measure the fish at its thickest part and allow 10 minutes per inch. A whole fish may take up to 12 minutes per inch. Never overcook! Fish is done when it turns opaque and just starts to flake when tested with a fork. Shrimp, crab, lobster and scallops also turn opaque; shellfish such as oysters, clams, and mussels open when cooked.*
- *Thin fillets are tricky on the grill. For best results, fold ends under for an even thickness and use a basket or perforated foil for cooking.*
- *Add extra flavor by tossing a handful of soaked fruitwoods, mesquite or whole sprigs of thyme, rosemary, dill, basil or oregano on the fire just before serving the fish.*

MONKFISH CASSOULET

MAKES 4 SERVINGS

$4\frac{1}{2}$ ounces dry white beans, soaked overnight
1 tablespoon + 1 teaspoon olive oil
1 cup sliced carrots ($\frac{1}{4}$" slices)
1 cup sliced leeks ($\frac{1}{2}$" slices)
1 cup sliced onions
4 ounces cooked Canadian bacon, diced
1 tablespoon minced garlic
One 8-ounce monkfish fillet, cut into cubes
1 cup chopped seeded peeled tomatoes
1 teaspoon salt
$\frac{1}{2}$ teaspoon freshly ground black pepper
2 bay leaves
4 fluid ounces ($\frac{1}{2}$ cup) dry white wine

1. In large saucepan of boiling water cook beans 1–$1\frac{1}{2}$ hours, until tender. Drain, rinse well and reserve.

2. Preheat oven to 350°F. In medium-size skillet, heat oil; add carrots, leeks, onions, bacon and garlic. Cook 5 minutes, until tender.

3. Place mixture in large ovenproof casserole; add monkfish, beans, tomatoes, salt, pepper and bay leaves. Pour white wine over mixture. Cover and bake 1 hour. To serve, remove bay leaves.

EACH SERVING (2 cups) PROVIDES: 1 Fat, 2 Vegetables, $1\frac{3}{4}$ Proteins, $1\frac{1}{2}$ Breads, 25 Optional Calories
PER SERVING: 312 Calories, 23 g Protein, 8 g Fat, 33 g Carbohydrate, 987 mg Sodium, 28 mg Cholesterol, 2 g Dietary Fiber

SALMON SALAD WITH HORSERADISH AND CHIVES

MAKES 4 SERVINGS

Four 3-ounce skinned and boned salmon fillets
$1\frac{1}{4}$ pounds small unpared white potatoes
1 cup diced yellow bell pepper
1 medium dill pickle, halved lengthwise, sliced
$\frac{1}{4}$ cup chopped fresh chives
$\frac{3}{4}$ cup nonfat plain yogurt
3 tablespoons grated drained fresh horseradish
2 tablespoons + 2 teaspoons reduced-calorie mayonnaise
$\frac{1}{2}$ teaspoon salt
$\frac{1}{4}$ teaspoon freshly ground black pepper
2 cups arugula or lettuce, washed

1. In large skillet, place salmon fillets in $\frac{1}{2}$ cup cold water. Bring to boil; reduce heat. Cover and poach 3–4 minutes, just until cooked and fish flakes easily when tested with a fork. Using slotted spoon, transfer to plate and cool completely.

2. In large saucepan of salted boiling water, cook potatoes until tender. Drain and cool completely.

3. Flake the salmon, coarsely chop potatoes and toss together in large bowl with bell pepper, dill pickle and chives.

4. In small bowl, mix together yogurt, horseradish, mayonnaise, salt and pepper. Pour over salmon mixture; toss to coat.

5. To serve, line large shallow bowl or platter with arugula; mound salad in the center.

EACH SERVING ($1\frac{1}{2}$ cups) PROVIDES: $\frac{1}{4}$ Milk, 1 Fat, 2 Vegetables, 2 Proteins, 1 Bread
PER SERVING: 315 Calories, 24 g Protein, 8 g Fat, 36 g Carbohydrate, 664 mg Sodium, 51 mg Cholesterol, 3 g Dietary Fiber

POACHED SALMON WITH DILL

For a simpler but equally delicious variation on this recipe (as shown), omit the rice and avocado. Subtract 1 Fat and ½ Bread from Selection Information.

MAKES 4 SERVINGS

2 cups low-sodium chicken broth
4 fluid ounces (½ cup) dry white wine
½ medium cucumber, pared, seeded and cut into
   1" strips
1 teaspoon grated lemon zest
1 cup cooked wild or long-grain rice
4 ounces diced pared avocado
2 tablespoons chopped fresh dill
¼ teaspoon freshly ground black pepper
Four 3-ounce skinned and boned salmon fillets

   1. In large skillet, bring chicken broth and wine to boil. Add cucumber and lemon zest; reduce heat and simmer 2 minutes, just until cucumber is tender.

   2. Stir in wild rice, avocado, dill and pepper.

   3. Place salmon fillets in the liquid in skillet. Cover and poach, 4–6 minutes, just until cooked and fish flakes when tested with a fork.

EACH SERVING (1 fillet and ¼ of the rice mixture) PROVIDES: 1 Fat, ¼ Vegetable, 2 Proteins, ½ Bread, 35 Optional Calories
PER SERVING: 247 Calories, 20 g Protein, 11 g Fat, 13 g Carbohydrate, 72 mg Sodium, 47 mg Cholesterol, 1 g Dietary Fiber

POACHED SALMON WITH GREEN SAUCE

MAKES 4 SERVINGS

½ vegetable bouillon cube
Four 3-ounce salmon fillets
4 fluid ounces (½ cup) dry white wine
1 cup torn spinach leaves
1 cup sorrel or spinach
1 cup watercress
¼ cup chopped chives
1 teaspoon salt
⅛ teaspoon freshly ground black pepper
½ cup nonfat sour cream

   1. In large skillet, bring ½ cup water to boil. Add bouillon cube; stir to dissolve. Add salmon fillets and poach 3–4 minutes, until fish is cooked and flakes when tested with a fork. Using a slotted spatula, transfer to serving platter; keep warm.

   2. Stir white wine into skillet; add spinach, sorrel, watercress and chives. Simmer 2 minutes, just until wilted. Place in blender or food processor; purée until smooth. Return to skillet; season with salt and pepper. Stir in sour cream; reheat over low heat, 1 minute, just until hot. Pour over fish.

EACH SERVING (1 fillet and ¼ of the sauce) PROVIDES: 1½ Vegetables, 2 Proteins, 45 Optional Calories
PER SERVING: 168 Calories, 20 g Protein, 5 g Fat, 3 g Carbohydrate, 739 mg Sodium, 47 mg Cholesterol, 1 g Dietary Fiber

Poached Salmon with Dill

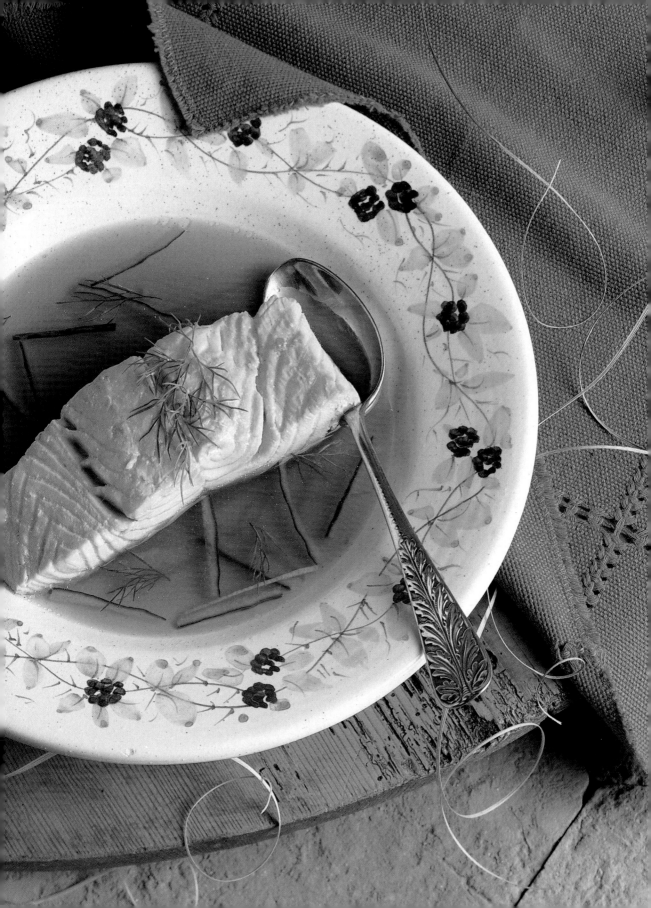

GRILLED SALMON WITH HERBS

If salmon is unavailable, you can substitute mackerel in this easy grilled fish recipe.

MAKES 4 SERVINGS

One 10-ounce salmon fillet
2 teaspoons reduced-calorie tub margarine
1 tablespoon fresh lemon juice
2 tablespoons minced fresh parsley
$\frac{1}{2}$ teaspoon garlic salt
$\frac{1}{2}$ teaspoon paprika
$\frac{1}{2}$ teaspoon freshly ground black pepper
3 or 4 sprigs fresh rosemary
3 or 4 sprigs fresh thyme

1. Spray grill rack with nonstick cooking spray. Place grill rack 5" from coals. Prepare the grill, according to manufacturer's directions.

2. Place salmon fillet on double sheet of heavy-duty foil, leaving a 6" border. Fold up edges to make foil pan.

3. Spread both sides of fillet with margarine; sprinkle with lemon juice. In small cup, mix pars-ley, garlic salt, paprika and pepper; sprinkle on both sides of fillet.

4. Drop rosemary and thyme sprigs directly on coals. Place foil pan containing fillet on grill rack. Cover grill, opening top and bottom flues slightly.

5. Grill fillet, covered, 15–20 minutes, until cooked through and fish flakes easily when tested with a fork. To serve, cut fillet into 4 equal pieces.

EACH SERVING (2 ounces fillet) PROVIDES: $\frac{1}{4}$ Fat, 2 Proteins
PER SERVING: 119 Calories, 14 g Protein, 6 g Fat, 2 g Carbohydrate, 231 mg Sodium, 39 mg Cholesterol, 0 g Dietary Fiber

BROILED SALMON WITH HERBS

1. Preheat broiler. Spread both sides of fillet with margarine; sprinkle with lemon juice. In small cup mix parsley, garlic, paprika, pepper, rosemary and thyme. Sprinkle on both sides of fillet. Place fillets on rack in broiler pan.

2. Broil fillet about 5 minutes or until fish flakes easily when tested with a fork. To serve, cut fillet into 4 equal pieces.

EACH SERVING PROVIDES: 2 Proteins, 10 Optional Calories
PER SERVING: 119 Calories, 14 g Protein, 6 g Fat, 26 g Carbohydrate, 231 mg Sodium, 39 mg Cholesterol, 0 g Dietary Fiber

---

Storing Seafood

◆

Here's a handy guide for storing fresh or frozen seafood.

Fish	*Refrigerator*	*Freezer*
Fillets or Steaks:		
Cod, Flounder, Haddock, Halibut	*3 days*	*6–8 months*
Pollock, Ocean Perch, Sea Trout, Rockfish	*3 days*	*4 months*
Mullet, Salmon	*3 days*	*Don't freeze*
Shellfish		
Crab	*5 days*	*6 months*
Surimi Seafoods	*2 weeks*	*9 months*
Shrimp	*4 days*	*5 months*
Oysters, shucked	*4–7 days*	*Don't freeze*
Clams, shucked	*5 days*	*Don't freeze*

SALMON WITH FENNEL AND TARRAGON

MAKES 4 SERVINGS

1 tablespoon + 1 teaspoon stick margarine
2 cups finely sliced fennel
1½ cups finely sliced leeks, with tops
½ cup finely chopped shallots
Four 3-ounce salmon fillets
1¼ cups low-sodium chicken broth
2 tablespoons dry white wine
½ teaspoon Dijon mustard
¼ teaspoon salt
Pinch freshly ground black pepper
2 tablespoons half-and-half
4 sprigs fennel tops to garnish (optional)

1. In large nonstick skillet, melt margarine. Add fennel, leeks and shallots; stir-fry, 2–3 minutes, just until golden brown. With slotted spoon, transfer to serving plater and keep warm. Add salmon fillets and cook 2 minutes on each side. Arrange salmon over fennel mixture; keep warm. Set aside; keep warm.

2. In same skillet, add broth, wine, mustard, salt and pepper. Bring to a boil; stir in half-and-half. Boil for 1 minute. Pour sauce over fillets and vegetables. Garnish with fennel tops, if desired.

EACH SERVING (2 cups) PROVIDES: 1 Fat, 2 Vegetables, 2 Proteins, 25 Optional Calories
PER SERVING: 227 Calories, 20 g Protein, 11 g Fat, 11 g Carbohydrate, 320 mg Sodium, 50 mg Cholesterol, 1 g Dietary Fiber

FETTUCCINE WITH SMOKED SALMON

If you like, you can use ½ cup chicken broth instead of the wine to reduce the Optional Calories to 35.

MAKES 4 SERVINGS

6 ounces uncooked fettuccine
1 cup clam-tomato juice
4 fluid ounces (½ cup) dry white wine
1 cup finely chopped red onion
2 cups chopped seeded peeled tomatoes
¼ cup light cream cheese
2 teaspoons pink or mixed peppercorns, bruised
¼ teaspoon salt
8 ounces smoked salmon, flaked
2 tablespoons chopped dill to garnish (optional)

1. In large pot of boiling water, cook fettuccine 8–10 minutes, until tender. Drain and place in serving bowl; keep warm.

2. In small saucepan, bring clam-tomato juice and wine to boil. Add onion; simmer, 3 minutes, until soft. Stir in tomatoes, cream cheese, peppercorns and salt; cook, stirring constantly, 2 minutes, until well blended.

3. Sprinkle salmon over fettuccine; add sauce and toss well. Garnish with dill, if desired.

EACH SERVING (2 cups) PROVIDES: 2 Vegetables, 2 Proteins, 2 Breads, 55 Optional Calories
PER SERVING: 348 Calories, 20 g Protein, 7 g Fat, 48 g Carbohydrate, 954 mg Sodium, 61 mg Cholesterol, 3 g Dietary Fiber

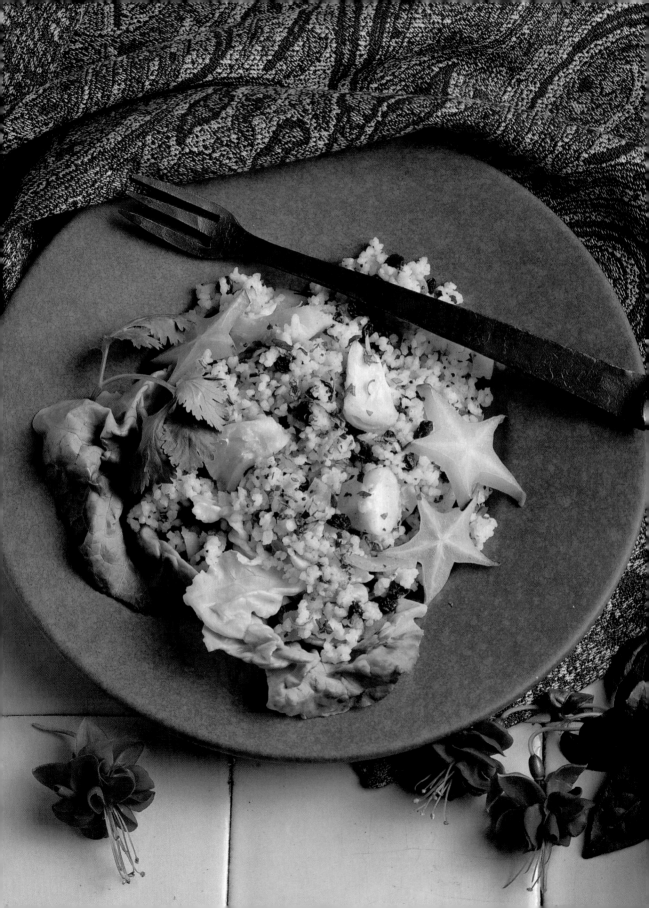

SPICED MONKFISH WITH COUSCOUS

MAKES 4 SERVINGS

6 ounces couscous
2 tablespoons olive oil
1 cup chopped red onion
1 tablespoon poppy seeds
2 teaspoons ground coriander
1 teaspoon ground cumin
$\frac{1}{2}$ cup chopped fresh mint
$\frac{1}{4}$ cup red wine vinegar
2 tablespoons fresh lemon juice
8 ounces cooked monkfish fillet, cut into bite-size pieces
$\frac{3}{4}$ cup fresh currants or 2 tablespoons dried
1 medium star fruit (carambola), sliced
4 fresh or dried dates, seeded and chopped
1 teaspoon salt
$\frac{1}{2}$ teaspoon freshly ground black pepper
2 cups shredded iceberg lettuce
2 sprigs fresh coriander leaves to garnish (optional)

1. Cook couscous according to package instructions; cool.

2. To prepare poppy-seed dressing, in small saucepan, heat oil; add onion, poppy seeds, ground coriander and cumin. Cook 1–2 minutes, until onion begins to soften. Cool slightly; stir in mint, vinegar and juice.

3. In large bowl, combine monkfish, couscous, currants, star fruit, dates, salt and pepper. Toss with poppy-seed dressing.

4. To serve, line a serving platter with shredded lettuce; mound salad in the center. Garnish with fresh coriander, if desired.

EACH SERVING (3 cups) PROVIDES: 1$\frac{1}{2}$ Fats, 1 Fruit, 1$\frac{1}{2}$ Vegetables, 1 Protein, 1$\frac{1}{2}$ Breads, 10 Optional Calories
PER SERVING: 379 Calories, 20 g Protein, 10 g Fat, 54 g Carbohydrate, 580 mg Sodium, 21 mg Cholesterol, 2 g Dietary Fiber

SEA BASS WITH POTATOES

MAKES 4 SERVINGS

$\frac{1}{2}$ cup low-sodium chicken broth
Four 5-ounce sea bass fillets
2 cups sliced mushrooms
3 tablespoons potato starch
1$\frac{1}{4}$ cups low-fat (1%) milk
4 fluid ounces ($\frac{1}{2}$ cup) dry white wine
1 tablespoon + 1 teaspoon reduced-calorie tub margarine
1 teaspoon salt
$\frac{1}{2}$ teaspoon freshly ground black pepper
5$\frac{1}{4}$ ounces dry instant mashed potatoes
1 tablespoon + 1 teaspoon grated Parmesan cheese
1 tablespoon chopped chives to garnish (optional)

1. In large skillet, bring chicken broth to a boil. Reduce heat; add sea bass fillets and mushrooms. Cover and poach 3–4 minutes, just until cooked and fish flakes when tested with a fork. Using slotted spoon, remove fillets and mushrooms; transfer to shallow 2-quart flameproof dish and keep warm.

2. Dissolve potato starch in milk; whisk into broth in skillet with wine, margarine, salt and pepper. Bring to a boil, stirring constantly; reduce heat and simmer 2–3 minutes, until thickened. Pour sauce over fish.

3. Preheat broiler. Mix instant mashed potatoes with boiling water to desired level of consistency. Spoon or pipe around the edges of the broilerproof dish. Sprinkle with Parmesan cheese and broil 6–10 minutes, until top is golden brown and bubbling.

4. Garnish with chopped chives, if desired.

EACH SERVING (1 fillet and $\frac{1}{4}$ of the sauce mixture and potatoes)
PROVIDES: $\frac{1}{4}$ Milk, $\frac{1}{2}$ Fat, 1 Vegetable, 2 Proteins, 2 Breads, 45 Optional Calories
PER SERVING: 382 Calories, 33 g Protein, 7 g Fat, 42 g Carbohydrate, 802 mg Sodium, 62 mg Cholesterol, 1 g Dietary Fiber

BAKED SCROD WITH RATATOUILLE

The fresh vegetables here add color as well as flavor to this satisfying baked fish.

MAKES 4 SERVINGS

1 cup chopped onions
2 teaspoon minced garlic
2 cups diced eggplant
1½ cups red, yellow or green diced bell peppers
1½ cups diced zucchini
1½ cups chopped seeded tomatoes
2 tablespoons minced fresh oregano
3 tablespoons shredded fresh basil
1 teaspoon salt
½ teaspoon freshly ground black pepper
Four 4-ounce scrod fillets
2 tablespoons tomato paste
1 tablespoon + 1 teaspoon olive oil
8 taco or tostada shells, crushed (4 ounces)
1½ ounces shredded cheddar cheese

1. Preheat oven to 350°F. Spray large skillet with nonstick cooking spray. Add onions and garlic; cook, stirring frequently, 5 minutes, until onions are softened. Add eggplant and bell peppers; cook, stirring frequently, 5 minutes, until peppers are tender-crisp. Stir in zucchini, tomatoes, oregano, basil, salt and pepper; continue cooking and stirring 5 minutes longer, until tender. Transfer half of the vegetables to a shallow 2-quart baking dish.

2. Arrange the scrod fillets over the vegetables. In small cup, mix tomato paste with oil and spread one-fourth of the mixture over each fillet. Top with remaining vegetables.

3. Sprinkle with crushed taco shells and cheese.

4. Bake 20–30 minutes, until the top is golden-brown and the fish flakes easily when tested with a fork.

EACH SERVING (1 fillet and ¾ cup ratatouille and toppings) PROVIDES: 1 Fat, 4 Vegetables, 2 Proteins, 1 Bread
PER SERVING: 311 Calories, 27 g Protein, 10 g Fat, 29 g Carbohydrate, 799 mg Sodium, 60 mg Cholesterol, 5 g Dietary Fiber

ASIAN SEA BASS

MAKES 4 SERVINGS

Four 4-ounce sea bass fillets
1 cup thin scallion strips
1 tablespoon finely chopped fresh ginger root
2 tablespoons reduced-calorie soy sauce
2 teaspoons sesame oil
4 scallion fans to garnish (optional)*
Cilantro sprigs to garnish (optional)
2 cups cooked regular long-grain white rice

1. In the center of an 18 × 12" piece of heavy-duty foil, place the fillets in a single layer. Sprinkle with the scallions, ginger root, 1 tablespoon of the soy sauce, and the sesame oil. Bring the sides of the foil together and fold over tightly to make packet.

2. Bring 1 inch of water to a boil in a large skillet. Place the foil packet in skillet; cover tightly, reduce heat and steam 10 minutes, until fillets flake easily when tested with a fork.

3. Transfer packet to a flat surface; open. With slotted spatula, transfer the fillets and scallions to warm serving platter. Pour cooking juices and the remaining 1 tablespoon soy sauce over the fillets.

4. Garnish platter with scallion fans and cilantro, if desired. Serve each portion with ½ cup rice.

*Make scallion fans by slitting the green tops of the scallions lengthwise into thin strips; place in cold water to curl.

EACH SERVING (1 fillet, ¼ scallion mixture and ½ cup rice) PROVIDES: ½ Fat, ½ Vegetable, 1½ Proteins, 1 Bread
PER SERVING: 276 Calories, 25 g Protein, 5 g Fat, 31 g Carbohydrate, 383 mg Sodium, 46 mg Cholesterol, 1 g Dietary Fiber

SALMON WITH CUCUMBER, DILL AND RICE

MAKES 4 SERVINGS

4 cups cooked regular long-grain rice
8 ounces drained canned pink salmon
1 cup diced unpared cucumber
1 cup radish slices, thinly sliced
$\frac{1}{4}$ cup white-wine vinegar
3 tablespoons fresh lemon juice
2 tablespoons chopped fresh dill
1 tablespoon + 1 teaspoon vegetable oil
1 tablespoon honey
1 teaspoon salt
1 teaspoon freshly ground black pepper
2 cups arugula or other lettuce leaves, washed

1. In large bowl, place rice, salmon, cucumber and radishes. Gently toss to combine.

2. In small bowl, whisk together vinegar, juice, dill, oil, honey, salt and pepper.

3. Line bottom of serving platter with arugula leaves. Mound salad in the center and drizzle dressing over the top.

EACH SERVING (2 cups) PROVIDES: 1 Fat, 2 Vegetables, 2 Proteins, 2 Breads, 15 Optional Calories
PER SERVING: 418 Calories, 19 g Protein, 8 g Fat, 66 g Carbohydrate, 846 mg Sodium, 22 mg Cholesterol, 2 g Dietary Fiber

STUFFED LOUISIANA RED SNAPPER

MAKES 4 SERVINGS

2 tablespoons + 2 teaspoons reduced-calorie tub margarine
1 cup finely chopped onions
1 tablespoon minced garlic
2 cups sliced mushrooms
1 cup chopped tomatoes
3 ounces plain dried bread crumbs
1 teaspoon salt
$\frac{1}{4}$ teaspoon ground red pepper
One 1 pound 8 ounce whole red snapper, pan dressed
8 fluid ounces (1 cup) dry white wine
2 sprigs fresh parsley
2 sprigs fresh thyme
4 whole allspice
2 whole cloves
2 bay leaves

1. Preheat oven to 375°F. In small nonstick skillet, melt margarine; add onions and garlic. Cook, stirring frequently, 5 minutes, until onions are tender. Add mushrooms and tomatoes; cook 3–4 minutes longer, until mushrooms are tender. Remove from heat. Stir in bread crumbs, salt and ground red pepper.

2. Stuff the cavity of the red snapper with stuffing mixture; place in shallow ovenproof dish. Fasten together in several places with toothpicks. Pour white wine and $\frac{1}{3}$ cup water over fish; surround fish with parsley, thyme, allspice, cloves and bay leaves.

3. Bake, uncovered, 25 minutes, until fish flakes easily when tested with a fork. Remove bay leaves. Cut into four equal pieces; serve each with $\frac{1}{4}$ of the stuffing.

EACH SERVING PROVIDES: 1 Fat, 2 Vegetables, 2 Proteins, 1 Bread, 50 Optional Calories
PER SERVING: 340 Calories, 34 g Protein, 7 g Fat, 25 g Carbohydrate, 908 mg Sodium, 52 mg Cholesterol, 3 g Dietary Fiber

SOLE POACHED WITH FENNEL

MAKES 4 SERVINGS

2 cups low-sodium chicken broth
1 cup julienned beets
1 cup julienned daikon (Japanese white radish)
   or red radishes
1 cup thin fennel slices
4 fluid ounces ($\frac{1}{2}$ cup) dry white wine
2 teaspoons finely chopped fresh thyme
1 teaspoon salt
$\frac{1}{2}$ teaspoon freshly ground black pepper
2 bay leaves
Four 5-ounce sole fillets
4 sprigs fennel tops to garnish (optional)

1. In large skillet, place broth, beets, daikon, fennel, wine, $\frac{1}{2}$ cup water, thyme, salt, pepper and bay leaves. Bring to boil. Reduce heat to low; simmer, covered, 5 minutes.

2. Roll up sole fillets, secure with 6" bamboo skewers and place, seam-side down, in skillet. Poach, covered, 5 minutes, until sole is cooked through and flakes easily when tested with a fork. Remove bay leaves.

3. Place each sole fillet in a shallow bowl and spoon one-fourth of the vegetables and poaching liquid over fish. Garnish each with 1 fennel sprig, if desired.

EACH SERVING PROVIDES: 1$\frac{1}{2}$ Vegetables, 2 Proteins, 35 Optional Calories
PER SERVING: 190 Calories, 29 g Protein, 3 g Fat, 7 g Carbohydrate, 750 mg Sodium, 68 mg Cholesterol, 1 g Dietary Fiber

PENNE WITH SALMON AND ASPARAGUS

MAKES 4 SERVINGS

6 ounces uncooked penne pasta
1 chicken bouillon cube
4 fluid ounces ($\frac{1}{2}$ cup) dry white wine
Four 3-ounce skinned and boned salmon fillets
2 cups 1" fresh asparagus pieces
1 cup nonfat sour cream
3 tablespoons prepared whole-grain low-sodium
   mustard
$\frac{3}{4}$ teaspoon salt
$\frac{1}{2}$ teaspoon freshly ground black pepper
$\frac{1}{4}$ cup chopped fresh chives

1. In large saucepan of boiling water, cook pasta 8–10 minutes, until tender. Drain, place in serving bowl and keep warm.

2. In large skillet, bring $\frac{1}{2}$ cup water to a boil. Add bouillon cube, stirring until dissolved; then add wine. Add salmon fillets and asparagus to skillet; poach 5 minutes, just until fish flakes when tested with a fork and asparagus is tender-crisp. Using a slotted spoon, remove salmon and asparagus to bowl with pasta. Reserve cooking liquid. Using a fork, flake salmon into bite-size pieces; keep warm.

3. In medium bowl, beat together sour cream, mustard, salt, pepper, 3 tablespoons of the chives and reserved cooking liquid. Pour over pasta-salmon mixture; gently toss to coat.

4. Sprinkle with remaining 1 tablespoon of chives.

EACH SERVING (2 cups) PROVIDES: 1 Vegetable, 2 Proteins, 2 Breads, 70 Optional Calories
PER SERVING: 364 Calories, 29 g Protein, 7 g Fat, 40 g Carbohydrate, 779 mg Sodium, 47 mg Cholesterol, 2 g Dietary Fiber

Penne with Salmon and Asparagus

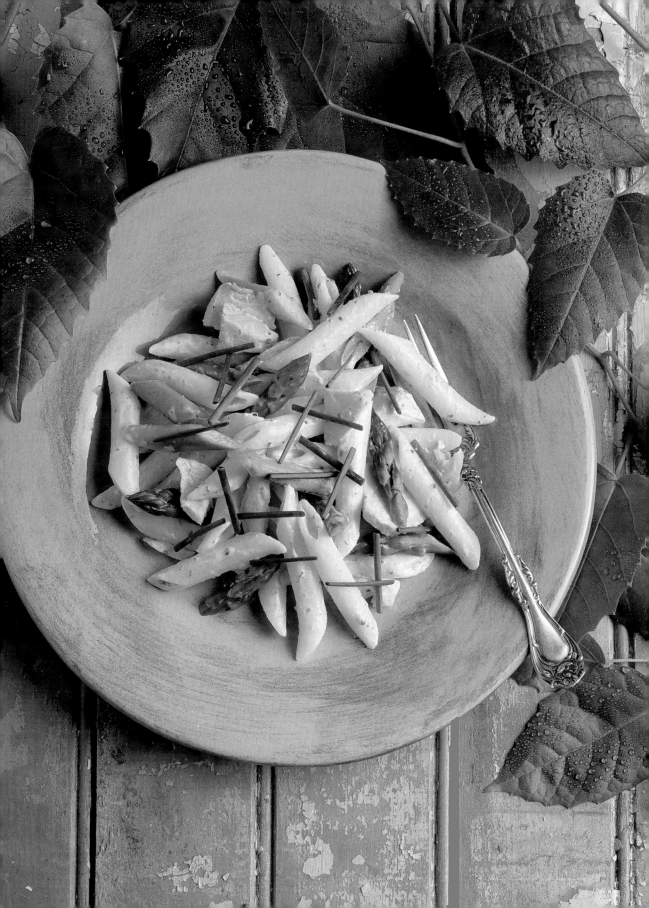

CAJUN RED SNAPPER

Cajun cooking hails from Louisiana and combines French flair with native southern ingredients. The spicing here is what gives the snapper its special Cajun flavor.

MAKES 4 SERVINGS

Four 5-ounce red snapper fillets
1 tablespoon paprika
1 teaspoon garlic powder
1 teaspoon onion powder
1 teaspoon freshly ground black pepper
1 teaspoon ground red pepper
1 teaspoon ground white pepper
1 teaspoon dried oregano leaves
$\frac{1}{2}$ teaspoon salt
$\frac{1}{2}$ teaspoon dried thyme leaves
1 tablespoon + 1 teaspoon reduced-calorie tub
  margarine
2 tablespoons fresh lemon juice
1 tablespoon chopped fresh chives
8 lemon wedges to garnish (optional)
Spicy brown mustard to taste

1. Place grill rack 5" from coals. Prepare grill according to manufacturer's directions.

2. Place snapper fillets on double sheet of heavy-duty foil, skin-side down, leaving a 6" border. Fold up edges to make foil pan.

3. In small cup, mix together paprika, garlic powder, onion powder, black pepper, ground red pepper, white pepper, oregano, salt and thyme.

4. Spread top of each fillet with one-fourth of the margarine; sprinkle each fillet with one-fourth of the spice mixture, $1\frac{1}{2}$ teaspoons juice and one-fourth of the chives.

5. Place foil pan containing fillet on grill rack. Cover grill, opening top and bottom flues slightly. (The cooker should only feel warm to the touch.)

6. Cook fillet, covered, 15–20 minutes or just until cooked and fish flakes easily when tested with a fork. Garnish each fillet with 2 lemon wedges, if desired, and serve with mustard.

EACH SERVING (1 fillet) PROVIDES: $\frac{1}{2}$ Fat, 2 Proteins
PER SERVING: 176 Calories, 30 g Protein, 4 g Fat, 4 g Carbohydrate, 402 mg Sodium, 52 mg Cholesterol, 0 g Dietary Fiber

BROILED CAJUN RED SNAPPER

1. Preheat broiler. In small cup, combine paprika, garlic powder, black pepper, ground red pepper, white pepper, oregano, salt and thyme. Arrange fillets in broiler pan.

2. Spread top of each fillet with 1 teaspoon margarine. Sprinkle each fillet with $1\frac{1}{2}$ teaspoons lemon juice, one-fourth of the spice mixture and one-fourth of the chives. Broil 3–4 minutes, until fish flakes easily when tested with a fork. Garnish each fillet with 2 lemon wedges, if desired, and serve with mustard.

FILLET OF SOLE WITH FRESH VEGETABLES

MAKES 4 SERVINGS

Four 5-ounce sole fillets
1 cup fish or vegetable broth
6 ounces angel hair pasta
2 cups broccoli florets
1 medium seeded pared cucumber, cut into strips
1 teaspoon grated lemon zest
2 tablespoons lemon juice
4–5 drops hot pepper sauce
½ teaspoon salt
½ teaspoon freshly ground black pepper
1 tablespoon + 1 teaspoon cornstarch
1½ cups plain nonfat yogurt
Lemon slices to garnish (optional)
Parsley sprigs to garnish (optional)

1. Cut each fillet diagonally into 4 equal pieces, making 16 pieces. Roll into 16 pinwheels; secure with toothpicks.

2. In large saucepan, bring broth to boil; add fillets. Reduce heat; poach 3–4 minutes, just until cooked through and fish flakes easily when tested with a fork. With a slotted spoon, remove fillets to plate; reserve broth. Keep fish warm.

3. In large pot of boiling water, cook pasta and broccoli 3 minutes, or until tender. Drain and place in serving bowl; keep warm.

4. In medium saucepan, bring reserved broth to a boil; add cucumber, zest, juice, hot pepper sauce, salt and pepper. In small cup, dissolve cornstarch in 1 tablespoon cold water; whisk into boiling broth. Reduce heat; cook, stirring constantly, 3 minutes, until thickened. Whisk in yogurt; cook just until heated through (do not boil).

5. Arrange pinwheels on top of pasta; remove toothpicks. Pour sauce over pinwheels. Garnish with lemon slices and parsley sprigs.

EACH SERVING (4 pinwheels and 1 cup vegetables/pasta) PROVIDES: ½ Milk, 1½ Vegetables, 2 Proteins, 2 Breads, 15 Optional Calories
PER SERVING: 372 Calories, 40 g Protein, 3 g Fat, 46 g Carbohydrate, 708 mg Sodium, 70 mg Cholesterol, 3 g Dietary Fiber

SOLE WITH CORN AND MUSHROOMS

MAKES 4 SERVINGS

1 tablespoon + 1 teaspoon sesame oil
2 cups baby corn ears
1 cup thin carrot strips
1 cup small shiitake mushrooms
1 cup minced scallions
1 cup snow peas, cut into 2" pieces
2 teaspoons minced garlic
2 tablespoons reduced-sodium soy sauce
1 tablespoon sesame seeds, toasted
½ teaspoon freshly ground black pepper
15 ounces sole fillet, cut into 2" strips
1 sprig fresh coriander to garnish (optional)
3 cups cooked regular long-grain rice

1. In large skillet, heat oil; add corn and carrots; stir-fry 2 minutes. Add mushrooms, scallions, snow peas and garlic to skillet. Cook 2 minutes longer, until tender-crisp. Using slotted spoon, transfer to serving dish; keep warm.

2. Pour soy sauce into skillet; add sesame seeds and pepper. Bring to a boil. Add fish to pan; reduce heat and cook 2–3 minutes, until fish is cooked and flakes easily when tested with a fork.

3. Using slotted spoon, transfer fish to serving dish with the vegetables. Toss gently to combine. Pour pan juices over fish and vegetables.

4. Garnish with coriander, if desired. Serve with cooked rice.

EACH SERVING (2 cups fish mixture and ¾ cup rice) PROVIDES: 1 Fat, 2 Vegetables, 1½ Proteins, 2 Breads, 10 Optional Calories
PER SERVING: 443 Calories, 31 g Protein, 8 g Fat, 61 g Carbohydrate, 425 mg Sodium, 51 mg Cholesterol, 6 g Dietary Fiber

SWORDFISH MEXICANA

*This zesty Mexican dish is also very nice
with turbot or bluefish.*

MAKES 4 SERVINGS

½ cup julienned carrots
½ cup fresh or thawed frozen corn kernels
½ cup thin slices onion
½ cup julienned green bell pepper
½ cup julienned red bell pepper
Four 5-ounce boneless swordfish steaks
1 cup drained and chopped canned peeled
   tomatoes
¼ cup fresh cilantro, minced
2 fresh medium chili peppers, seeded and finely
   chopped
1 tablespoon + 1 teaspoon vegetable oil
1 teaspoon salt
4 fresh lime slices to garnish (optional)
4 fresh cilantro sprigs to garnish (optional)

1. Preheat oven to 425°F. In medium saucepan, bring 1 inch water to a boil; add carrots, corn, onion and green and red bell peppers. Reduce heat; steam, covered, 1–2 minutes, until slightly wilted, but still crunchy; drain.

2. Cut out four 12" squares of baking parchment paper; fold each 2 times into a 6" square. Unfold and lay out flat on clean surface.

3. Place one-fourth of the vegetables on the top left-hand square of each paper.

4. Top each vegetable mound with a swordfish steak, then one-fourth of the chopped tomato, 1 tablespoon of the cilantro, one-half of a chili pepper, 1 teaspoon of the oil and ¼ teaspoon of the salt.

5. Fold the bottom right-hand corner of each paper over to meet the top left-hand corner, forming 4 triangular packets. Close each packet tightly, overlapping folds along the 2 opened sides, making semicircular packets.

6. Place on 2 baking sheets and bake 7–9 minutes. Place each parcel on serving plate. Standing back to avoid the steam, cut each packet open slightly in the center. Garnish each serving with 1 lime slice and 1 cilantro sprig, if desired.

EACH SERVING (1 fillet and ¾ cup vegetables) PROVIDES: 1 Fat, 1½ Vegetables, 2 Proteins, ¼ Bread
PER SERVING: 270 Calories, 30 g Protein, 11 g Fat, 13 g Carbohydrate, 693 mg Sodium, 55 mg Cholesterol, 3 g Dietary Fiber

JAMAICAN JERKED GRILLED SWORDFISH

*The hot seasonings typical of the islands are what
makes a dish "jerked." Catfish or whitefish can be
substituted for the swordfish.*

MAKES 4 SERVINGS

½ cup chopped onion
¼ cup chopped scallions
1 small fresh chili pepper, seeded
1 teaspoon hot pepper sauce
1 teaspoon salt
1 teaspoon chopped fresh thyme
½ teaspoon ground allspice
½ teaspoon freshly ground black pepper
¼ teaspoon cinnamon
⅛ teaspoon ground nutmeg
Four 5-ounce boneless swordfish steaks

1. To prepare marinade, in blender or food processor, place onion, scallions, chili pepper, hot pepper sauce, salt, thyme, allspice, black pepper, cinnamon and nutmeg. Purée until smooth; scrape into a gallon-size sealable plastic bag; add swordfish steaks. Seal bag, squeezing out air; turn to coat fillets. Refrigerate 6–8 hours, turning bag occasionally.

2. Spray grill rack with nonstick cooking spray. Place grill rack 5" from coals. Prepare grill according to manufacturer's directions.

3. Place swordfish fillets on grill rack. Cook 10–12 minutes, turning once, or until cooked through and fish flakes when tested with a fork.

EACH SERVING (1 steak) PROVIDES: ½ Vegetable, 2 Proteins
PER SERVING: 189 Calories, 29 g Protein, 6 g Fat, 3 g Carbohydrate, 713 mg Sodium, 55 mg Cholesterol, 1 g Dietary Fiber

JAMAICAN JERKED BROILED SWORDFISH

Prepare fish as in step 1.

Preheat broiler. Spray rack with nonstick cooking spray. Broil 5" from heat 2 minutes on each side.

◆

TROUT WITH RASPBERRIES AND MINT

MAKES 4 SERVINGS

Four 6-ounce whole trout, pan-dressed
$^3/_4$ cup fresh raspberries, washed
$^1/_2$ cup chopped fresh mint
2 tablespoons raspberry vinegar
2 tablespoons fresh lemon juice
1 tablespoon + 1 teaspoon walnut oil
1 teaspoon salt
$^1/_2$ teaspoon freshly ground black pepper
4 fresh mint sprigs to garnish (optional)

1. Using a sharp pointed knife, diagonally make three 3 × $^1/_4$" deep cuts across each fish on both sides and place in a shallow ovenproof dish.

2. In small bowl, toss raspberries with $^1/_4$ cup of the chopped mint. Fill each fish cavity with one-fourth of the raspberry mixture.

3. In small bowl, whisk together vinegar, juice, oil, salt, pepper and the remaining $^1/_4$ cup chopped mint. Pour into shallow ovenproof dish; add trout; cover and refrigerate 2–4 hours, turning trout once.

4. Preheat oven to 450°F. Place fish and marinade mixture on lowest oven rack; bake 20 minutes, or until fish flakes when tested with a fork. To serve, top each fish with a mint sprig, if desired.

EACH SERVING (1 trout) PROVIDES: 1 Fat, $^1/_4$ Fruit, 1$^1/_2$ Proteins
PER SERVING: 225 Calories, 24 g Protein, 12 g Fat, 4 g Carbohydrate, 611 mg Sodium, 66 mg Cholesterol, 1 g Dietary Fiber

BAKED TROUT WITH TOMATO AND CHERVIL

MAKES 4 SERVINGS

2 cups arugula or other lettuce, washed, torn and shredded
Four 5-ounce trout fillets
2 cups chopped seeded peeled tomatoes
$^1/_4$ cup tomato juice
$^1/_4$ cup Worcestershire sauce
1 tablespoon + 1 teaspoon chopped fresh chervil or thyme
$^1/_2$ teaspoon salt
$^1/_2$ teaspoon freshly ground black pepper
1 tablespoon + 1 teaspoon reduced-calorie tub margarine
4 fresh chervil sprigs to garnish (optional)
4 lemon wedges to garnish (optional)

1. Preheat oven to 425°F. Spray 2 baking sheets with nonstick cooking spray.

2. Cut out four 12" squares of baking parchment paper. Fold each 2 times into a 6" square. Unfold and lay out flat on clean surface.

3. Place $^1/_2$ cup arugula on the top left-hand square of each paper. Place 1 trout fillet on top of each mound of arugula.

4. Top each fillet with $^1/_2$ cup tomato, 1 tablespoon tomato juice, 1 tablespoon Worcestershire sauce, 1 teaspoon chervil, $^1/_4$ of the salt and $^1/_4$ of pepper. Top each stack with 1 teaspoon margarine. Fold into tightly sealed triangle, starting at one corner, making tiny overlapping folds $^1/_4$" apart, and tucking the ends under.

5. Place on prepared baking sheets and bake 5 minutes. Place each parcel on a serving plate. Standing back to avoid the steam, cut each packet open slightly in the center. Garnish each with a chervil sprig and lemon wedge, if desired.

EACH SERVING (1 fillet and $^1/_4$ of the tomato mixture) PROVIDES: $^1/_2$ Fat, 2 Vegetables, 2 Proteins
PER SERVING: 266 Calories, 32 g Protein, 12 g Fat, 8 g Carbohydrate, 619 mg Sodium, 82 mg Cholesterol, 2 g Dietary Fiber

TROUT FLORENTINE

When a dish is called Florentine, it means that it is made with spinach. Here, a luscious spinach-and-cheese mixture is rolled up in the trout fillets.

MAKES 4 SERVINGS

2 cups cooked spinach, well drained and chopped
$\frac{1}{4}$ cup part-skim ricotta cheese
2 tablespoons chopped chives
$\frac{1}{2}$ teaspoon grated lemon zest
1 teaspoon salt
$\frac{1}{2}$ teaspoon freshly ground black pepper
$\frac{1}{4}$ teaspoon freshly grated nutmeg
Four 5-ounce trout fillets
2 cups skim milk
$\frac{1}{4}$ cup + $1\frac{1}{2}$ teaspoons all-purpose flour
1 slice reduced-calorie bread, made into crumbs
1 tablespoon + 1 teaspoon grated Parmesan cheese
1 cup fresh watercress

1. Preheat oven to 375°F. Spray an 8" square ovenproof dish with nonstick cooking spray. In medium bowl, combine spinach, ricotta cheese, chives, lemon zest, $\frac{1}{2}$ teaspoon of the salt, $\frac{1}{4}$ teaspoon of the pepper and the nutmeg.

2. Spread one-fourth of the spinach mixture over each trout fillet and roll up. Place in prepared dish, seam-side down.

3. In medium saucepan, whisk together milk, flour, the remaining $\frac{1}{2}$ teaspoon salt and $\frac{1}{4}$ teaspoon pepper over low heat 5 minutes, until sauce thickens. Pour over fillets.

4. In small bowl, toss together bread crumbs with Parmesan cheese; sprinkle on top of fillets. Bake 30 minutes, until fish flakes when tested with a fork and is golden brown. Top with watercress.

EACH SERVING (1 fillet stuffed with $\frac{1}{4}$ spinach mixture, sauce and watercress) PROVIDES: $\frac{1}{2}$ Milk, $1\frac{1}{2}$ Vegetables, $2\frac{1}{4}$ Proteins, $\frac{1}{2}$ Bread, 10 Optional Calories
PER SERVING: 354 Calories, 40 g Protein, 12 g Fat, 20 g Carbohydrate, 832 mg Sodium, 91 mg Cholesterol, 3 g Dietary Fiber

TROUT ALMONDINE

Almonds add the special touch to this quick and easy dish.

MAKES 4 SERVINGS

4 fluid ounces ($\frac{1}{2}$ cup) dry white wine
$\frac{1}{4}$ cup minced fresh parsley
4 lemon slices
$\frac{1}{4}$ cup fresh lemon juice
1 teaspoon salt
$\frac{1}{2}$ teaspoon freshly ground black pepper
Four 5-ounce trout fillets
2 ounces sliced almonds, toasted
4 sprigs fresh Italian parsley to garnish (optional)

1. In large deep skillet, combine white wine, parsley, lemon slices, juice, salt and pepper. Bring to a boil.

2. Arrange trout fillets in single layer in skillet; reduce heat. Poach, covered, 4–6 minutes, until cooked through and fish flakes when tested with a fork. Transfer each fillet to a serving plate; pour $\frac{1}{4}$ poaching liquid over each.

3. Sprinkle with toasted almonds and garnish with parsley, if desired.

EACH SERVING (1 fillet) PROVIDES: 1 Fat, $2\frac{1}{2}$ Proteins, 25 Optional Calories
PER SERVING: 322 Calories, 33 g Protein, 17 g Fat, 6 g Carbohydrate, 629 mg Sodium, 82 mg Cholesterol, 1 g Dietary Fiber

GRILLED TUNA WITH CITRUS SALSA

MAKES 4 SERVINGS

1 medium pink grapefruit
2 small navel oranges
$\frac{1}{2}$ cup chopped fresh mint
1 teaspoon honey
$\frac{1}{4}$ teaspoon hot pepper sauce
$\frac{1}{4}$ cup fresh lemon juice
$\frac{1}{4}$ cup orange juice
2 tablespoons fresh lime juice
Four 5-ounce boneless tuna steaks
1 cup fresh watercress

1. To prepare salsa, over small bowl peel grapefruit and oranges; remove membrane. Using a serrated knife, cut fruits into bite-size pieces; place in bowl. Stir in $\frac{1}{4}$ cup of the mint, the honey and hot pepper sauce. Cover with plastic wrap; refrigerate 1 hour, or until chilled.

2. To prepare marinade, in a gallon-size sealable plastic bag, combine the lemon, orange and lime juices and remaining $\frac{1}{4}$ cup mint. Add tuna steaks. Seal bag, squeezing out air; turn to coat fillets. Refrigerate 30 minutes, turning bag several times. Remove steaks from marinade; discard marinade.

3. Spray grill rack with nonstick cooking spray. Place grill rack 5" from coals. Prepare grill according to manufacturer's directions.

4. Grill tuna steaks on rack 10–12 minutes, turning once, until fish flakes when tested with a fork.

5. Line serving platter with watercress; arrange tuna steaks on top. Serve with citrus salsa.

EACH SERVING (1 steak and $\frac{1}{4}$ cup salsa) PROVIDES: 1 Fruit, $\frac{1}{2}$ Vegetable, 2 Proteins, 15 Optional Calories
PER SERVING: 272 Calories, 34 g Protein, 7 g Fat, 17 g Carbohydrate, 68 mg Sodium, 54 mg Cholesterol, 2 g Dietary Fiber

BROILED TUNA WITH CITRUS SALSA

Preheat broiler. Spray rack with nonstick cooking spray. Place fish on rack 5" from source of heat and broil 2 minutes on each side.

STIR-FRIED TUNA

MAKES 4 SERVINGS

1 tablespoon + 1 teaspoon olive oil
1 cup scallions
1 small orange, peeled and sectioned
$1\frac{1}{4}$ pounds fresh boneless tuna, cut into 2" strips
2 cups drained cooked lima beans
2 tablespoons prepared horseradish
$\frac{1}{2}$ cup fresh orange juice
$\frac{1}{2}$ cup low-sodium chicken broth
$1\frac{1}{2}$ teaspoons julienned orange zest
1 teaspoon salt
2 teaspoons fresh chopped rosemary
$\frac{1}{2}$ teaspoon freshly ground black pepper
1 sprig fresh rosemary to garnish (optional)

1. In large nonstick skillet, heat oil; add scallions and orange sections. Cook 2 minutes, until slightly softened. Add tuna, lima beans and horseradish. Quickly stir-fry 3 minutes, just until tuna is cooked and flakes when tested with a fork.

2. Stir in orange juice, broth, orange zest, salt, rosemary and pepper. Bring to a boil. Transfer to serving plate; garnish with rosemary sprig, if desired.

EACH SERVING ($1\frac{1}{2}$ cups) PROVIDES: 1 Fat, $\frac{1}{2}$ Fruit, $\frac{1}{2}$ Vegetable, 2 Proteins, 1 Bread, 3 Optional Calories
PER SERVING: 408 Calories, 40 g Protein, 12 g Fat, 34 g Carbohydrate, 638 mg Sodium, 54 mg Cholesterol, 6 g Dietary Fiber

TUNA-NOODLE CASSEROLE

This all-time favorite casserole is perfect on a cold, dreary night or when you've had a stressful day.

MAKES 4 SERVINGS

$4\frac{1}{2}$ ounces medium egg noodles
1 cup chopped onions
1 cup chopped celery
1 cup chopped bell peppers (green, red and yellow)
1 cup sliced mushrooms
$\frac{1}{2}$ cup frozen sweet corn, thawed
One 10.5-ounce can reduced-calorie undiluted mushroom soup (70 calories per can)
8 ounces drained canned chunk light tuna packed in water, flaked
$\frac{1}{2}$ cup skim milk
Few drops hot pepper sauce
2 tablespoons minced parsley
$\frac{1}{2}$ teaspoon freshly ground black pepper
2 slices reduced-calorie fresh whole-wheat bread, made into crumbs
1 tablespoon + 1 teaspoon grated Parmesan cheese
2 medium tomatoes, sliced

1. Preheat oven to 350°F. Spray shallow 2-quart casserole with nonstick cooking spray. In large pot of boiling water, cook noodles 8 minutes, until tender. Drain; keep warm.

2. Meanwhile, spray a large saucepan with nonstick cooking spray. Add onions and celery; cook, stirring frequently, about 2 minutes, until tender-crisp. Add bell peppers, mushrooms and corn. Continue cooking and stirring, 5 minutes longer, until tender.

3. Stir in soup, tuna, milk, hot pepper sauce, parsley and pepper.

4. Remove from heat; stir in noodles. Transfer to prepared casserole.

5. Sprinkle with bread crumbs and Parmesan cheese; bake 15–20 minutes, until crumbs are golden brown and crisp. Top with fresh tomato slices. Serve hot.

EACH SERVING (1½ cups) PROVIDES: 3 Vegetables, 1 Protein, 2 Breads, 40 Optional Calories
PER SERVING: 342 Calories, 27 g Protein, 5 g Fat, 50 g Carbohydrate, 597 mg Sodium, 56 mg Cholesterol, 6 g Dietary Fiber

TUNA WITH FUSILLI AND FRUIT

MAKES 4 SERVINGS

2 cups cooked fusilli pasta
8 ounces drained canned chunk light tuna packed in water, flaked
1 cup drained pineapple chunks in unsweetened juice
2 medium kiwi fruit, pared, halved and sliced crosswise
1 cup red bell pepper strips
1 cup chopped, unpared cucumber
$\frac{3}{4}$ cup plain nonfat yogurt
2 tablespoons + 2 teaspoons reduced-calorie mayonnaise
2 tablespoons chopped fresh mint
$\frac{1}{2}$ teaspoon salt
$\frac{1}{2}$ teaspoon freshly ground black pepper
2 cups fresh spinach leaves, washed, torn and patted dry
4 fresh mint sprigs to garnish (optional)

1. In large bowl, toss together pasta, tuna, pineapple, kiwi fruit, bell pepper and cucumber.

2. In small bowl, whisk yogurt, mayonnaise, chopped mint, salt and pepper. Drizzle over pasta mixture; toss to coat.

3. Line large serving plate with spinach leaves; mound the pasta mixture in the center; garnish with mint sprigs, if desired.

EACH SERVING (1½ cups) PROVIDES: ¼ Milk, 1 Fat, 1 Fruit, 2 Vegetables, 1 Protein, 1 Bread
PER SERVING: 308 Calories, 25 g Protein, 4 g Fat, 44 g Carbohydrate, 589 mg Sodium, 28 mg Cholesterol, 5 g Dietary Fiber

MEDITERRANEAN-STYLE SALAD WITH SUN-DRIED TOMATOES

An elegant salad that is particularly nice for dinner in sultry weather.

MAKES 4 SERVINGS

6 sun-dried tomato halves (not packed in oil)
1 cup low-sodium chicken broth
1 cup finely diced tomatoes (reserve juice)
1 tablespoon + 1 teaspoon red wine vinegar
1 teaspoon chopped fresh rosemary
$\frac{1}{4}$ teaspoon freshly ground black pepper
3 cups mixed greens, torn into bite-size pieces
1 cup cut green beans (2" pieces), steamed until tender-crisp
1 medium green bell pepper, sliced into thin rings
8 ounces drained canned water-packed tuna, broken into chunks
8 ounces pared cooked potatoes, sliced
$\frac{1}{2}$ cup thinly sliced red onion
12 large black olives
4 anchovy fillets, chopped

1. To prepare dressing, in small saucepan, combine sun-dried tomato halves, broth and $\frac{1}{4}$ cup water; bring to a boil. Reduce heat to low; simmer 5 minutes. Remove from heat; let stand 20 minutes.

2. Transfer broth mixture to blender or food processor; add diced tomatoes with juice, vinegar, rosemary and pepper; purée until smooth. Set aside.

3. To serve, arrange greens evenly on 4 plates; top each with one-fourth of the green beans, bell pepper, tuna, potato, onion and olives. Drizzle with one-fourth of the dressing and sprinkle with one-fourth of the anchovies.

EACH SERVING PROVIDES: $\frac{1}{2}$ Fat, 4 Vegetables, 1 Protein, $\frac{1}{2}$ Bread, 15 Optional Calories
PER SERVING: 207 Calories, 22 g Protein, 3 g Fat, 24 g Carbohydrate, 662 mg Sodium, 26 mg Cholesterol, 5 g Dietary Fiber

SALAD NIÇOISE

MAKES 4 SERVINGS

1 pound, 4 ounces small red potatoes, scrubbed
2 cups trimmed green beans
8 ounces drained canned chunk light tuna packed in water, flaked
24 cherry tomatoes, halved
4 cups romaine or other lettuce leaves, washed and thinly sliced
2 large hard-cooked eggs, peeled and quartered
6 large pitted black olives, rinsed and sliced crosswise
8 flat anchovy fillets, rinsed
$\frac{1}{4}$ cup red-wine vinegar
2 tablespoons fresh lemon juice
1 tablespoon olive oil
$\frac{1}{4}$ teaspoon salt
$\frac{1}{4}$ teaspoon freshly ground black pepper

1. In large pan of boiling water, cook potatoes 15–20 minutes, until tender. Remove with slotted spoon. Rinse with cold water; drain. Coarsely chop and place in a large bowl.

2. Add green beans to the water; cook 3 minutes, just until bright green and tender-crisp. Rinse with cold water, drain.

3. Toss the green beans, tuna and tomatoes with the potatoes.

4. Line large serving plate with lettuce leaves; mound the tuna-potato mixture in the center.

5. Decoratively arrange the egg quarters, olives and anchovy fillets on top of tuna-potato mixture.

6. In small bowl, whisk vinegar, juice, oil, salt and pepper. Drizzle over salad; serve immediately.

EACH SERVING (1$\frac{1}{2}$ cups) PROVIDES: 1 Fat, 4 Vegetables, 1$\frac{1}{2}$ Proteins, 1 Bread, 15 Optional Calories
PER SERVING: 325 Calories, 27 g Protein, 8 g Fat, 35 g Carbohydrate, 747 mg Sodium, 134 mg Cholesterol, 5 g Dietary Fiber

TURBOT À LA NAGE

Nage means "swimming" in French, and here turbot "swims" in a lovely poaching broth of white wine flavored with carrots, celery, leeks, parsley, tarragon and other spices.

MAKES 4 SERVINGS

8 fluid ounces (1 cup) dry white wine
1 cup finely diced carrots
1 cup finely diced celery
1 cup very thinly sliced leeks, split lengthwise
1 cup finely diced turnips
5 parsley sprigs
4 tarragon sprigs
2 tablespoons white wine vinegar
2 bay leaves
1 teaspoon salt
1 teaspoon black peppercorns
Four 5-ounce turbot fillets
1 teaspoon Dijon mustard
1 tablespoon julienned lemon zest, to garnish (optional)
2 tablespoons julienned chives, to garnish (optional)

1. In large deep skillet place 2 cups water, the wine, vinegar, carrots, celery, leeks, turnips, parsley, tarragon, vinegar, bay leaves, salt and peppercorns. Cover and bring to a boil; reduce heat and simmer 30 minutes.

2. Place turbot fillets in pan; cover and poach over lowest heat, 3–5 minutes, until fish is cooked and flakes easily when tested with a fork.

3. To prepare sauce, strain poaching liquid and reduce to $\frac{1}{3}$ cup. Mix with the mustard.

4. Top fillets with sauce; garnish with lemon zest and chives, if desired.

EACH SERVING (1 fillet) PROVIDES: 2 Vegetables, 2 Proteins, 50 Optional Calories
PER SERVING: 354 Calories, 22 g Protein, 20 g Fat, 12 g Carbohydrate, 768 mg Sodium, 65 mg Cholesterol, 2 g Dietary Fiber

GREEK KABOBS WITH TURBOT

MAKES 4 SERVINGS

Four 5-ounce turbot fillets
2 cups whole medium mushrooms
2 cups thawed frozen artichoke hearts
4 small plum tomatoes, halved
20 fresh bay leaves
$\frac{1}{4}$ cup lemon juice
2 tablespoons chopped fresh oregano
1 tablespoon + 1 teaspoon olive oil
1 teaspoon garlic powder
$\frac{1}{4}$ teaspoon salt
1 teaspoon freshly ground black pepper
4 large pita breads (8 ounces)
8 lemon wedges to garnish (optional)
2 tablespoons chives, cut into 1" strips to garnish (optional)

1. Spray grill rack with nonstick cooking spray. Place grill rack 5" from coals. Prepare grill according to manufacturer's directions.

2. Meanwhile, prepare the kabobs: cut each turbot fillet into 5 pieces. Onto four 12" kabob sticks, alternately thread the fish, mushrooms, artichoke hearts, plum tomatoes and bay leaves.

3. In small bowl, whisk together juice, oregano, oil, garlic powder, salt and pepper.

4. Grill kabobs, 12–15 minutes, turning and basting frequently with lemon mixture, until fish is cooked through and vegetables are tender. Grill pita breads during the last 3 minutes, turning once.

5. Arrange kabobs and pita bread on serving platter. Garnish with lemon wedges and fresh chives, if desired.

EACH SERVING (1 kabob) PROVIDES: $2\frac{1}{2}$ Vegetables, 2 Proteins, 2 Breads, 40 Optional Calories
PER SERVING: 532 Calories, 29 g Protein, 26 g Fat, 47g Carbohydrate, 601 mg Sodium, 65 mg Cholesterol, 5 g Dietary Fiber

BROILED KABOBS

Preheat broiler. Broil kabobs 6" from heat for 7 minutes, or until fish flakes easily when tested with fork.

NEW ENGLAND STEAMED CLAMS

Steamed clams are a summer treat, especially when served with new potatoes and fresh corn on the cob in this easy version of the clam bake.

MAKES 4 SERVINGS

24 medium littleneck or cherrystone clams, in
 their shells
1 tablespoon powdered mustard
$1\frac{1}{4}$ pounds small new potatoes
4 small ears of corn, 5" long
2 tablespoons + 2 teaspoons reduced-calorie tub
 margarine
8 lemon wedges to garnish (optional)

1. In large pot, place $2\frac{1}{4}$ cups cold water, the clams and mustard; let stand 30 minutes to rid clams of their sand. Rinse well.

2. In large saucepan of boiling water, cook potatoes 7–9 minutes, until tender. Using slotted spoon, transfer to serving platter; keep warm.

3. To same pot of boiling water, add corn on the cob; cook, covered, 4 minutes, until tender. Using slotted spoon, transfer to serving platter; keep warm.

4. To same pot of boiling water, add clams; cook, with lid slightly askew, 4 minutes, until clams open. Transfer to serving platter. Strain broth and reserve to dunk clams. Drizzle melted margarine over potatoes and corn. Serve with lemon wedges, if desired.

EACH SERVING (6 clams, 4 ounces potatoes and 1 ear corn) PROVIDES: 1 Fat, 1 Protein, 2 Breads
PER SERVING: 270 Calories, 13 g Protein, 6 g Fat, 43 g Carbohydrate, 129 mg Sodium, 19 mg Cholesterol, 5 g Dietary Fiber

SPAGHETTI VONGOLE

MAKES 4 SERVINGS

1 tablespoon + 1 teaspoon olive oil
2 cups canned stewed tomatoes
$1\frac{1}{2}$ cups chopped onions
2 tablespoons tomato paste
2 teaspoons minced garlic
$\frac{1}{2}$ teaspoon dried basil leaves
$\frac{1}{2}$ teaspoon dried oregano leaves
$\frac{1}{2}$ teaspoon dried parsley leaves
6 ounces uncooked spaghetti
15 ounces minced fresh clams (without shells) or
 12 ounces drained canned minced clams
$\frac{1}{2}$ teaspoon freshly ground black pepper
$\frac{1}{4}$ teaspoon salt
1 sprig fresh basil to garnish (optional)

1. In large nonstick skillet, heat oil; add tomatoes, onions, tomato paste, garlic, basil, oregano and parsley; cook, stirring frequently, 5 minutes, until tender. Reduce heat. Simmer, uncovered, until a thick sauce forms.

2. In large pot of boiling water, cook spaghetti 8–10 minutes, until done. Drain and place on serving platter; keep warm.

3. Stir clams into tomato sauce. Season with pepper and salt. Cook 5 minutes longer.

4. Spoon sauce over spaghetti. Garnish with fresh basil, if desired.

EACH SERVING ($1\frac{1}{2}$ cups sauce, using fresh clams, and 1 cup spaghetti)
PROVIDES: 1 Fat, 2 Vegetables, $1\frac{1}{2}$ Proteins, 2 Breads
PER SERVING: 343 Calories, 21 g Protein, 7 g Fat, 50 g Carbohydrate, 588 mg Sodium, 36 mg Cholesterol, 5 g Dietary Fiber

ITALIAN CALAMARI SALAD

Calamari—or squid—is an Italian treat. If it's not available in the fish section of your supermarket, look for it in a fish store.

MAKES 4 SERVINGS

12 ounces cooked calamari, sliced $\frac{1}{4}$" thick
2 cups sliced roasted red bell peppers (2" strips)
1 cup frozen thawed artichoke hearts
1 cup sliced scallions
20 small pitted black olives, halved
8 sun-dried tomato halves (not packed in oil)
$\frac{1}{2}$ cup shredded fresh basil
2 teaspoons minced garlic
$\frac{1}{2}$ teaspoon salt
$\frac{1}{2}$ teaspoon freshly ground black pepper
2 tablespoons red-wine vinegar
2 teaspoons olive oil
2 cups arugula or lettuce

1. In large bowl, combine calamari, roasted bell peppers, artichokes, scallions, olives, tomatoes, basil, garlic, salt and pepper. Add vinegar and oil; toss to coat thoroughly. Cover with plastic wrap and refrigerate 2–4 hours, stirring occasionally.

2. To serve, line large serving plate with arugula; mound salad in center.

EACH SERVING (2 cups) PROVIDES: 1 Fat, 4 Vegetables, 1$\frac{1}{2}$ Proteins
PER SERVING: 209 Calories, 20 g Protein, 6 g Fat, 21 g Carbohydrate, 481 mg Sodium, 248 mg Cholesterol, 5 g Dietary Fiber

MARYLAND CRAB CAKES

Maryland is justifiably famous for its crab cakes, and with this easy recipe, you'll be able to make delicious crab cakes no matter where you live.

MAKES 4 SERVINGS

1 pound cooked crab meat, picked through for shells and cartilage
3 ounces fresh bread crumbs
$\frac{1}{2}$ cup minced scallions
$\frac{1}{4}$ cup low-fat (1%) milk
2 tablespoons + 2 teaspoons reduced-calorie mayonnaise
2 tablespoons fresh minced parsley
$\frac{1}{2}$ teaspoon salt
$\frac{1}{4}$ teaspoon white pepper
3 tablespoons all-purpose flour
1 tablespoon + 1 teaspoon reduced-calorie tub margarine
2$\frac{1}{2}$ cups mixed green lettuce leaves

1. In large bowl, combine crab meat, bread crumbs, scallions, milk, mayonnaise, parsley, salt and white pepper.

2. With moistened hands, form into 8 small round cakes; refrigerate 1 hour.

3. On sheet of wax paper, spread flour; lightly dust each cake on both sides.

4. In large skillet, melt margarine; cook crab cakes 4–5 minutes on each side, until golden-brown and crispy. Line serving platter with greens; arrange crab cakes on top.

EACH SERVING (2 cakes) PROVIDES: 1$\frac{1}{2}$ Fats, 1$\frac{1}{2}$ Vegetables, 2 Proteins, 1 Bread, 5 Optional Calories
PER SERVING: 257 Calories, 27 g Protein, 8 g Fat, 19 g Carbohydrate, 800 mg Sodium, 118 mg Cholesterol, 1 g Dietary Fiber

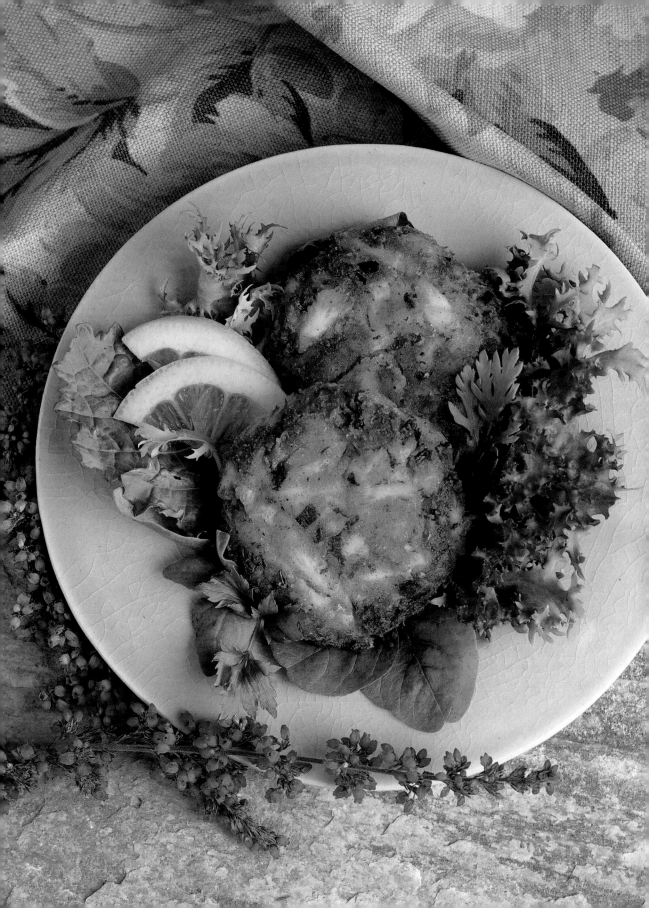

BROILED STUFFED LOBSTER

You can buy bouquet garni pre-made or make your own. In a small square of cheesecloth, place parsley, thyme and bay leaf; tie cheesecloth tightly.

MAKES 4 SERVINGS

2 cups low-fat (1%) milk
4 fluid ounces ($\frac{1}{2}$ cup) dry white wine
1 bouquet garni
$\frac{1}{4}$ cup all-purpose flour
2 cups sliced mushrooms
2 tablespoons + 2 teaspoons reduced-calorie tub margarine
1 teaspoon Dijon mustard
1 large egg yolk, slightly beaten
2 tablespoons minced fresh parsley
2 teaspoons fresh lemon juice
$\frac{1}{2}$ teaspoon salt
$\frac{1}{2}$ teaspoon freshly ground black pepper
Four 1-pound live lobsters
2 slices bread, made into crumbs
1 tablespoon + 1 teaspoon grated Parmesan cheese
4 lemon wedges to garnish (optional)
4 sprigs fresh parsley to garnish (optional)

1. In medium saucepan, heat milk and wine with bouquet garni. Bring to a boil; remove from heat. Leave to infuse 30 minutes. Remove bouquet garni.

2. Add mushrooms, flour, margarine and mustard. Stir over low heat 3 minutes, until sauce has thickened and mushrooms are cooked. Remove from heat. Beat in egg yolk, parsley, lemon juice, salt and pepper.

3. In large pot of boiling water, cook lobsters about 10–11 minutes, until bright red. Using tongs, transfer to cutting board; remove meat from tails, leaving shells intact.

4. Preheat broiler. Cut lobster meat into 1" cubes. Pour one-fourth of the sauce into bottom of each lobster's body cavity and tail. Refill with lobster meat. Sprinkle each lobster with $\frac{1}{2}$ ounce bread crumbs and 1 teaspoon Parmesan cheese. Place on flameproof pan.

5. Broil, 4" from heat, 3–4 minutes, until golden brown and heated through. Place on serving platter; garnish each with 1 lemon wedge and 1 parsley sprig, if desired.

EACH SERVING PROVIDES: $\frac{1}{2}$ Milk, 1 Fat, 1 Vegetable, 2 Proteins, $\frac{3}{4}$ Bread, 60 Optional Calories
PER SERVING: 317 Calories, 31 g Protein, 9 g Fat, 23 g Carbohydrate, 989 mg Sodium, 141 mg Cholesterol, 1 g Dietary Fiber

SUMMER STEAMED LOBSTER

MAKES 4 SERVINGS

$\frac{1}{4}$ cup reduced-calorie tub margarine
1 tablespoon fresh lemon juice
$1\frac{1}{2}$ teaspoons minced fresh parsley
$1\frac{1}{2}$ teaspoons minced fresh tarragon or $\frac{1}{2}$ teaspoon dried leaves
$1\frac{1}{2}$ teaspoons finely chopped watercress
$\frac{1}{4}$ teaspoon salt
$\frac{1}{4}$ teaspoon freshly ground black pepper
Four 1-pound live lobsters
4 lemon wedges to garnish (optional)
4 sprigs fresh parsley to garnish (optional)

1. To prepare herb butter, in small bowl, beat together margarine, juice, parsley, tarragon, watercress, salt and pepper. Cover with plastic wrap and refrigerate.

2. In large pot of boiling water, cook lobsters 10–11 minutes, until bright red. Using tongs, transfer lobsters to serving platter. Serve with herb butter. Garnish with lemon and parsley, if desired.

EACH SERVING (1 lobster and $\frac{1}{4}$ herb butter) PROVIDES: $1\frac{1}{2}$ Fats, 2 Proteins
PER SERVING: 163 Calories, 23 g Protein, 7 g Fat, 2 g Carbohydrate, 677 mg Sodium, 82 mg Cholesterol, 0 g Dietary Fiber

LOBSTER SALAD

Oranges, grapefruit, cantaloupe and mango give this lobster salad an adventurous new flavor.

MAKES 4 SERVINGS

1 small orange
1 medium pink grapefruit
1 pound cooked lobster meat
1½ cups cantaloupe balls
1 cup mango slices
2 cups stemmed watercress leaves, rinsed and drained
½ cup nonfat sour cream
2 tablespoons + 2 teaspoons reduced-calorie mayonnaise
2 teaspoons grated orange zest
¼ cup orange juice
½ teaspoon freshly ground black pepper
2 tablespoons chopped chives to garnish (optional)

1. Peel orange and grapefruit over small bowl to catch juices; section, seed and coarsely chop.

2. In large bowl, combine lobster, orange, grapefruit, cantaloupe and mango.

3. Line large serving platter with watercress. Mound lobster mixture in center.

4. In small bowl, whisk together sour cream and mayonnaise; whisk in orange zest and juice. Pour over salad. Sprinkle with black pepper.

5. Garnish with chopped chives, if desired.

EACH SERVING (2 cups) PROVIDES: 1 Fat, 1¾ Fruits, 1 Vegetable, 2 Proteins, 10 Optional Calories
PER SERVING: 248 Calories, 27 g Protein, 4 g Fat, 26 g Carbohydrate, 519 mg Sodium, 85 mg Cholesterol, 2 g Dietary Fiber

SCALLOPS WITH LIME AND HERBS

This scallop stir-fry is very nice over rice.

MAKES 4 SERVINGS

1 tablespoon + 1 teaspoon sesame oil
2 cups sliced green beans, 2" slices
2 teaspoons minced garlic
2 cups sliced summer squash
1 cup thawed frozen peas
1 tablespoon minced fresh parsley
1 tablespoon minced fresh cilantro
1½ teaspoons minced fresh thyme or ½ teaspoon dried leaves
15 ounces bay scallops
½ cup low-sodium chicken broth
¼ cup fresh lime juice
1 teaspoon salt
½ teaspoon freshly ground black pepper
1 lime, sliced

1. In large skillet, heat oil; add green beans and garlic. Cook, stirring constantly, 1 minute, until beans begin to soften. Add summer squash, peas, parsley, cilantro and thyme. Stir-fry 3–4 minutes longer, until almost tender-crisp.

2. Add scallops to pan; cook 1 minute longer. Pour in broth, juice, salt and pepper. Bring to a boil; add lime slices to pan.

EACH SERVING (1½ cups) PROVIDES: 1 Fat, 2 Vegetables, 1½ Proteins, ½ Bread, 3 Optional Calories
PER SERVING: 208 Calories, 22 g Protein, 6 g Fat, 18 g Carbohydrate, 774 mg Sodium, 35 mg Cholesterol, 3 g Dietary Fiber

TAGLIATELLE WITH SCALLOPS

Tagliatelle is a long, thin, flat pasta. You can substitute fettuccine for the tagliatelle if you like.

MAKES 4 SERVINGS

1 teaspoon saffron strands (optional)
4 cups cooked tagliatelle pasta (hot)
1 pound, 4 ounces scallops
2 tablespoons + 2 teaspoons reduced-calorie tub
    margarine
1 cup finely chopped onions
1 cup low-sodium chicken broth
$\frac{1}{2}$ cup half-and-half
$\frac{1}{2}$ teaspoon salt
Black pepper to taste
1 tablespoon cornstarch
2 cups chopped seeded peeled tomatoes
2 tablespoons finely chopped chervil to garnish
    (optional)

1. In small bowl, pour 1 tablespoon boiling water over saffron strands, if using; let stand 15 minutes to infuse.

2. Line serving bowl with cooked pasta; keep hot.

3. Using sharp knife, slice each scallop horizontally into 3 thin slices.

4. In large nonstick skillet, melt margarine; add onions. Cook over low heat, 2 minutes, until softened. Add scallop mixture and broth; simmer uncovered 1–2 minutes, until opaque. Using slotted spoon, transfer scallops to serving dish with pasta. Discard liquid.

5. In medium saucepan, mix half-and-half, saffron with soaking water, if using, salt and pepper. In cup, dissolve cornstarch in 1 tablespoon cold water; add to half-and-half mixture. Bring to a boil; add tomatoes. Simmer, stirring constantly, 3 minutes, until thickened.

6. Pour sauce over pasta and scallops. Toss together. Garnish with chervil, if desired.

EACH SERVING (2 cups) PROVIDES: 1 Fat, 1$\frac{1}{2}$ Vegetables, 2 Proteins, 2 Breads, 55 Optional Calories
PER SERVING: 636 Calories, 40 g Protein, 11 g Fat, 93 g Carbohydrate, 618 mg Sodium, 58 mg Cholesterol, 4 g Dietary Fiber

SCALLOP STIR-FRY

MAKES 4 SERVINGS

4$\frac{1}{2}$ ounces Chinese noodles
2 cups sugar snap peas
1 cup red bell pepper strips
15 ounces sea scallops, sliced into halves
$\frac{1}{2}$ medium fresh pineapple, cut into bite-size pieces
1$\frac{1}{2}$ cups drained canned water chestnuts
1 teaspoon grated orange zest
$\frac{1}{2}$ cup fresh orange juice
1 teaspoon grated lemon zest
2 tablespoons fresh lemon juice
1 tablespoon grated fresh ginger root
1 teaspoon garlic powder
1 teaspoon salt
$\frac{1}{2}$ teaspoon coriander seeds, crushed
$\frac{1}{2}$ teaspoon freshly ground black pepper
1 sprig fresh coriander leaves to garnish (optional)

1. Cook noodles according to directions; drain and keep warm.

2. Spray large skillet with nonstick cooking spray. Add sugar snap peas and bell pepper; stir-fry 1 minute.

3. To skillet, add scallops, pineapple, water chestnuts, orange zest, orange juice, lemon zest, lemon juice, ginger, garlic powder, salt, coriander seeds and pepper. Cook 3–4 minutes, turning frequently, until scallops are cooked and vegetables are tender-crisp.

4. Add noodles to skillet. Toss thoroughly to combine. Garnish with fresh coriander, if desired.

EACH SERVING (2 cups) PROVIDES: 1$\frac{1}{4}$ Fruits, 1$\frac{1}{2}$ Vegetables, 1$\frac{1}{2}$ Proteins, 2 Breads
PER SERVING: 355 Calories, 25 g Protein, 2 g Fat, 59 g Carbohydrate, 735 mg Sodium, 35 mg Cholesterol, 6 g Dietary Fiber

SHRIMP SCAMPI

*A lower-calorie version of the Italian classic,
with all the great flavor!*

MAKES 4 SERVINGS

1 tablespoon + 1 teaspoon olive oil
1 pound, 4 ounces shelled and deveined medium
  shrimp, tails left on
1 tablespoon minced garlic
$\frac{1}{2}$ cup low-sodium chicken broth
4 fluid ounces ($\frac{1}{2}$ cup) dry white wine
$\frac{1}{4}$ cup fresh lemon juice
$\frac{1}{4}$ cup minced parsley
$\frac{1}{4}$ teaspoon salt
$\frac{1}{4}$ teaspoon freshly ground black pepper
4 fresh lemon slices to garnish (optional)
1 tablespoon minced fresh parsley to garnish
  (optional)

1. In large skillet, heat oil. Add shrimp and cook, stirring constantly, over high heat, 2 minutes, or just until pink. Add garlic and cook, stirring constantly, about 30 seconds. Using slotted spoon, transfer shrimp to serving platter; keep hot.

2. To same skillet, add broth, wine, lemon juice, parsley, salt and pepper. Increase heat to high. Boil, uncovered, until sauce is reduced by half. Spoon over shrimp. Coat lemon slices with parsley; arrange on platter to garnish, if desired.

EACH SERVING (4 ounces shrimp and $\frac{1}{4}$ of the sauce) PROVIDES: 1 Fat, 2 Proteins, 30 Optional Calories
PER SERVING: 223 Calories, 29 g Protein, 7 g Fat, 4 g Carbohydrate, 355 mg Sodium, 215 mg Cholesterol, 0 g Dietary Fiber

SHRIMP CREOLE

MAKES 4 SERVINGS

1 tablespoon + 1 teaspoon olive oil
1 cup chopped onions
1 cup chopped red bell pepper
2 teaspoons minced garlic
24 medium deveined shrimp, tails removed
3 cups canned low-sodium stewed tomatoes
2 cups sliced fresh or frozen okra
$\frac{1}{2}$ teaspoon salt
$\frac{1}{2}$ teaspoon chili powder
$\frac{1}{2}$ teaspoon freshly ground black pepper
$\frac{1}{2}$ teaspoon dried thyme leaves
$\frac{1}{8}$ teaspoon mace
2 whole allspice
2 whole cloves
1 bay leaf
1 tablespoon cornstarch
2 cups cooked regular long-grain rice
Parsley sprigs to garnish (optional)

1. In large saucepan, heat oil; add onions, bell pepper and garlic. Cook, stirring frequently, 5 minutes, until tender. Add shrimp, tomatoes, okra, salt, chili powder, pepper, thyme, mace, allspice, cloves and bay leaf. Cover and simmer 20 minutes. Remove bay leaf.

2. Mix cornstarch with 2 tablespoons cold water. Stir into pan; cook 1–2 minutes, stirring until thickened.

3. Spread rice around edge of serving plate. Spoon shrimp mixture in center and garnish with parsley, if desired.

EACH SERVING (1$\frac{1}{4}$ cups shrimp and $\frac{1}{2}$ cup rice) PROVIDES: 1 Fat, 3$\frac{1}{2}$ Vegetables, 1$\frac{1}{2}$ Proteins, 1 Bread, 10 Optional Calories
PER SERVING: 366 Calories, 24 g Protein, 7 g Fat, 54 g Carbohydrate, 445 mg Sodium, 129 mg Cholesterol, 8 g Dietary Fiber

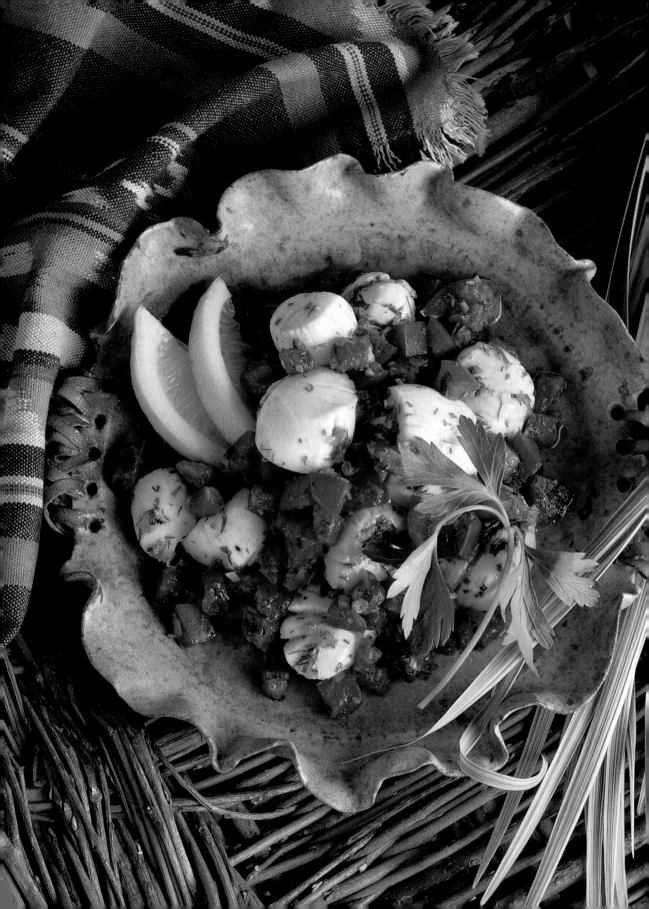

SCALLOPS SEVICHE

You can buy garlic oil, or make your own by adding several crushed garlic cloves to a bottle of vegetable oil.

MAKES 4 SERVINGS

10 ounces sea scallops
2 cups low-sodium chicken broth
$\frac{1}{2}$ cup fresh lemon juice
$1\frac{1}{2}$ cups chopped seeded peeled tomatoes
$\frac{1}{2}$ cup finely minced scallions
1 tablespoon + 1 teaspoon garlic oil
1 tablespoon finely chopped fresh chives
1 tablespoon finely chopped fresh dill
1 tablespoon finely chopped fresh parsley
1 tablespoon finely chopped fresh tarragon
$\frac{1}{4}$ teaspoon finely ground black pepper
$\frac{1}{8}$ teaspoon salt
4 parsley sprigs to garnish (optional)
4 lemon slices to garnish (optional)

1. Wash the scallops in cold water and pat dry with paper towels. In medium skillet, bring the chicken broth to a simmer over medium-high heat. Add scallops; cover and poach for 2–3 minutes or until opaque. Transfer to a colander and rinse with cold water. Slice horizontally $\frac{1}{4}$" thick.

2. Pour the juice into a gallon-size sealable plastic bag; add scallops. Seal bag, squeezing out air; turn to coat scallops. Refrigerate for 24 hours, turning bag occasionally.

3. When ready to serve, drain off liquid from the scallops and discard. Stir in tomatoes, scallions, oil, chives, dill, parsley, tarragon, pepper and salt.

4. Spoon the scallops onto four serving plates. Garnish each serving with a parsley sprig and lemon slice, if desired.

EACH SERVING ($\frac{3}{4}$ cup) PROVIDES: 1 Fat, 1 Vegetable, 1 Protein, 10 Optional Calories
PER SERVING: 125 Calories, 13 g Protein, 5 g Fat, 7 g Carbohydrate, 258 mg Sodium, 23 mg Cholesterol, 1 g Dietary Fiber

SHRIMP ÉTOUFFÉE

MAKES 4 SERVINGS

2 tablespoons vegetable oil
3 tablespoons all-purpose flour
1 cup chopped celery
1 cup chopped onions
1 cup chopped green bell pepper
1 cup sliced scallions
1 tablespoon minced garlic
2 cups low-sodium chicken broth, hot
1 tablespoon minced fresh parsley
1 teaspoon salt
1 teaspoon fresh lemon juice
$\frac{1}{4}$ teaspoon freshly ground black pepper
$\frac{1}{8}$ teaspoon ground red pepper
15 ounces shelled and deveined shrimp, tails removed
$3\frac{1}{2}$ cups cooked regular long-grain rice

1. In heavy small saucepan, heat 1 tablespoon + 1 teaspoon oil. Add flour, stirring constantly. Cook over low heat, about 15 minutes, until medium-brown.

2. In large saucepan, heat remaining 2 teaspoons oil. Sauté celery, onions, bell pepper, scallions and garlic for 15 minutes, stirring frequently, until tender.

3. Whisk broth into flour mixture until smooth. Add broth mixture to vegetable mixture. Mix in parsley, salt, juice, black pepper and red pepper. Simmer 5 minutes.

4. Add shrimp and simmer 5 minutes, until shrimp are opaque.

5. Serve over cooked rice.

EACH SERVING (1 cup shrimp mixture and heaping $\frac{3}{4}$ cup rice) PROVIDES: $1\frac{1}{2}$ Fats, 2 Vegetables, $1\frac{1}{2}$ Proteins, 2 Breads, 10 Optional Calories
PER SERVING: 480 Calories, 30 g Protein, 10 g Fat, 65 g Carbohydrate, 771 mg Sodium, 162 mg Cholesterol, 3 g Dietary Fiber

CARIBBEAN SHRIMP CURRY

MAKES 4 SERVINGS

1 tablespoon + 1 teaspoon vegetable oil
1 cup sliced carrots
1 cup sliced onions
1 tablespoon curry powder
15 ounces peeled and deveined medium shrimp, tails removed
2 small pared chopped apples
1 cup cauliflower florets
$\frac{1}{2}$ cup sliced plantain
1 tablespoon cornstarch dissolved in 1$\frac{1}{4}$ cups cold water
$\frac{1}{4}$ cup mango chutney
$\frac{1}{2}$ vegetable bouillon cube
$\frac{1}{2}$ teaspoon salt
3 cups cooked basmati or white rice
1 tablespoon + 1 teaspoon toasted, unsweetened shredded coconut
2 sprigs fresh coriander leaves to garnish (optional)

1. In large nonstick skillet, heat oil; add carrots, onions and curry. Stir-fry over medium-low heat 15 minutes, stirring often, until vegetables begin to soften. Add shrimp, apple, cauliflower and plantain; continue to cook, stirring frequently, 2 minutes, until shrimp begin to turn pink. Add cornstarch mixture, chutney and bouillon cube; bring to a simmer and cook, stirring, over low heat.

2. Line serving platter with rice; spoon curry mixture in center. Sprinkle with coconut; garnish with coriander.

EACH SERVING (2 cups) PROVIDES: 1 Fat, $\frac{1}{2}$ Fruit, 1$\frac{1}{2}$ Vegetables, 1$\frac{1}{2}$ Proteins, 1$\frac{3}{4}$ Breads, 45 Optional Calories
PER SERVING: 510 Calories, 28 g Protein, 8 g Fat, 80 g Carbohydrate, 857 mg Sodium, 162 mg Cholesterol, 4 g Dietary Fiber

ASIAN STIR-FRIED SHRIMP

Hoisin sauce gives this enticing stir-fry its unique spicing. It's generally available in the international section of the supermarket.

MAKES 4 SERVINGS

1 tablespoon + 1 teaspoon sesame oil
1 cup oyster mushrooms, sliced
1 cup thinly sliced red bell pepper strips
1 cup chopped scallions
1 tablespoon minced garlic
1$\frac{1}{2}$ teaspoons grated fresh ginger root
1 pound 4 ounces peeled and deveined medium shrimp, tails removed
1 cup bean sprouts
1 cup snow peas
$\frac{3}{4}$ cup canned water chestnuts
3 tablespoons hoisin sauce
2 teaspoons rice vinegar
$\frac{1}{2}$ teaspoon salt
2$\frac{1}{2}$ cups cooked rice noodles
2 cucumber twists to garnish (optional)
2 radish flowers to garnish (optional)

1. In wok or large deep skillet, heat oil; add mushrooms, bell peppers, scallions, garlic and ginger. Stir-fry over high heat 1 minute, until vegetables begin to soften. Add shrimp, bean sprouts, snow peas and water chestnuts. Stir-fry 2–3 minutes, just until shrimp turn opaque.

2. Stir in hoisin sauce, rice vinegar and salt, and stir-fry 1 minute more, just until sauce bubbles.

3. Line serving dish with noodles; spoon shrimp mixture in center. Garnish with cucumber and radishes, if desired.

EACH SERVING (2 cups) PROVIDES: 1 Fat, 2$\frac{1}{2}$ Vegetables, 2 Proteins, 1$\frac{1}{2}$ Breads, 25 Optional Calories
PER SERVING: 363 Calories, 34 g Protein, 7 g Fat, 39 g Carbohydrate, 880 mg Sodium, 216 mg Cholesterol, 2 g Dietary Fiber

SHRIMP TERIYAKI ON THE GRILL

MAKES 4 SERVINGS

1 pound 4 ounces peeled and deveined large
  shrimp, tails left on
$\frac{1}{4}$ cup + 2 tablespoons teriyaki sauce
$\frac{1}{2}$ medium fresh pineapple, cut into 1" cubes
2 medium red bell peppers, cored, seeded and cut
  into 1" cubes
4 cups cooked regular long-grain rice
1 cup julienned scallions

1. Spray grill rack with nonstick cooking spray. Place grill rack 5" from coals. Soak eight wooden skewers in cold water. Prepare grill according to manufacturer's directions.

2. Meanwhile, marinate the shrimp: Place them in a gallon-size sealable plastic bag and pour in $\frac{1}{4}$ cup teriyaki sauce. Seal, squeezing out the air; turn to coat shrimp. Refrigerate at least 2 hours, turning bag occasionally.

3. Drain shrimp. Discard teriyaki sauce. On eight soaked wooden skewers, alternately thread shrimp, pineapple and bell pepper.

4. Grill kabobs 12–15 minutes, turning frequently, until cooked through.

5. Serve on a bed of steamed rice. Sprinkle with remaining 2 tablespoons teriyaki sauce, if desired. Garnish with scallions.

EACH SERVING (2 kabobs and 1 cup rice) PROVIDES: 1 Fruit, 1$\frac{1}{2}$ Vegetables, 2 Proteins, 2 Breads, 30 Optional Calories
PER SERVING: 496 Calories, 37 g Protein, 4 g Fat, 77 g Carbohydrate, 910 mg Sodium, 215 mg Cholesterol, 3 g Dietary Fiber

BROILED SHRIMP TERIYAKI

Spray broiler rack with nonstick cooking spray. Preheat broiler. On eight 12" metal skewers, alternately thread shrimp, pineapple and bell pepper. Arrange skewers on rack in broiler pan. Broil about 5" from heat about 6 minutes, until shrimp are opaque, turning once.

Nothing Fishy!

When buying fresh fish and shellfish, use your nose—there should be no fishy odor. Whole fish should have bright, nonsunken eyes and shiny, resilient skin. Look for compact and moist fresh fillets with no dryness around the edges. Shrimp should be clear and pinkish. Both shrimp and scallops should have a firm texture and a sweet smell.

When you get your fish home, wrap it in an air-tight package and keep it in the coldest part of the refrigerator; use within three days. Clams, mussels and oysters should be tightly closed; when shucked, their meat should be plump and juicy. If any shells don't open after cooking, discard them.

PAPARDELLE WITH SHRIMP

Papardelle are long, flat egg noodles cut with a pretty crimped edge. If you like, you can substitute egg noodles for the papardelle.

MAKES 4 SERVINGS

6 ounces uncooked papardelle pasta or wide noodles

2 tablespoons + 2 teaspoons reduced-calorie tub margarine

13 ounces peeled and deveined medium shrimp, tails removed

$1\frac{1}{2}$ teaspoons curry powder

2 fluid ounces ($\frac{1}{4}$ cup) dry white wine

$\frac{3}{4}$ cup low-sodium chicken broth

2 large eggs

$\frac{3}{4}$ ounce grated Parmesan cheese

3 tablespoons finely chopped mint

$\frac{1}{2}$ teaspoon salt

$\frac{1}{4}$ teaspoon freshly ground black pepper

4 fresh lime slices to garnish (optional)

4 fresh mint sprigs to garnish (optional)

1. In large pot of boiling water, cook pasta 8–9 minutes, until tender. Drain and keep warm.

2. In large nonstick skillet, melt margarine; add shrimp and curry powder; cook 2–3 minutes, just until shrimp begin to turn opaque. Add wine; bring to a boil, then add broth. In small bowl, beat together eggs and cheese; gradually whisk $\frac{1}{2}$ cup hot broth mixture into egg mixture. Pour egg mixture into skillet, whisking constantly. Reduce heat and stir in pasta. Stir over low heat, 2–3 minutes, until sauce thickens and pasta is heated through.

3. Sprinkle with chopped mint, salt and pepper. Toss to combine thoroughly. Garnish with lime slices and mint, if desired.

EACH SERVING (2 cups) PROVIDES: 1 Fat, 2 Proteins, 2 Breads, 15 Optional Calories
PER SERVING: 379 Calories, 31 g Protein, 12 g Fat, 33 g Carbohydrate, 635 mg Sodium, 291 mg Cholesterol, 2 g Dietary Fiber

---

Catch of the Day

◆

All fish are not created equal, as you see at a glance at the chart below. When cooking fish, you'll find it helpful to keep their fat content in mind when planning meals.

	Calories	Protein (grams)	Fat (grams)	Sodium (mg)	Cholesterol (mg)
Bluefish	180	29	6	87	85
Cod	118	26	1	88	63
Haddock	127	27	1	99	84
Halibut	159	30	3	79	47
Orange Roughy	100	21	1	92	29
Perch, Ocean	132	28	1	89	130
Rockfish (Snapper)	137	27	2	87	51
Sea Bass	140	27	3	99	60
Swordfish	176	29	6	130	57
Tuna, Yellowfin	157	34	1	53	65

(per 4-ounce cooked, edible portion)

CURRIED SHRIMP AND RICE SALAD

MAKES 4 SERVINGS

1 cup finely chopped onions
$\frac{1}{2}$ cup low-sodium chicken broth
1 tablespoon curry powder
2 tablespoons apricot spreadable fruit
2 tablespoons golden raisins
4 ounces white or basmati rice
2 small unpared McIntosh apples
2 medium bananas, peeled and cut into $\frac{1}{4}$"-thick slices
1 tablespoon fresh lemon juice
12 ounces cooked, peeled and deveined medium shrimp
1 cup chopped celery
$1\frac{1}{2}$ cups plain nonfat yogurt
2 tablespoons + 2 teaspoons reduced-calorie mayonnaise
$\frac{1}{2}$ teaspoon salt
2 cups Boston, bibb or other lettuce leaves
Lime slices to garnish (optional)
Cilantro to garnish (optional)

1. In small saucepan, bring onions, broth and curry powder to a gentle boil. Reduce heat; simmer until onions are soft, about 5–7 minutes. Remove from heat. Stir in spreadable fruit and raisins; cool completely.

2. Cook rice until tender, according to package directions. Rinse, drain and refrigerate.

3. Core apples and cut into 1" cubes. In medium bowl, toss apples with banana slices and juice. Stir in shrimp, celery and rice. In medium bowl, whisk together the broth mixture with the yogurt, mayonnaise and salt. Pour over the fruit and shrimp mixture and stir gently to coat.

4. Serve on bed of lettuce leaves; garnish with fresh lime slices and cilantro leaves, if desired.

EACH SERVING ($1\frac{1}{2}$ cups) PROVIDES: $\frac{1}{2}$ Milk, 1 Fat, $2\frac{1}{4}$ Fruits, 2 Vegetables, $1\frac{1}{2}$ Proteins, 1 Bread, 3 Optional Calories
PER SERVING: 413 Calories, 27 g Protein, 5 g Fat, 67 g Carbohydrate, 622 mg Sodium, 171 mg Cholesterol, 4 g Dietary Fiber

SHRIMP ZITI

MAKES 4 SERVINGS

1 tablespoon + 1 teaspoon olive oil
2 cups grated unpared zucchini
10 ounces peeled and deveined medium shrimp
1 cup tomato sauce
$\frac{1}{4}$ cup Neufchâtel cheese
$\frac{1}{2}$ teaspoon salt
$\frac{1}{2}$ teaspoon freshly ground black pepper
4 cups cooked ziti pasta (hot)
Fresh basil leaves to garnish (optional)

1. In large nonstick skillet, heat oil; add zucchini. Cook, stirring frequently, 1–2 minutes, just until tender. Stir in shrimp, tomato sauce, cheese, salt and pepper. Cook, stirring, 3–4 minutes, until shrimp are pink and mixture is well blended.

2. Place hot pasta in heated serving bowl and pour shrimp mixture over it. Toss to thoroughly combine.

3. Garnish with fresh basil, if desired.

EACH SERVING (2 cups) PROVIDES: 1 Fat, 2 Vegetables, 1 Protein, 2 Breads, 35 Optional Calories
PER SERVING: 377 Calories, 24 g Protein, 10 g Fat, 47 g Carbohydrate, 807 mg Sodium, 119 mg Cholesterol, 4 g Dietary Fiber

SEAFOOD LASAGNA

MAKES 4 SERVINGS

8 ounces uncooked lasagna noodles
2½ cups canned plum tomatoes, well drained
1½ cups chopped watercress
1 cup sliced mushrooms
1 cup chopped onion
2 tablespoons low-sodium tomato paste
¾ teaspoon salt
½ teaspoon freshly ground black pepper
8 ounces haddock fillet, cubed
8 peeled and deveined medium shrimp, tails removed
1½ cups plain nonfat yogurt
⅔ cup low-fat cottage cheese
1 large egg, lightly beaten
¼ teaspoon freshly ground nutmeg
2 tablespoons + 2 teaspoons Parmesan cheese
½ cup fresh watercress
1 sliced medium tomato

1. Preheat oven to 375°F. Spray a 9 × 9" ovenproof dish with nonfat cooking spray. In large pot of boiling water, cook lasagna noodles 9 minutes, just until tender. Rinse with cold water; lay flat on paper towels to drain.

2. In medium saucepan, bring tomatoes, watercress, mushrooms, onions, tomato paste, ½ teaspoon of the salt and ¼ teaspoon of the pepper to a boil. Reduce heat; simmer 5 minutes. Add haddock and shrimp; simmer 3–4 minutes longer, just until shrimp turns opaque.

3. In medium bowl, beat together yogurt, cottage cheese, egg, the remaining ¼ teaspoon salt, the remaining ¼ teaspoon pepper and the nutmeg.

4. In ovenproof dish, layer one-third of the fish sauce, one-third of the yogurt-cheese mixture and one-third of the lasagna noodles; repeat 2 times, ending with lasagna noodles. Sprinkle with Parmesan cheese; bake 1 hour.

5. Top with watercress and fresh tomato slices.

EACH SERVING (13½ ounces) PROVIDES: ½ Milk, 4 Vegetables, 2 Proteins, 2½ Breads, 35 Optional Calories
PER SERVING: 498 Calories, 45 g Protein, 6 g Fat, 65 g Carbohydrate, 871 mg Sodium, 177 mg Cholesterol, 5 g Dietary Fiber

PAELLA

Paella is a traditional Spanish dish that includes various meats and fish in a rice base. Our paella features chicken instead of meat, combined with shrimp and mussels in saffron-flavored rice.

MAKES 4 SERVINGS

1 tablespoon + 1 teaspoon olive oil
1 cup thinly sliced red onion
1 cup coarsely chopped red bell pepper
2 tablespoons minced garlic
6 ounces regular long-grain rice
5 ounces thin-sliced chicken cutlets
3 cups low-sodium chicken broth
10 ounces peeled and deveined medium shrimp, tails left on
Pinch saffron strands (optional)
12 medium mussels, cooked
4 ounces drained canned garbanzo beans
2 tablespoons minced fresh parsley
½ teaspoon salt
¼ teaspoon freshly ground black pepper

1. In large skillet, heat oil; add onion, bell pepper and garlic. Cook, stirring frequently, 5 minutes, until tender. Stir in rice and chicken. Continue to cook, 2 minutes, until chicken is lightly browned.

2. Stir in broth, shrimp and saffron, if using. Bring to a gentle boil; reduce heat, cover and simmer until most of the liquid is absorbed. Stir in mussels, garbanzo beans, parsley, salt and pepper.

3. Continue to cook, covered, until all liquid is absorbed.

EACH SERVING (3 cups) PROVIDES: 1 Fat, 1 Vegetable, 2½ Proteins, 2 Breads, 15 Optional Calories
PER SERVING: 422 Calories, 34 g Protein, 9 g Fat, 49 g Carbohydrate, 587 mg Sodium, 136 mg Cholesterol, 3 g Dietary Fiber

CALIFORNIA SEAFOOD SALAD

MAKES 4 SERVINGS

¼ cup clam-tomato juice or tomato juice
¼ cup fresh lemon juice
1 tablespoon + 1 teaspoon olive oil
1 tablespoon Worcestershire sauce
¼ teaspoon salt
¼ teaspoon freshly grated black pepper
4 cups romaine or other lettuce, washed and torn into bite-size leaves
4 ounces cooked crab meat
8 medium cooked shrimp, tails left on
12 cherry tomatoes, halved
2 ounces avocado, sliced
2 medium oranges, peeled and sliced into semicircles
2 ounces Croutons (page 357)

1. To make dressing, in small bowl, whisk together clam-tomato juice, lemon juice, oil, Worcestershire sauce, salt and pepper. Cover and refrigerate.

2. Line serving platter with lettuce; mound crab meat in center. Alternately arrange shrimp and tomato halves in a circle around the crab, then avocado and orange slices in a second circle around the outside.

3. Pour dressing over salad. Sprinkle with croutons and serve.

EACH SERVING PROVIDES: 1½ Fats, ½ Fruit, 2¾ Vegetables, 1 Protein, ½ Bread
PER SERVING: 250 Calories, 21 g Protein, 9 g Fat, 23 g Carbohydrate, 546 mg Sodium, 139 mg Cholesterol, 4 g Dietary Fiber

SEAFOOD EN PAPILLOTTE

MAKES 4 SERVINGS

24 medium unpeeled shrimp
12 medium mussels, scrubbed
5 ounces sea scallops
½ cup chopped chives
4 fluid ounces (½ cup) dry white wine
1 tablespoon + 1 teaspoon olive oil
1 tablespoon minced garlic
1 teaspoon salt
½ teaspoon freshly ground black pepper
8 lemon slices
8 sprigs parsley

1. Spray grill rack with nonstick cooking spray. Place grill rack 5" from coals. Prepare grill according to manfacturer's directions.

2. Cut four 18" squares of double-thickness heavy-duty foil. Lay out on flat surface.

3. Arrange shrimp, mussels and scallops evenly in center of each square of foil. Sprinkle evenly with chives, wine, oil, garlic, salt and pepper; top with lemon slices and parsley.

4. Fold bottom right-hand corner of foil over to meet top left-hand corner, forming a large triangular packet. Close the packet tightly by making overlapping folds along the two opened sides.

5. Place foil packets on grill; cook 30 minutes. Carefully transfer packets to serving plates. To serve, cut open in center, avoiding the steam.

EACH SERVING (2 cups) PROVIDES: 1 Fat, 2½ Proteins, 25 Optional Calories
PER SERVING: 183 Calories, 21 g Protein, 7 g Fat, 4 g Carbohydrate, 775 mg Sodium, 166 mg Cholesterol, 0 g Dietary Fiber

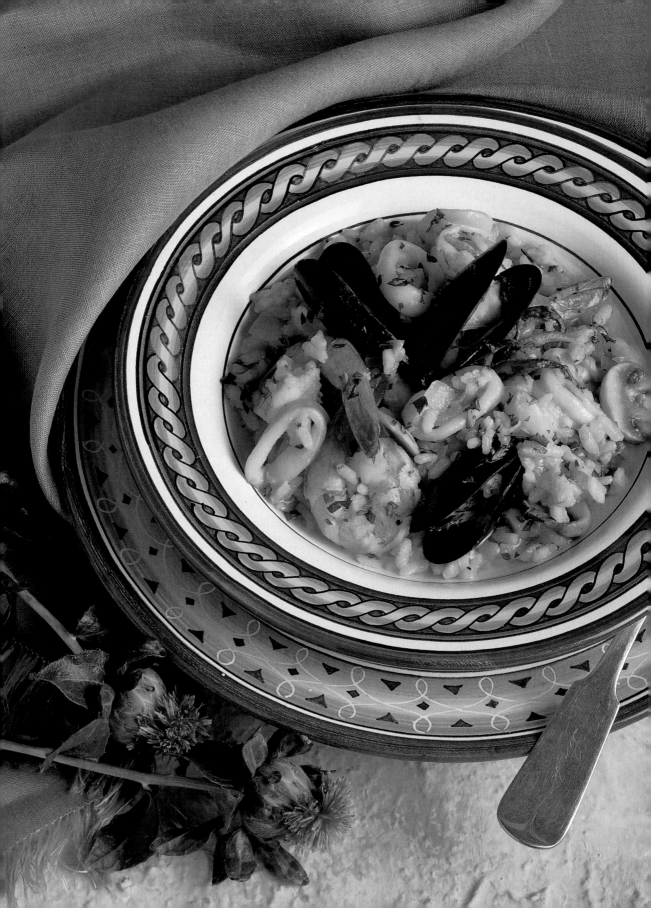

SEAFOOD RISOTTO

If you like, substitute fish or vegetable bouillon for the white wine, and reduce your Optional Calories to 20.

MAKES 4 SERVINGS

1 tablespoon + 1 teaspoon olive oil
1 cup chopped onion
2 teaspoons minced garlic
8 ounces arborio or other short-grain rice
1 fish or vegetable bouillon cube
3 cups boiling water
8 fluid ounces (1 cup) dry white wine
2 teaspoons dried mixed herbs
10 ounces cleaned calamari
2 cups sorrel or spinach leaves
1 cup sliced mushrooms
$\frac{3}{4}$ teaspoon salt
$\frac{1}{2}$ teaspoon freshly ground black pepper
12 medium mussels in their shells
8 ounces shelled, deveined and cooked medium
  shrimp
1 tablespoon + 1 teaspoon grated Parmesan cheese
2 tablespoons fresh minced parsley

1. In large, deep skillet, heat oil; add onions and garlic; cook, stirring frequently, 5 minutes, until tender. Add rice. Continue cooking and stirring 2 minutes longer.

2. In large measuring cup, dissolve bouillon cube in boiling water. Stir in wine. Pour 1 cup of the liquid over rice mixture in skillet; add mixed herbs. Bring to a gentle boil, stirring until all the liquid is absorbed. Repeat with another cup of liquid.

3. Add calamari and 1 more cup of the bouillon mixture to the rice mixture in skillet, cooking gently until liquid is absorbed. Stir in sorrel, mushrooms, salt and pepper.

4. Meanwhile, in medium-size saucepan, bring remaining cup liquid to a boil. Add the mussels; steam, covered, 4–5 minutes, until their shells open; drain. Add to the rice mixture. Stir in shrimp. Continue to cook, covered, until the liquid has been absorbed and shrimp are heated through.

5. Remove from heat; stir in cheese. Sprinkle with parsley and serve immediately.

EACH SERVING (2 cups) PROVIDES: 1 Fat, 2 Vegetables, 2½ Proteins, 2 Breads, 65 Optional Calories
PER SERVING: 464 Calories, 32 g Protein, 8 g Fat, 55 g Carbohydrate, 919 mg Sodium, 285 mg Cholesterol, 2 g Dietary Fiber

JAMBALAYA

MAKES 4 SERVINGS

1 tablespoon vegetable oil
1 cup chopped onion
2 tablespoons minced garlic
8 ounces regular long-grain rice
2 cups low-sodium chicken broth
2 cups low-sodium chopped drained canned peeled
    tomatoes
2 ounces lean ham, diced
2 teaspoons chopped fresh thyme leaves
$\frac{1}{2}$ teaspoon salt
$\frac{1}{8}$–$\frac{1}{4}$ teaspoon dried, crushed chili pepper
$\frac{1}{4}$ teaspoon ground white pepper
15 ounces peeled and deveined medium shrimp,
    tails removed
1 tablespoon chopped fresh parsley to garnish
    (optional)

1. In large saucepan, heat oil; add onions and garlic. Cook, stirring frequently, 5 minutes, until tender. Add rice; cook, 1 minute, stirring constantly. Stir in broth, tomatoes, ham, thyme, salt, chili pepper and white pepper.

2. Bring to boil; reduce heat; cover. Simmer 10 minutes; add shrimp and cook 5 or 10 minutes, until rice is soft. Garnish with parsley, if desired.

EACH SERVING (1$\frac{3}{4}$ cups) PROVIDES: $\frac{3}{4}$ Fat, 1$\frac{1}{2}$ Vegetables, 2 Proteins, 2 Breads, 10 Optional Calories
PER SERVING: 431 Calories, 31 g Protein, 7 g Fat, 58 g Carbohydrate, 681 mg Sodium, 168 mg Cholesterol, 2 g Dietary Fiber

Shrimp and Vegetable Rice (page 288)

CHAPTER TEN

PASTA, GRAINS AND RICE

ANGEL HAIR PASTA WITH FRESH TOMATO SAUCE

MAKES 6 SERVINGS

5 cups chopped ripe tomatoes
1 cup chopped onions
$\frac{1}{2}$ cup chopped fresh basil
$\frac{1}{4}$ cup red wine vinegar
2 tablespoons olive oil
3 garlic cloves, minced
1 teaspoon granulated sugar
$4\frac{1}{2}$ ounces uncooked angel hair pasta
12 ounces grated part-skim mozzarella cheese

1. In large bowl, combine tomatoes, onions, basil, vinegar, oil, garlic and sugar; stir to mix well. Cover with plastic wrap; let stand at room temperature at least 4 hours.

2. Meanwhile, in large pot of boiling water, cook pasta 2 minutes, until tender; drain. Transfer pasta to large serving bowl; top with prepared sauce and cheese. Gently toss to mix well.

EACH SERVING PROVIDES: 1 Fat, 2 Vegetables, 2½ Proteins, 1 Bread, 15 Optional Calories
PER SERVING: 314 Calories, 18 g Protein, 14 g Fat, 29 g Carbohydrate, 281 mg Sodium, 33 mg Cholesterol, 3 g Dietary Fiber

ROSEMARY-ZUCCHINI PASTA

MAKES 6 SERVINGS

1 tablespoon margarine
3 garlic cloves, minced
2 cups sliced zucchini
2 cups sliced yellow summer squash
1 cup red bell pepper strips
1 cup canned crushed tomatoes
$\frac{1}{2}$ cup orange juice
1 tablespoon fresh rosemary leaves
2 teaspoons chicken bouillon granules
3 cups cooked pasta wheels (hot)
$\frac{1}{4}$ cup chopped fresh parsley

1. In large nonstick skillet, heat margarine over low heat; add garlic. Cook, stirring frequently, 5 minutes. Add zucchini, squash and bell pepper; sauté 2–3 minutes.

2. Stir in tomatoes, juice, $\frac{1}{2}$ cup water, the rosemary, and bouillon; stir to combine. Reduce heat to low; simmer 5 minutes, or until vegetables are tender-crisp. Remove from heat.

3. Stir in pasta; transfer to large serving bowl. Sprinkle with parsley.

EACH SERVING PROVIDES: ½ Fat, 2 Vegetables, 1 Bread, 15 Optional Calories
PER SERVING: 159 Calories, 5 g Protein, 3 g Fat, 29 g Carbohydrate, 393 mg Sodium, 1 mg Cholesterol, 3 g Dietary Fiber

RIGATONI WITH HOT VEGETABLE SAUCE

MAKES 6 SERVINGS

$5\frac{1}{2}$ cups frozen broccoli, cauliflower and carrot medley (two 16-ounce bags)
1 tablespoon instant minced onion
3 chicken bouillon cubes
$1\frac{1}{2}$ teaspoons garlic powder
1 teaspoon dried basil leaves
$\frac{1}{8}$ teaspoon freshly ground black pepper
2 tablespoons cornstarch, dissolved in $\frac{1}{4}$ cup water
3 cups cooked rigatoni (hot)

1. To prepare sauce, in large saucepan, combine vegetable medley, 1 cup water, the minced onion, bouillon, garlic powder, basil and black pepper; bring to a boil.

2. Reduce heat to low; simmer 5–10 minutes, until vegetables are heated through. Return to a boil; stir in dissolved cornstarch. Cook 2–3 minutes, stirring constantly, until thickened.

3. Add rigatoni; toss to mix well.

EACH SERVING PROVIDES: $1\frac{3}{4}$ Vegetables, 1 Bread, 15 Optional Calories
PER SERVING: 163 Calories, 7 g Protein, 1 g Fat, 33 g Carbohydrate, 599 mg Sodium, 0 mg Cholesterol, 5 g Dietary Fiber

ORZO WITH GARLIC-GINGERED SPRING VEGETABLES

Orzo is a tiny, rice-shaped pasta—a perfect pair with brilliant spring vegetables.

MAKES 6 SERVINGS

$4\frac{1}{2}$ ounces uncooked orzo
1 tablespoon olive oil
2 tablespoons minced fresh ginger root
3 garlic cloves, crushed
2 cups sliced baby carrots
2 cups sliced baby zucchini
1 cup chopped red bell pepper
1 cup chopped yellow bell pepper
1 teaspoon chicken bouillon granules, dissolved in $\frac{3}{4}$ cup boiling water
$\frac{1}{8}$ teaspoon freshly ground black pepper, or to taste

1. In medium saucepan, bring 3 cups water to a boil; stir in orzo. Reduce heat to low; simmer 8–10 minutes, or until orzo is tender. Drain; set aside.

2. In wok or large skillet, heat oil; add ginger and garlic. Cook over low heat, stirring frequently, 5 minutes.

3. Increase heat to high; add carrots. Stir-fry, adding zucchini, red bell pepper, yellow bell pepper and dissolved boullion granules. Cook, stirring occasionally, 3 minutes, until vegetables are tender-crisp.

4. Add cooked orzo and black pepper; toss to mix well. Serve immediately.

EACH SERVING PROVIDES: $\frac{1}{2}$ Fat, 2 Vegetables, 1 Bread, 2 Optional Calories
PER SERVING: 134 Calories, 4 g Protein, 3 g Fat, 24 g Carbohydrate, 177 mg Sodium, 0 mg Cholesterol, 2 g Dietary Fiber

CHINESE NOODLES IN SESAME-SOY SAUCE

MAKES 6 SERVINGS

2 tablespoons reduced-sodium soy sauce
1 tablespoon dark sesame oil
1 teaspoon granulated sugar
1 teaspoon white wine vinegar
4 cups julienned pared cucumbers
3 cups cooked vermicelli or rice noodles (hot)
$\frac{1}{2}$ cup chopped scallions (green portion only)

1. To prepare sauce, in small bowl, combine soy sauce, sesame oil, sugar and vinegar; stir to mix well. Set aside.

2. In large bowl, combine cucumbers, vermicelli and prepared sauce; toss to mix well. Transfer to serving platter; sprinkle with scallions.

EACH SERVING PROVIDES: $\frac{1}{2}$ Fat, $1\frac{1}{2}$ Vegetables, 1 Bread, 3 Optional Calories
PER SERVING: 140 Calories, 4 g Protein, 3 g Fat, 25 g Carbohydrate, 208 mg Sodium, 0 mg Cholesterol, 2 g Dietary Fiber

ORIENTAL RICE NOODLES AND SCALLIONS IN CILANTRO SAUCE

MAKES 6 SERVINGS

6 ounces uncooked rice noodles
$\frac{1}{4}$ cup chopped fresh cilantro
3 tablespoons soy sauce
1 tablespoon creamy peanut butter
1 tablespoon white wine vinegar
$1\frac{1}{2}$ cups diagonally sliced scallions

1. In small saucepan, bring $2\frac{1}{2}$ cups water to a boil; add rice noodles. Remove from heat; cover and let stand 5–7 minutes, until noodles are tender. Pour into strainer; rinse under running cold water. Drain well.

2. Meanwhile, in food processor or blender, combine 2 tablespoons of the cilantro, the soy sauce, peanut butter and vinegar; process until smooth.

3. In large bowl, combine cooked rice noodles, the remaining 2 tablespoons cilantro and the scallions. Pour cilantro sauce over noodle mixture; gently toss to coat.

EACH SERVING PROVIDES: $\frac{1}{2}$ Fat, $\frac{1}{2}$ Vegetable, 1 Bread
PER SERVING: 131 Calories, 3 g Protein, 1 g Fat, 26 g Carbohydrate, 535 mg Sodium, 0 mg Cholesterol, 1 g Dietary Fiber

---

Low-Fat Pasta

Pasta has always been a low-fat favorite, but the sauce on pasta can be a high-fat trap. To keep your pasta high on flavor and low on fat, follow these tasty sauce suggestions.

- *Make tomato or vegetable-based sauces, such as Rigatoni with Hot Vegetable Sauce (page 269).*
- *For cream sauces, use low-fat milk or evaporated skimmed milk; nonfat yogurt; fat-free mayonnaise; or low-fat or fat-free sour cream—see Lemon-Dilled Pasta Salad (page 276).*
- *Top pasta with your favorite herbs and spices and a light sprinkle of Parmesan cheese.*
- *When preparing a meaty pasta dish, choose skinless poultry, lean cuts of meat or fish.*
- *Add beans or lentils to pasta for a protein punch.*

MULTI-MUSHROOM CHINESE SPAGHETTI

Vermicelli takes on the woodsy aroma and meaty flavor of wild mushrooms with intriguing undertones in this rich and satisfying sauce.

MAKES 6 SERVINGS

1 tablespoon margarine
2" pared fresh ginger root, minced
4 garlic cloves, finely minced
$\frac{1}{4}$ cup minced onion
3 cups sliced cremini mushrooms
3 cups sliced shiitake mushrooms
1 tablespoon chicken bouillon granules
1 tablespoon fresh lemon juice
$\frac{1}{2}$ teaspoon ground red pepper
2 tablespoons cornstarch, dissolved in $\frac{1}{4}$ cup water
3 cups bean sprouts
3 cups cooked vermicelli (hot)
$\frac{1}{4}$ cup chopped scallions (green portion only)

1. In large nonstick skillet, melt margarine over low heat; add ginger and garlic. Cook, stirring frequently, 5–7 minutes. Increase heat to medium; add onion. Sauté until browned; add cremini and shiitake mushrooms. Sauté 2–3 minutes.

2. Add 1 cup water, the bouillon granules, juice and red pepper. Reduce heat to low; simmer, stirring occasionally, 10 minutes.

3. Stir in dissolved cornstarch; increase heat to medium. Cook, stirring frequently, 2–3 minutes, or until thickened. Reduce heat to low; stir in bean sprouts. Cook, covered, 2–3 minutes, or just until bean sprouts are wilted.

4. In large serving bowl, combine vermicelli and mushroom mixture; toss to mix well. Sprinkle with scallions.

EACH SERVING PROVIDES: $\frac{1}{2}$ Fat, 3 Vegetables, 1 Bread, 15 Optional Calories
PER SERVING: 171 Calories, 7 g Protein, 3 g Fat, 31 g Carbohydrate, 480 mg Sodium, 1 mg Cholesterol, 3 g Dietary Fiber

EASY SPAGHETTI WITH MEAT SAUCE

MAKES 6 SERVINGS

1 spaghetti squash ($2\frac{1}{2}$ to 3 pounds)
1 cup chopped onions
2 cups tomato sauce
12 ounces broiled ground beef, crumbled
1 cup drained canned whole tomatoes
$\frac{1}{2}$ cup tomato paste
1 teaspoon Italian seasoning
$\frac{1}{4}$ teaspoon garlic powder
$\frac{1}{4}$ teaspoon salt
$\frac{1}{8}$ teaspoon crushed red pepper flakes
Pinch ground black pepper
3 cups cooked spaghetti (hot)

1. Preheat oven to 350°F.

2. With tines of a fork, pierce squash in several places; arrange on baking sheet. Bake 1 hour, or until tender. Cut squash into halves lengthwise; remove and discard seeds. Into medium bowl, scoop out pulp; set aside. Keep warm.

3. To prepare sauce, heat large nonstick skillet sprayed with nonstick cooking spray over medium heat; add onions. Cook, stirring frequently, 2–3 minutes, or until onions are browned.

4. Add tomato sauce, ground beef, whole tomatoes, tomato paste, Italian seasoning, garlic powder, salt, red pepper flakes and black pepper; stir to mix well. Reduce heat to low; simmer, covered, stirring occasionally, 30–60 minutes.

5. Meanwhile, in large bowl, combine prepared spaghetti squash and spaghetti; toss to mix well. Pour sauce over spaghetti mixture.

EACH SERVING PROVIDES: 4 Vegetables, 2 Proteins, 1 Bread
PER SERVING: 365 Calories, 21 g Protein, 12 g Fat, 44 g Carbohydrate, 893 mg Sodium, 49 mg Cholesterol, 4 g Dietary Fiber

FOUR-CHEESE MACARONI

MAKES 6 SERVINGS

9 ounces uncooked pasta wheels
1 cup skim milk
3 ounces reduced-fat sharp cheddar cheese, grated
3 ounces reduced-fat Monterey Jack cheese, grated
1½ ounces American cheese, grated
1½ ounces reduced-fat mozzarella cheese, grated
½ teaspoon white pepper

1. In large pot of boiling water, cook pasta wheels 8–10 minutes, until tender. Drain and return to pot.

2. Add milk, cheddar cheese, Monterey Jack cheese, American cheese, mozzarella cheese and white pepper. Cook over low heat, stirring constantly, about 5 minutes, until cheeses are melted.

EACH SERVING PROVIDES: 2 Proteins, 2 Breads, 15 Optional Calories
PER SERVING: 299 Calories, 18 g Protein, 9 g Fat, 35 g Carbohydrate, 353 mg Sodium, 30 mg Cholesterol, 1 g Dietary Fiber

---

Perfect Pasta

◆

You can make perfect pasta every time by following the pointers below:

- *Use at least a quart of water for every 4 ounces of dry pasta.*
- *Bring water to a fast boil. Add pasta in small amounts—be sure the water remains boiling at all times.*
- *Cook uncovered, and stir frequently for even cooking.*
- *Test for doneness after about 5 minutes. Pasta should be tender but still firm when you eat it, what the Italians call* al dente.
- *Fresh pasta cooks in approximately 2 to 3 minutes, so check it carefully to be sure it does not overcook.*
- *When pasta is* al dente, *drain immediately and serve.*

SPINACH FETTUCCINE IN CHEESE SAUCE

MAKES 6 SERVINGS

1¼ cups part-skim ricotta cheese
1 cup skim milk
6 ounces low-fat mozzarella cheese, grated
1½ ounces grated nonfat Parmesan cheese
2 tablespoons margarine
4 garlic cloves, crushed
4 cups drained thawed frozen chopped spinach (two 10-ounce packages)
3 cups cooked spinach fettuccine noodles (hot)

1. In food processor, combine ricotta cheese, milk, mozzarella cheese and Parmesan cheese; purée until smooth. Set aside.

2. In large skillet, melt margarine over medium heat; add garlic. Cook over low heat, 5 minutes.

3. Add cheese mixture and spinach to skillet; cook, stirring, until heated through. Add pasta; toss gently to mix well.

EACH SERVING PROVIDES: 1 Fat, 1¼ Vegetables, 2½ Proteins, 1 Bread, 15 Optional Calories
PER SERVING: 335 Calories, 26 g Protein, 13 g Fat, 30 g Carbohydrate, 462 mg Sodium, 57 mg Cholesterol, 2 g Dietary Fiber

CHEESE-STUFFED MANICOTTI

MAKES 6 SERVINGS

1 teaspoon olive oil
3 garlic cloves, crushed
3 cups low-sodium tomato sauce
1 tablespoon Italian seasoning
$\frac{1}{4}$ teaspoon ground black pepper
$1\frac{1}{2}$ cups part-skim ricotta cheese
$4\frac{1}{2}$ ounces part-skim mozzarella cheese, grated
$\frac{3}{4}$ cup grated Parmesan cheese
1 egg, lightly beaten
$\frac{1}{4}$ cup chopped fresh flat-leaf parsley
12 cooked manicotti shells ($\frac{3}{4}$ ounce each)

1. In large nonstick skillet, heat oil; add garlic. Sauté over medium heat 2 minutes, or just until golden. Add tomato sauce, Italian seasoning and pepper; stir to mix well. Reduce heat to low; simmer, covered, stirring occasionally, about 15 minutes.

2. Preheat oven to 350°F. Spray a 13 × 9" baking pan with nonstick cooking spray.

3. Meanwhile, in medium bowl, combine ricotta cheese, mozzarella cheese, Parmesan cheese, egg and parsley. Fill each manicotti shell with an equal amount of cheese mixture; arrange shells in prepared baking pan.

4. Pour prepared sauce over stuffed shells. Bake 30–40 minutes.

EACH SERVING PROVIDES: 2 Vegetables, 2 Proteins, 2 Breads, 75 Optional Calories
PER SERVING: 409 Calories, 24 g Protein, 14 g Fat, 46 g Carbohydrate, 410 mg Sodium, 75 mg Cholesterol, 3 g Dietary Fiber

CRAB AND PASTA RUFFLES IN LEMON-HORSERADISH SAUCE

Horseradish and lemon spike the crab dressing, all nestled in deeply ruffled pasta.

MAKES 6 SERVINGS

$\frac{3}{4}$ cup nonfat mayonnaise
   (10 calories per tablespoon)
$\frac{1}{4}$ cup fresh lemon juice
1 tablespoon + $1\frac{1}{2}$ teaspoons drained horseradish
3 cups cooked pasta ruffles
12 ounces well-drained thawed frozen cooked crabmeat or imitation crabmeat, cubed
$1\frac{1}{2}$ cups diagonally sliced carrots
1 cup diagonally sliced celery
$\frac{1}{2}$ cup diagonally sliced scallions
$\frac{1}{2}$ cup chopped red onion
$\frac{1}{4}$ medium red onion, thinly sliced and separated into rings

1. To prepare dressing, in small bowl, combine mayonnaise, juice and horseradish; stir to mix well.

2. In large bowl, combine pasta, crabmeat, carrots, celery, scallions and red onion. Pour mayonnaise mixture over pasta mixture; toss to coat. Garnish with onion rings.

3. Refrigerate, covered, at least 1 hour, until well chilled.

EACH SERVING PROVIDES: $1\frac{1}{4}$ Vegetables, 1 Protein, 1 Bread, 20 Optional Calories
PER SERVING: 205 Calories, 16 g Protein, 2 g Fat, 31 g Carbohydrate, 402 mg Sodium, 57 mg Cholesterol, 3 g Dietary Fiber

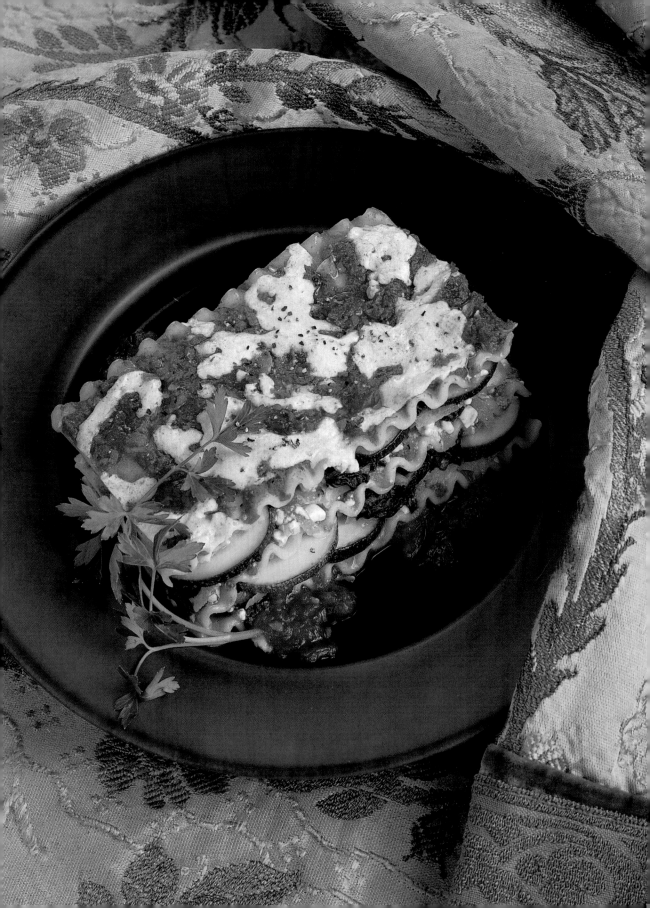

VEGETABLE LASAGNA

MAKES 6 SERVINGS

4 cups thawed frozen spinach (two 10-ounce packages)
3 cups sliced zucchini
3 cups nonfat unsalted cottage cheese
2 cups sliced mushrooms
2 cups finely grated carrots
1 cup chopped onions
2 eggs, lightly beaten
$\frac{1}{4}$ cup grated Parmesan cheese
$3\frac{1}{2}$ cups low-sodium tomato sauce
9 cooked lasagna noodles (1 ounce each)
$4\frac{1}{2}$ ounces grated part-skim mozzarella cheese

1. Preheat oven to 350°F. Spray a 13 × 9" baking pan with nonstick cooking spray.

2. In large bowl, combine spinach, zucchini, cottage cheese, mushrooms, carrots, onions, eggs and Parmesan cheese; stir to mix well. Set aside.

3. In bottom of prepared pan, with spatula, evenly spread $\frac{1}{2}$ cup of the tomato sauce; arrange 3 lasagna noodles over sauce. Spread with half of the vegetable mixture; top with 1 cup of the remaining sauce. Repeat procedure, ending with 3 lasagna noodles, then the remaining 1 cup of sauce. Cover with foil; bake 45 minutes. Uncover; evenly top with mozzarella cheese. Bake, uncovered, 15 minutes, until cheese is melted. Let stand 15–20 minutes before cutting.

EACH SERVING PROVIDES: $6\frac{1}{4}$ Vegetables, $2\frac{1}{4}$ Proteins, 2 Breads, 25 Optional Calories
PER SERVING: 363 Calories, 20 g Protein, 8 g Fat, 55 g Carbohydrate, 300 mg Sodium, 86 mg Cholesterol, 7 g Dietary Fiber

CUCUMBERS AND BOW-TIE PASTA IN SOUR CREAM-CHIVE DRESSING

MAKES 6 SERVINGS

$\frac{3}{4}$ cup nonfat sour cream
$\frac{1}{4}$ cup chopped chives
2 tablespoons white wine vinegar
1 teaspoon granulated sugar
$\frac{1}{4}$ teaspoon freshly ground black pepper
3 cups cooked bow-tie pasta
3 cups sliced English cucumbers, quartered
$\frac{1}{4}$ cup sliced radishes

1. To prepare dressing, in medium bowl, combine sour cream, chives, vinegar, sugar and pepper; stir to mix well.

2. In large serving bowl, combine pasta and cucumbers. Pour dressing over pasta mixture; gently toss to coat. Top with radish slices. Refrigerate, covered, until well chilled.

EACH SERVING PROVIDES: 1 Vegetable, 1 Bread, 25 Optional Calories
PER SERVING: 130 Calories, 6 g Protein, 1 g Fat, 24 g Carbohydrate, 23 mg Sodium, 0 mg Cholesterol, 2 g Dietary Fiber

Vegetable Lasagna

TRICOLOR PASTA SALAD

MAKES 6 SERVINGS

3 cups cooked tricolor pasta
1 cup chopped green bell pepper
1 cup chopped red bell pepper
1 cup chopped yellow bell pepper
$\frac{1}{4}$ cup chopped onion
$\frac{1}{4}$ cup chopped scallions
$\frac{1}{2}$ cup fat-free ranch dressing
8 iceberg lettuce leaves

1. In large bowl, combine cooked pasta, green bell pepper, red bell pepper, yellow bell pepper, onion and scallions; gently toss to coat. Pour ranch dressing over pasta mixture; toss gently to mix well.

2. Line serving bowl with lettuce leaves; arrange pasta salad in bowl. Refrigerate, covered, until well chilled.

EACH SERVING PROVIDES: 1$\frac{1}{2}$ Vegetables, 1 Bread, 25 Optional Calories
PER SERVING: 142 Calories, 4 g Protein, 1 g Fat, 28 g Carbohydrate, 204 mg Sodium, 0 mg Cholesterol, 2 g Dietary Fiber

LEMON-DILLED PASTA SALAD

Nonfat yogurt, brightened with fresh lemon juice and accented with dill, is the base of the creamy, almost fat-free dressing in this pasta salad.

MAKES 6 SERVINGS

$\frac{3}{4}$ cup plain nonfat yogurt
$\frac{1}{2}$ cup + 2 tablespoons fresh lemon juice
$\frac{1}{3}$ cup finely chopped fresh dill
3 cups cooked macaroni shells
3 cups small broccoli florets, steamed until tender-crisp
3 cups small cauliflower florets, steamed until tender-crisp

1. To prepare dressing, in small bowl, combine yogurt, juice and dill; stir to mix well.

2. In large serving bowl, combine macaroni shells, broccoli and cauliflower. Pour yogurt mixture over macaroni mixture; toss gently until thoroughly mixed.

3. Refrigerate, covered, at least 1 hour, until well chilled.

EACH SERVING PROVIDES: 2 Vegetables, 1 Bread, 15 Optional Calories
PER SERVING: 137 Calories, 8 g Protein, 1 g Fat, 27 g Carbohydrate, 47 mg Sodium, 1 mg Cholesterol, 4 g Dietary Fiber

BULGUR PILAF

Best known for its use in Middle Eastern tabbouleh, bulgur lends a mild wheaty taste to this pilaf, where it stands in for rice.

MAKES 6 SERVINGS

2 cups sliced mushrooms
1 cup chopped onions
6 ounces uncooked bulgur
3 ounces chopped dried apricots
$\frac{1}{2}$ cup chopped fresh parsley
1$\frac{1}{2}$ ounces dark raisins
3 ounces slivered almonds

1. In medium saucepan, combine mushrooms, onions, bulgur, apricots, parsley and raisins. Stir in 3 cups water; bring to a boil.

2. Reduce heat to low; simmer, covered, 15–20 minutes, until liquid is absorbed and bulgur is tender. Stir in almonds.

EACH SERVING PROVIDES: 1 Fat, 1 Fruit, 1 Vegetable, $\frac{1}{2}$ Protein, 1 Bread
PER SERVING: 253 Calories, 8 g Protein, 8 g Fat, 42 g Carbohydrate, 12 mg Sodium, 0 mg Cholesterol, 8 g Dietary Fiber

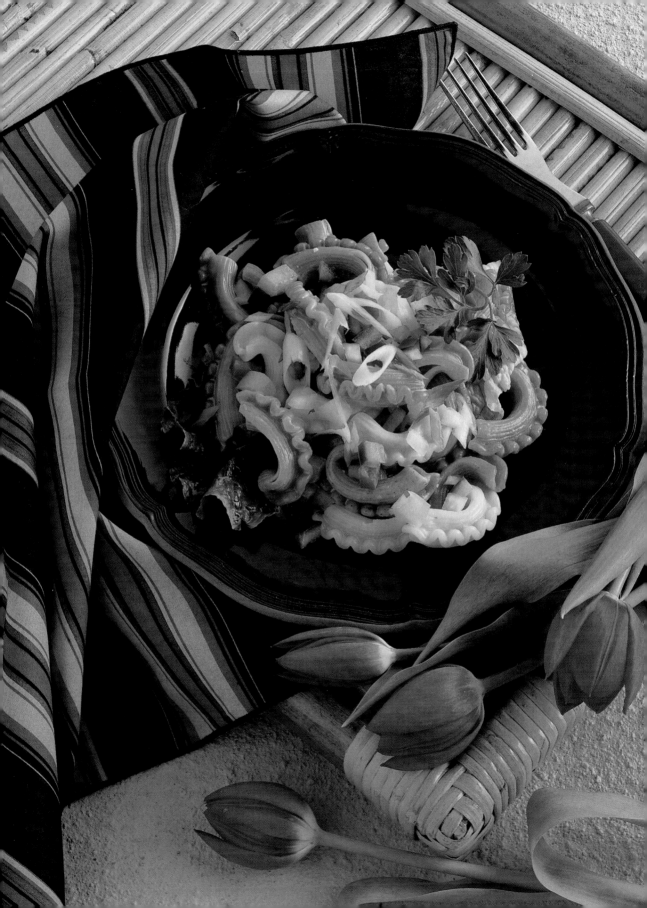

COUSCOUS WITH LIME-GINGER SAUCE

Although couscous looks and acts like a grain, it is actually pasta. The ultimate convenience food: just pour boiling water over the couscous and let it stand 5 minutes.

MAKES 6 SERVINGS

6 ounces uncooked couscous
1 teaspoon dark sesame oil
$\frac{1}{4}$ teaspoon salt
1 cup finely chopped red bell pepper
1 cup coarsely grated carrots
1 cup finely chopped scallions
$\frac{1}{2}$ cup fresh lime juice
$\frac{1}{4}$ cup finely chopped fresh parsley
$\frac{1}{4}$ teaspoon ground ginger
$\frac{1}{8}$ teaspoon freshly ground black pepper

1. In medium saucepan, bring $1\frac{1}{2}$ cups water to a boil; add couscous, oil and salt. Remove from heat; cover and let stand, stirring occasionally, 5–10 minutes, until water is absorbed.

2. In large bowl, combine bell pepper, carrots, scallions, juice, parsley, ginger and black pepper. Add cooked couscous; toss gently to mix well.

3. Refrigerate, covered, at least 3 hours, until thoroughly chilled.

EACH SERVING PROVIDES: 1 Vegetable, 1 Bread, 5 Optional Calories
PER SERVING: 138 Calories, 4 g Protein, 1 g Fat, 28 g Carbohydrate, 103 mg Sodium, 0 mg Cholesterol, 1 g Dietary Fiber

KASHA VARNISHKES

The classic combination of buckwheat groats and bow-tie pasta comes into a health-conscious age, without chicken fat.

MAKES 6 SERVINGS

3 ounces uncooked buckwheat groats (kasha)
1 egg, lightly beaten
1 tablespoon vegetable oil
1 medium onion, thinly sliced
1 teaspoon chicken bouillon granules, dissolved in 2 tablespoons water
2 cups thinly sliced mushrooms
$1\frac{1}{2}$ cups cooked bow-tie pasta
1 teaspoon paprika
$\frac{1}{8}$ teaspoon freshly ground black pepper

1. In small bowl, combine groats and egg; stir until groats are coated. Set aside.

2. In large nonstick skillet, heat oil; add groat mixture. Cook over low heat, stirring constantly, 5 minutes, or until groats are dry and grains are separated.

3. In small saucepan, combine cooked groat mixture and $\frac{1}{2}$ cup water; bring to a boil. Reduce heat to low; simmer, covered, 10–15 minutes.

4. Meanwhile, spray same large nonstick skillet with nonstick cooking spray; add onion and dissolved bouillon granules. Cook over medium heat, stirring constantly, adding water if needed, about 5 minutes, or until onion is browned.

5. Add mushrooms; sauté 2–3 minutes. Reduce heat to low; add cooked groats, pasta, $\frac{3}{4}$ teaspoon of the paprika and the pepper; toss to mix well.

6. Transfer groat mixture to serving bowl; sprinkle with the remaining $\frac{1}{4}$ teaspoon paprika.

EACH SERVING PROVIDES: $\frac{1}{2}$ Fat, $\frac{3}{4}$ Vegetable, 1 Bread, 10 Optional Calories
PER SERVING: 147 Calories, 5 g Protein, 4 g Fat, 24 g Carbohydrate, 174 mg Sodium, 35 mg Cholesterol, 3 g Dietary Fiber

MILLET WITH CARROTS AND PRUNES

*The crunchy, nutlike texture of millet
provides a nice counterpoint to the citrus-
infused tender carrots and prunes.*

MAKES 6 SERVINGS

3 cups diced carrots
4½ ounces uncooked millet
½ cup orange juice
1 cup chopped fresh parsley
4½ ounces chopped pitted prunes
1 tablespoon dry sherry

1. In medium saucepan, combine carrots, 1½ cups water, the millet and juice; bring to a boil. Reduce heat to low; simmer, covered, 20 minutes.

2. Remove from heat; stir in parsley, prunes and sherry.

EACH SERVING PROVIDES: 1 Fruit, 1 Vegetable, 1 Bread, 10 Optional Calories
PER SERVING: 171 Calories, 4 g Protein, 1 g Fat, 38 g Carbohydrate, 25 mg Sodium, 0 mg Cholesterol, 6 g Dietary Fiber

SPANISH-STYLE HOMINY

*Hearty hominy, dished out onto Southern
breakfast plates, takes on vegetables, tomato
and cheese in this spicy casserole.*

MAKES 6 SERVINGS

3 cups drained canned golden hominy
1 cup finely chopped green bell pepper
1 cup sliced mushrooms
1 cup finely chopped onion
1 cup tomato sauce
½ cup tomato paste
2½ teaspoons chili powder
1 teaspoon ground cumin
⅛ teaspoon freshly ground black pepper
3 ounces shredded reduced-fat Monterey Jack cheese
3 ounces shredded reduced-fat sharp cheddar cheese

1. Preheat oven to 350°F. Spray a 2-quart casserole with nonstick cooking spray.

2. In prepared casserole, combine hominy, bell pepper, mushrooms, onions, tomato sauce, tomato paste, chili powder, cumin and black pepper; stir to mix well.

3. Sprinkle Monterey Jack cheese and cheddar cheese evenly over hominy mixture. Bake 30 minutes, or until cheeses are bubbly.

EACH SERVING PROVIDES: 2¼ Vegetables, 1¼ Proteins, 1 Bread, 5 Optional Calories
PER SERVING: 196 Calories, 11 g Protein, 6 g Fat, 24 g Carbohydrate, 789 mg Sodium, 20 mg Cholesterol, 5 g Dietary Fiber

CORNMEAL-CHEESE SOUFFLÉ

Some cooks prefer stone-ground meal, as stone mills are gentler than steel mills and less likely to overgrind, heat or damage the grains. Stone-ground meal is available in health food stores.

MAKES 6 SERVINGS

$4\frac{1}{2}$ ounces uncooked stone-ground cornmeal
2 cups skim milk
6 eggs
1 tablespoon granulated sugar
$4\frac{1}{2}$ ounces grated reduced-fat cheddar cheese

1. Preheat oven to 325°F. Spray a 2-quart soufflé dish with nonstick cooking spray.

2. In large saucepan, bring $2\frac{1}{4}$ cups water to a boil; stir in cornmeal and return to a boil. Reduce heat to low; cook, stirring constantly, 2–3 minutes, until mixture is smooth and thickened. Transfer to large bowl.

3. Add milk, eggs and sugar to cornmeal mixture. With mixer on medium speed, beat 3–4 minutes; stir in cheese. Pour mixture into prepared soufflé dish.

4. Bake 35–40 minutes, until knife inserted in center comes out clean. Serve immediately.

EACH SERVING PROVIDES: $\frac{1}{4}$ Milk, 2 Proteins, 1 Bread, 15 Optional Calories
PER SERVING: 258 Calories, 17 g Protein, 9 g Fat, 24 g Carbohydrate, 256 mg Sodium, 229 mg Cholesterol, 1 g Dietary Fiber

POLENTA WITH FONTINELLA-MUSHROOM SAUCE

Instant polenta reduces the cooking and stirring time to just 5 minutes. Fontinella is an Italian hard cheese; if you can't find it, substitute Romano.

MAKES 6 SERVINGS

$4\frac{1}{2}$ ounces uncooked instant polenta
$\frac{1}{8}$ teaspoon salt
2 tablespoons margarine
$\frac{1}{8}$ teaspoon freshly ground black pepper
2 tablespoons all-purpose flour
$1\frac{1}{2}$ cups skim milk
$4\frac{1}{2}$ ounces grated fontinella cheese
$\frac{1}{2}$ cup grated Parmesan cheese
3 cups sliced mushrooms

1. Spray a tall, round 1-quart container or a clean 4-cup yogurt or cottage cheese container and a 13 × 9" baking dish with nonstick cooking spray.

2. In small saucepan, bring $2\frac{1}{2}$ cups water to a boil; with whisk, stir in polenta and salt. Reduce heat to low; cook, whisking constantly, 5 minutes. Transfer to prepared container; refrigerate, covered, 1 hour or until polenta is cold.

3. Preheat oven to 350°F. Remove solidified polenta from container; cut crosswise into 6 equal slices; arrange in prepared baking dish.

4. In small saucepan, melt margarine over medium-high heat; stir in pepper. Sprinkle flour over margarine mixture; whisk quickly to combine. Whisk in milk, fontinella cheese and Parmesan cheese; stir in mushrooms.

5. Pour mushroom sauce over polenta slices; bake 30 minutes.

EACH SERVING PROVIDES: $\frac{1}{4}$ Milk, 1 Fat, 1 Vegetable, 1 Protein, 1 Bread, 50 Optional Calories
PER SERVING: 267 Calories, 14 g Protein, 13 g Fat, 24 g Carbohydrate, 504 mg Sodium, 29 mg Cholesterol, 2 g Dietary Fiber

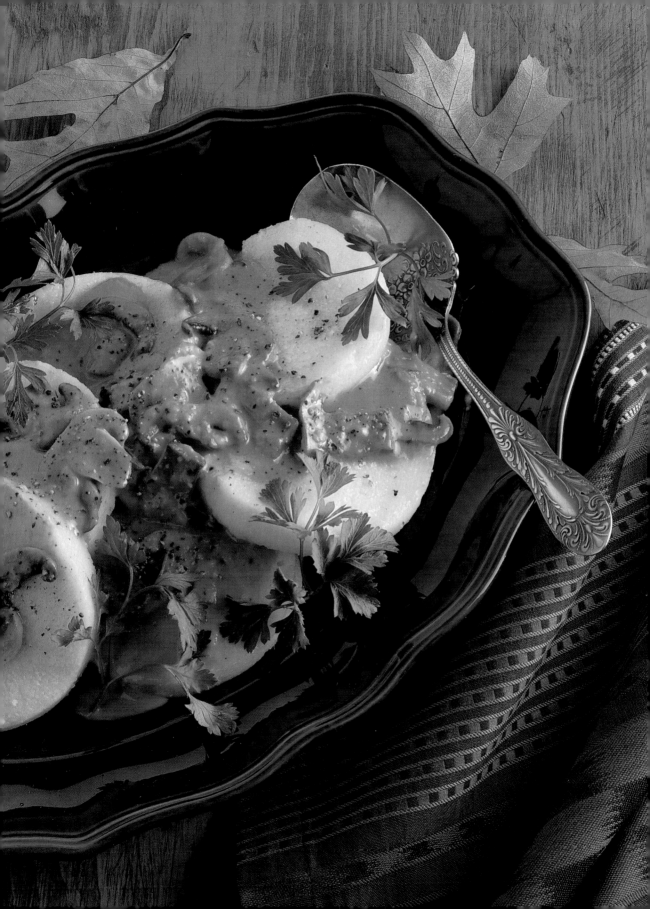

TABBOULEH

MAKES 6 SERVINGS

½ cup fresh lemon juice
6 ounces uncooked bulgur
1 tablespoon olive oil
1 teaspoon freshly ground black pepper
¼ teaspoon salt
3 cups chopped ripe tomatoes
1 cup chopped fresh flat-leaf parsley
½ cup chopped red onion
¼ cup chopped scallions (green part only)
2 garlic cloves, crushed
1 sliced lemon to garnish (optional)

1. In medium saucepan, bring juice and 1½ cups water to a boil; add bulgur, oil, pepper and salt. Remove from heat; cover and let stand 20–25 minutes.

2. In large bowl combine tomatoes, parsley, red onion, scallions and garlic; toss to mix well. Add bulgur mixture; toss to mix well.

3. Transfer bulgur mixture to large serving bowl; refrigerate, covered, at least 3 hours, until thoroughly chilled. To serve, garnish with lemon slices, if desired.

EACH SERVING PROVIDES: ½ Fat, 1¼ Vegetables, 1 Bread
PER SERVING: 150 Calories, 5 g Protein, 3 g Fat, 29 g Carbohydrate, 106 mg Sodium, 0 mg Cholesterol, 7 g Dietary Fiber

---

Rice Rules

◆

Below are the basic guidelines for cooking rice. However, if you are cooking a specialty rice, be sure to follow the directions on the package.

Combine 1 cup of rice and the amount of water listed in the chart below in a 2-to-3-quart saucepan. Heat to boiling; stir once or twice. Lower heat to simmer; cover and cook for the time specified in the chart. If rice is not quite tender, or if liquid is not absorbed, replace lid and cook 2 to 4 minutes longer. Fluff with fork and serve.

1 Cup Uncooked Rice	Liquid	Cooking Time
Regular-milled Long Grain	1¾ to 2 cups	15 minutes
Regular-milled Medium or Short Grain	1½ cups	15 minutes
Brown	2 to 2½ cups	45 to 50 minutes

STUFFED PEPPERS

MAKES 6 SERVINGS

3 large green bell peppers (about 7 ounces each)
3 large red bell peppers (about 7 ounces each)
3 cups cooked regular long-grain rice
12 ounces ground turkey
$\frac{3}{4}$ cup chopped fresh parsley
$\frac{1}{2}$ cup chopped onion
2 eggs, lightly beaten
2 tablespoons Worcestershire sauce
1 teaspoon paprika
$\frac{1}{4}$ teaspoon ground red pepper
$\frac{1}{4}$ teaspoon salt
$3\frac{1}{2}$ cups canned crushed tomatoes

1. Preheat oven to 350°F. Spray baking pan with nonstick cooking spray. Cut tops from green and red bell peppers; remove seeds. Set aside.

2. In large bowl, combine rice, turkey, parsley, onion, eggs, Worcestershire sauce, paprika, ground red pepper and salt; stir to mix well.

3. Stuff an equal amount of rice mixture into each prepared bell pepper; arrange peppers in prepared baking pan.

4. Bake $1\frac{1}{2}$ hours, basting frequently.

EACH SERVING PROVIDES: $2\frac{1}{2}$ Vegetables, $1\frac{1}{2}$ Proteins, 1 Bread, 20 Optional Calories
PER SERVING: 325 Calories, 18 g Protein, 7 g Fat, 48 g Carbohydrate, 456 mg Sodium, 112 mg Cholesterol, 5 g Dietary Fiber

WILD RICE ASPARAGUS SALAD WITH WINE VINEGAR VINAIGRETTE

MAKES 6 SERVINGS

2 teaspoons chicken bouillon granules
3 ounces uncooked regular long-grain rice
3 ounces uncooked wild rice
4 cups diagonally sliced asparagus, steamed until tender-crisp
1 cup chopped red onion
1 cup chopped red bell pepper
$\frac{1}{2}$ cup chopped fresh parsley
$\frac{1}{2}$ cup white wine vinegar
1 tablespoon olive oil
1 teaspoon granulated sugar
$\frac{1}{8}$ teaspoon freshly ground black pepper
12 red-tipped lettuce leaves
$\frac{1}{2}$ medium red onion, thinly sliced and separated into rings

1. In medium saucepan, bring $2\frac{3}{4}$ cups water and the bouillon granules to a boil; add long-grain and wild rice. Reduce heat to low; simmer, covered, 20–30 minutes, until rice is tender. Remove from heat.

2. In large bowl, combine asparagus, chopped red onion, bell pepper, parsley, vinegar, oil, sugar and black pepper. Add cooked rice; toss to mix well.

3. Line serving platter with lettuce leaves; arrange rice mixture on platter. Top with onion rings. Refrigerate, covered, until well chilled.

EACH SERVING PROVIDES: $\frac{1}{2}$ Fat, $2\frac{1}{2}$ Vegetables, 1 Bread, 5 Optional Calories
PER SERVING: 172 Calories, 7 g Protein, 3 g Fat, 32 g Carbohydrate, 311 mg Sodium, 1 mg Cholesterol, 3 g Dietary Fiber

RASPBERRY-RICE SALAD

MAKES 6 SERVINGS

1½ cups raspberries (reserve 8 berries)
¼ cup orange juice
2 tablespoons white vinegar
1 teaspoon granulated sugar
3 cups cooked regular long-grain rice
2 cups canned mandarin orange sections
¾ cup chopped scallions (green portion only)
2 tablespoons chopped fresh flat-leaf parsley
2 tablespoons chopped fresh chives
12 red-tipped lettuce leaves

1. To prepare dressing, in food processor, combine raspberries, juice, vinegar and sugar; purée until smooth.

2. In large bowl, combine rice, orange sections, ½ cup of the scallions, the parsley and chives; toss gently to mix well. Pour dressing over rice mixture; toss gently to coat.

3. Line serving platter with lettuce leaves; arrange rice mixture on platter. Top with reserved berries; sprinkle with remaining ¼ cup scallions. Refrigerate, covered, until well chilled.

EACH SERVING PROVIDES: 1 Fruit, ¾ Vegetable, 1 Bread, 10 Optional Calories
PER SERVING: 193 Calories, 4 g Protein, 1 g Fat, 44 g Carbohydrate, 10 mg Sodium, 0 mg Cholesterol, 2 g Dietary Fiber

ORIENTAL FRIED RICE

MAKES 6 SERVINGS

1 cup thinly sliced baby carrots
1 cup finely chopped scallions
1 cup sliced mushrooms
1 cup bean sprouts
1 tablespoon chicken bouillon granules, dissolved in ¾ cup boiling water
3 eggs, slightly beaten
¼ cup dry sherry
3 cups cooked long-grain rice (hot)

1. Heat large nonstick skillet sprayed with nonstick cooking spray; add carrots, scallions, mushrooms, bean sprouts and dissolved bouillon granules. Stir-fry 2–3 minutes, until vegetables are tender-crisp. Transfer vegetables to bowl; keep warm.

2. Spray same skillet with nonstick cooking spray; add eggs and sherry and stir to combine. Cook over medium heat, stirring to break up eggs into tiny pieces, about 2 minutes, until eggs are set.

3. Add cooked vegetables and rice to egg mixture; toss to combine. Cook, stirring frequently, 1–2 minutes, until heated through.

EACH SERVING PROVIDES: 1¼ Vegetables, ½ Protein, 1 Bread, 15 Optional Calories
PER SERVING: 198 Calories, 7 g Protein, 3 g Fat, 35 g Carbohydrate, 525 mg Sodium, 106 mg Cholesterol, 2 g Dietary Fiber

SPANISH RICE

MAKES 6 SERVINGS

3 cups chopped canned tomatoes
6 ounces uncooked instant brown rice
1 cup chopped green bell pepper
1 cup chopped onions
6 slices crisp cooked bacon, crumbled
$\frac{1}{2}$ teaspoon ground cumin
$\frac{1}{2}$ teaspoon garlic powder

1. In large nonstick skillet sprayed with non-stick cooking spray, combine tomatoes, rice, bell pepper, onions, bacon, cumin and garlic powder; bring to a boil.

2. Reduce heat to low; simmer, covered, stirring occasionally, 30–35 minutes.

EACH SERVING PROVIDES: 1$\frac{3}{4}$ Vegetables, 1 Bread, 35 Optional Calories
PER SERVING: 174 Calories, 6 g Protein, 5 g Fat, 31 g Carbohydrate, 310 mg Sodium, 5 mg Cholesterol, 3 g Dietary Fiber

---

Microwave Magic

◆

Rice cooks very nicely in a microwave—for confirmation of this, try our Microwave Risotto, page 286! Use the instructions below to cook basic rice.

- *Combine 1 cup rice and liquid (see chart on page 282) in a 2-to-3-quart microwavable baking dish.*
- *Cover and cook on HIGH for 5 minutes, or until boiling.*
- *Reduce setting to medium and cook 15 minutes for regular white rice, 20 minutes for parboiled rice and 30 minutes for brown rice.*

HERBED INSTANT BROWN RICE

In this speedy but special dish, you can enjoy in short order the nutritious benefits of brown rice enhanced with vegetables and herbs.

MAKES 6 SERVINGS

1 tablespoon margarine
$\frac{1}{2}$ cup chopped onion
3 garlic cloves, minced
1 cup finely chopped red bell pepper
$\frac{1}{2}$ cup finely chopped celery
6 ounces uncooked instant brown rice
$\frac{1}{4}$ teaspoon ground marjoram
$\frac{1}{2}$ cup chopped fresh flat-leaf parsley

1. In large nonstick skillet, melt margarine over medium-high heat; add onion and garlic. Sauté 2–3 minutes, until garlic is lightly browned. Add bell pepper and celery; sauté 2–3 minutes.

2. Add 1$\frac{1}{2}$ cups water, the rice and marjoram; bring to a boil. Reduce heat to low; simmer, covered, 5 minutes. Remove from heat; stir in parsley. Let stand 5 minutes.

EACH SERVING PROVIDES: $\frac{1}{2}$ Fat, $\frac{3}{4}$ Vegetable, 1 Bread
PER SERVING: 128 Calories, 3 g Protein, 3 g Fat, 26 g Carbohydrate, 46 mg Sodium, 0 mg Cholesterol, 2 g Dietary Fiber

CURRIED BASMATI RICE

Considered a luxury food in India and Pakistan, where it was originally grown, this aromatic rice was named basmati, *queen of fragrance.*

MAKES 6 SERVINGS

1 cup sliced mushrooms
1 cup chopped onions
½ cup chopped red bell pepper
½ cup chopped green bell pepper
6 ounces uncooked basmati rice
1½ teaspoons curry powder
¼ teaspoon salt

1. In large Dutch oven sprayed with nonstick cooking spray, combine mushrooms, onions, red bell pepper and green bell pepper; sauté over medium-high heat 3–4 minutes.

2. Add 1½ cups water, the rice, curry powder and salt; stir to mix well. Reduce heat to low; simmer, covered, 15–20 minutes.

EACH SERVING PROVIDES: 1 Vegetable, 1 Bread
PER SERVING: 117 Calories, 4 g Protein, 1 g Fat, 26 g Carbohydrate, 104 mg Sodium, 0 mg Cholesterol, 1 g Dietary Fiber

MICROWAVE RISOTTO

With the aid of a food processor and microwave oven, this savory risotto can be cooked in less than 30 minutes!

MAKES 6 SERVINGS

1 cup fresh basil
2 ounces pine nuts
¾ cup dry white wine
4 garlic cloves
1 tablespoon + 2 teaspoons olive oil
6 ounces uncooked arborio or other short-grain rice
3 cups chicken broth
12 sun-dried tomato halves (not packed in oil)
¼ cup grated Parmesan cheese

1. To prepare pesto, in food processor, combine basil, pine nuts, ¼ cup of the wine, garlic cloves and 2 teaspoons of the oil; process 4–5 minutes, stopping occasionally to scrape blade. Set aside.

2. In a 2½-quart casserole, microwave the remaining tablespoon oil on High 1 minute; stir in rice. Add 2 cups of the broth, the remaining ½ cup wine and ½ cup water; stir to mix well. Microwave on High 12 minutes.

3. Add prepared pesto, the remaining 1 cup broth and the sun-dried tomatoes to rice mixture; stir to mix well. Microwave on High 8 minutes. Sprinkle with Parmesan cheese.

EACH SERVING PROVIDES: 1½ Fats, 1 Vegetable, ¼ Protein, 1 Bread, 60 Optional Calories
PER SERVING: 259 Calories, 8 g Protein, 11 g Fat, 31 g Carbohydrate, 566 mg Sodium, 3 mg Cholesterol, 1 g Dietary Fiber

Microwave Risotto

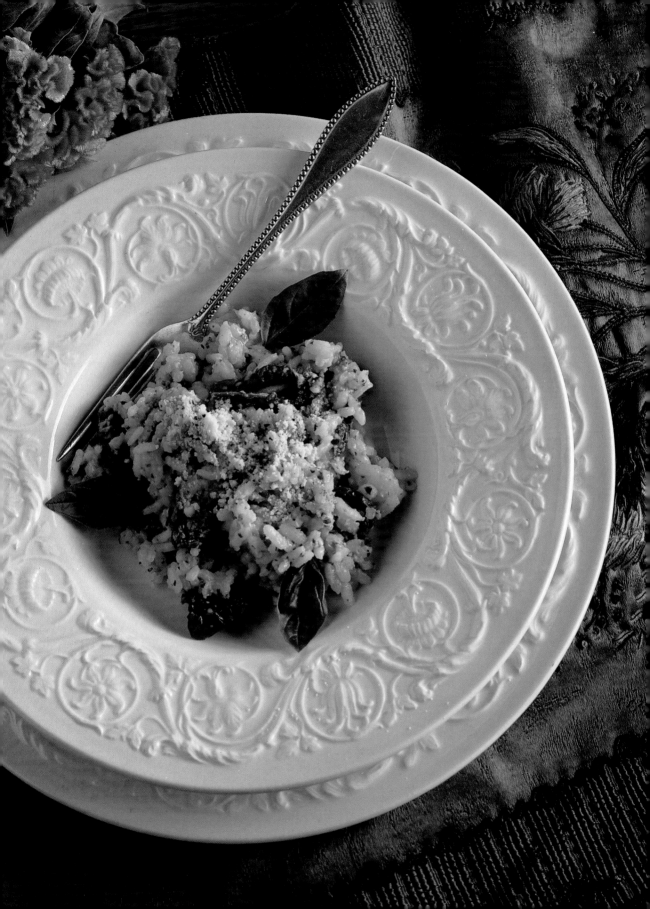

SHRIMP AND VEGETABLE RICE

MAKES 6 SERVINGS

1¼ cups chicken broth (¼ cup chilled)
2 tablespoons cornstarch
1 teaspoon vegetable oil
2 cups diced carrots
2 cups snow peas
3 tablespoons reduced-sodium soy sauce
2 teaspoons dark sesame oil
1 pound 3 ounces peeled and deveined large
   shrimp
3 cups cooked regular long-grain rice

1. In small bowl, combine ¼ cup cold chicken broth and cornstarch; stir until cornstarch is dissolved. Set aside.

2. In large skillet, heat oil; add carrots and ⅓ cup of the remaining broth. Cook over medium heat 2 minutes. Add snow peas, ⅓ cup of the remaining broth, the soy sauce and sesame oil; stir gently to combine. Reduce heat to low; simmer, covered, 5 minutes, until snow peas are tender-crisp.

3. Add shrimp and the remaining ⅓ cup of broth; cook, stirring occasionally, 3–4 minutes, just until shrimp turn pink.

4. Increase heat to high; bring mixture to a boil. Add dissolved cornstarch. Cook, stirring frequently, 2 minutes, or until thickened. Add rice; stir to combine.

EACH SERVING PROVIDES: ½ Fat, 1¼ Vegetables, 1¼ Proteins, 1 Bread, 15 Optional Calories
PER SERVING: 284 Calories, 20 g Protein, 4 g Fat, 40 g Carbohydrate, 627 mg Sodium, 108 mg Cholesterol, 3 g Dietary Fiber

Vegetarian Bean Chili (page 290)

CHAPTER ELEVEN

POTATOES, LEGUMES AND BEANS

VEGETARIAN BEAN CHILI

You don't have to be a vegetarian to appreciate this hearty, delicious chili!

MAKES 4 SERVINGS

1 tablespoon + 1 teaspoon olive oil
1 cup chopped onions
1 cup chopped carrot
1 cup seeded and diced red, green or yellow bell pepper
1 cup chopped celery
1 tablespoon finely chopped garlic
2 teaspoons finely chopped seeded jalapeño pepper
1 tablespoon + 1 teaspoon chili powder
1½ teaspoons ground cumin
1 teaspoon dried oregano leaves
¼ teaspoon ground cloves
1 pound rinsed drained cooked pinto or red beans
6 ounces rinsed drained dried lentils
2 cups chopped canned plum tomatoes with juice
1 packet instant vegetable broth and seasoning mix
2–4 tablespoons chopped fresh cilantro (to taste)
¼ cup nonfat sour cream
¼ cup chopped red onion
2 tablespoons chopped fresh cilantro

1. In large heavy saucepan, heat oil over medium heat; add onions, carrot, bell pepper, celery, garlic and jalapeño pepper. Sauté, stirring occasionally, until vegetables are wilted, about 10 minutes. Add chili powder, cumin, oregano and cloves; sauté, stirring, another minute.

2. Add beans and lentils; stir to combine. Add tomatoes and broth mix. Cover with 2¾ cups water. Bring to a boil over high heat; cover, reduce heat and simmer, stirring occasionally, until lentils are tender, about 30 minutes. When lentils are tender, uncover pot and cook over medium heat, stirring occasionally, until beans and lentils are falling apart and chili has achieved desired consistency, about 15 minutes. Stir in cilantro.

3. Divide evenly among four bowls and top each with ¼ of the sour cream, red onion and cilantro.

EACH SERVING (1¾ cups) PROVIDES: 1 Fat, 3 Vegetables, 2 Proteins, 2 Breads, 15 Optional Calories
PER SERVING: 435 Calories, 25 g Protein, 7 g Fat, 73 g Carbohydrate, 498 mg Sodium, 0 mg Cholesterol, 14 g Dietary Fiber

◆

MEXICAN BLACK BEANS

MAKES 4 SERVINGS

1 tablespoon + 1 teaspoon olive oil
½ cup finely chopped onion
½ cup finely chopped green bell pepper
½ small jalapeño pepper, seeded and finely chopped
1 tablespoon finely chopped garlic
1 teaspoon chili powder
2 bay leaves
1 teaspoon ground cumin
1 teaspoon dried oregano leaves
1 pound rinsed drained cooked black beans
1 cup low-sodium chicken broth
Salt and freshly ground black pepper to taste
2 tablespoons chopped fresh cilantro

1. In medium saucepan, heat oil over medium heat; add onion, bell pepper, jalapeño and garlic. Sauté, stirring occasionally, until vegetables are wilted, about 8 minutes. Add chili powder, bay leaves, cumin and oregano; sauté, stirring, 1 minute.

2. Add beans, broth, salt and pepper. Increase heat to high; bring to a boil and lower heat to medium-low. Gently simmer, stirring occasionally, until creamy and tender, about 30 minutes. Remove bay leaves; stir in cilantro and serve.

EACH SERVING (½ cup) PROVIDES: 1 Fat, ½ Vegetable, 2 Proteins, 5 Optional Calories
PER SERVING: 219 Calories, 11 g Protein, 6 g Fat, 32 g Carbohydrate, 23 mg Sodium, 0 mg Cholesterol, 3 g Dietary Fiber

SOUTHWESTERN BLACK BEAN SALAD

MAKES 4 SERVINGS

1 pound rinsed drained cooked black beans
1 cup diced seeded roasted red bell pepper
$\frac{1}{2}$ cup cooked corn kernels
$\frac{1}{2}$ cup finely chopped red onion
$\frac{1}{2}$ cup chopped fresh cilantro
4 medium scallions, thinly sliced
1 medium jalapeño pepper, finely chopped
1 tablespoon + 1 teaspoon fresh lime juice
1 tablespoon + 1 teaspoon olive oil
2 garlic cloves, finely chopped
Salt and freshly ground black pepper to taste

In large mixing bowl, combine all ingredients. Toss well and serve.

EACH SERVING (1$\frac{1}{2}$ cups) PROVIDES: 1 Fat, 1 Vegetable, 2 Proteins, $\frac{1}{4}$ Bread
PER SERVING: 237 Calories, 12 g Protein, 5 g Fat, 38 g Carbohydrate, 10 mg Sodium, 0 mg Cholesterol, 4 g Dietary Fiber

---

Lowdown on Legumes

◆

What exactly are legumes? They are food that comes from plants with seed pods, and that means lentils, split peas, and kidney, pinto, lima, mung or black beans. Bursting with protein, legumes are virtually fat free, inexpensive and high in fiber. When served with any grain or a small amount of protein, they become a complete protein.

Legumes are a staple all over the world, and we have our favorite legume dishes, such as Red Beans and Rice (page 292) or Baked Beans (page 292). You'll enjoy expanding your legume repertoire with the exciting recipes here, such as Vegetarian Bean Chili (page 290), Italian-Style White Beans (page 293) or Spicy Chick-Pea Stew (page 294).

BLACK BEANS AND RICE

While we often think of beans and rice as side dishes, the combination makes a very satisfying dinner when you add a simple salad. And if you're a red bean fan, just use the recipe on page 292.

MAKES 4 SERVINGS

1 tablespoon + 1 teaspoon olive oil
$\frac{1}{2}$ cup finely chopped onion
1 cup finely chopped green bell pepper
1 tablespoon finely chopped garlic
1 pound rinsed drained cooked black beans
1 cup low-sodium chicken broth + $\frac{1}{2}$ cup water
1$\frac{1}{2}$ cups coarsely chopped canned plum tomatoes with juice
1 teaspoon chopped fresh thyme or $\frac{1}{2}$ teaspoon dried leaves
1 bay leaf
1 tablespoon + 1 teaspoon dry sherry
$\frac{1}{4}$ teaspoon dried oregano leaves
$\frac{1}{4}$ teaspoon hot pepper sauce
1 tablespoon chopped fresh cilantro
Salt and freshly ground pepper to taste
4 cups cooked regular long-grain rice
1 tablespoon chopped fresh flat-leaf parsley to garnish (optional)

1. In medium saucepan, heat oil over medium-low heat; add onion, bell pepper and garlic. Sauté, stirring occasionally, 15 minutes.

2. Add beans, broth and water, tomatoes, thyme, bay leaf, sherry, oregano and hot pepper sauce. Over high heat, bring to a boil. Reduce heat; simmer 45 minutes, stirring occasionally, until sauce thickens and vegetables are tender. If mixture becomes too thick, add hot water to thin to desired consistency. Stir in cilantro; season with salt and pepper. Remove bay leaf. Serve over rice, sprinkled with parsley, if desired.

EACH SERVING (1 cup) PROVIDES: 1 Fat, 1$\frac{1}{2}$ Vegetables, 2 Proteins, 2 Breads, 10 Optional Calories
PER SERVING: 507 Calories, 18 g Protein, 6 g Fat, 93 g Carbohydrate, 176 mg Sodium, 0 mg Cholesterol, 4 g Dietary Fiber

RED BEANS AND RICE

MAKES 4 SERVINGS

1 tablespoon + 1 teaspoon olive oil
1 cup finely chopped onions
2 teaspoons finely chopped garlic
1 pound rinsed drained cooked kidney beans
2 ounces diced lean smoked ham or turkey
1 cup low-sodium chicken broth
1 cup chopped canned plum tomatoes with juice
$\frac{1}{2}$ cup thinly sliced scallions
1 teaspoon chopped fresh thyme or $\frac{1}{2}$ teaspoon
   dried leaves
1 large or 2 small bay leaves
$\frac{1}{4}$ teaspoon hot pepper sauce
Salt and freshly ground pepper to taste
4 cups cooked regular long-grain rice

1. In medium saucepan, heat oil over medium heat; add onion and garlic. Sauté stirring, until onions are wilted, 6–7 minutes.

2. Add beans, ham, broth, tomatoes, scallions, thyme, bay leaves and hot pepper sauce; mix well. Over high heat, bring to a boil. Reduce heat; simmer 40 minutes, stirring occasionally, until beans are creamy. Season with salt and pepper. Remove bay leaf. Serve over rice.

EACH SERVING ($\frac{3}{4}$ cup) PROVIDES: 1 Fat, 1$\frac{1}{4}$ Vegetables, 2$\frac{1}{2}$ Proteins, 2 Breads, 5 Optional Calories
PER SERVING: 512 Calories, 20 g Protein, 7 g Fat, 92 g Carbohydrate, 300 mg Sodium, 8 mg Cholesterol, 6 g Dietary Fiber

BAKED BEANS

Classic baked beans were a colonial staple.
Our updated version keeps the nutrition and
the taste, minus the salt pork and without a
lot of extra sweetening.

MAKES 4 SERVINGS

$\frac{1}{2}$ cup finely chopped onion
2 tablespoons ketchup
1 tablespoon cider vinegar
2$\frac{1}{2}$ teaspoons dark brown sugar
2$\frac{1}{2}$ teaspoons maple syrup
2$\frac{1}{2}$ teaspoons molasses
$\frac{3}{4}$ teaspoon powdered mustard
$\frac{1}{4}$ teaspoon ground ginger
$\frac{1}{4}$ teaspoon freshly ground black pepper
Pinch ground cloves
1 pound rinsed drained cooked navy or great
   northern beans
Salt to taste

1. Preheat oven to 275°F. In 2$\frac{1}{2}$-quart flameproof casserole, combine all ingredients except beans and salt. Add 1 cup water; stir to combine. Bring to a boil over medium-high heat. Reduce heat to medium-low; simmer, stirring occasionally, until mixture has thickened, about 20 minutes.

2. Stir in beans and salt; cover and bake 1 hour, stirring occasionally. Add a tablespoon or two of water, if needed, to keep beans from drying out. If there is too much liquid after 1 hour, uncover and continue to bake, stirring occasionally, until excess liquid is absorbed by beans.

EACH SERVING ($\frac{1}{2}$ cup) PROVIDES: $\frac{1}{4}$ Vegetable, 2 Proteins, 35 Optional Calories
PER SERVING: 213 Calories, 10 g Protein, 1 g Fat, 42 g Carbohydrate, 95 mg Sodium, 0 mg Cholesterol, 4 g Dietary Fiber

ITALIAN-STYLE WHITE BEANS

MAKES 4 SERVINGS

1 tablespoon + 1 teaspoon olive oil
1 garlic clove, finely chopped
2 teaspoons chopped fresh sage
1 teaspoon chopped fresh rosemary
1 cup drained chopped canned plum tomatoes
1 pound rinsed drained cooked cannellini (white kidney) beans
Salt to taste
Freshly ground black pepper to taste
1 tablespoon chopped fresh flat-leaf parsley
1 teaspoon red wine vinegar

1. In heavy small saucepan, heat oil over medium-low heat; add garlic, sage and rosemary. Sauté, stirring, until garlic turns pale gold, about 5 minutes. Add tomatoes; increase heat to medium; cook another 5 minutes, stirring occasionally.

2. Add beans, salt and pepper; reduce heat to low. Simmer, stirring occasionally, about 5 minutes. Stir in parsley and vinegar.

EACH SERVING (1½ cups) PROVIDES: 1 Fat, ½ Vegetable, 2 Proteins
PER SERVING: 198 Calories, 10 g Protein, 5 g Fat, 29 g Carbohydrate, 101 mg Sodium, 0 mg Cholesterol, 5 g Dietary Fiber

BAKED BROWN RICE AND LENTILS

Once you've tried this tasty vegetarian casserole, you may find that it becomes one of your staple family casseroles.

MAKES 4 SERVINGS

1 tablespoon +1 teaspoon vegetable or olive oil
1 cup diced onion
½ cup diced red bell pepper
2 finely chopped garlic cloves
2 teaspoons finely chopped fresh thyme or 1 teaspoon dried leaves
Pinch crushed red pepper flakes
1 cup thinly sliced carrots, lightly steamed
1 cup broccoli florets, lightly steamed
Salt and freshly ground black pepper to taste
2 cups cooked brown rice
8 ounces cooked lentils
6 ounces shredded nonfat Monterey Jack cheese

1. Preheat oven to 350°F. In a 10" nonstick skillet, heat oil over medium heat; add onion and bell pepper. Sauté, stirring, until wilted, about 5 minutes. Add garlic, thyme and red pepper flakes. Sauté, stirring, about 3 minutes. Add steamed carrots and broccoli; season with salt and pepper. Sauté, stirring, 2 minutes; reserve. Combine rice and lentils.

2. Spray a 2-quart ovenproof casserole with nonstick cooking spray. Place a layer of half the rice-lentil mixture in casserole, then a layer of half the vegetables, then a layer of half the cheese. Repeat, ending with cheese. Bake until heated through and cheese is melted, about 15–20 minutes. Place under broiler about 2 minutes to brown cheese.

EACH SERVING (1½ cups) PROVIDES: 1 Fat, 1¾ Vegetables, 2 Proteins, 1 Bread
PER SERVING: 309 Calories, 21 g Protein, 6 g Fat, 43 g Carbohydrate, 385 mg Sodium, 8 mg Cholesterol, 6 g Dietary Fiber

SPICY CHICK-PEA STEW

MAKES 4 SERVINGS

4 cups cubed eggplant ($\frac{1}{2}$–$\frac{3}{4}$" cubes)
1 teaspoon salt
1 tablespoon + 1 teaspoon olive oil
1 tablespoon finely chopped onion
1 tablespoon finely chopped carrot
1 tablespoon finely chopped celery
1 tablespoon finely chopped fresh ginger root
3 garlic cloves, finely chopped
1 tablespoon raisins
1 teaspoon ground cumin
$\frac{1}{4}$ teaspoon cinnamon
2 cups chopped canned plum tomatoes with juice
$\frac{1}{4}$ teaspoon hot pepper sauce
1 pound rinsed drained cooked chick-peas
$\frac{1}{2}$ cup fresh or frozen green peas
2 tablespoons chopped fresh flat-leaf parsley to
    garnish (optional)
$1\frac{1}{2}$ cups cooked couscous

    1. Toss eggplant cubes with salt and place in a mesh strainer or colander; drain for 30 minutes. Press out excess liquid with wooden spoon.

    2. In large nonstick skillet, heat oil over medium heat; add onion, carrot and celery. Sauté, stirring occasionally, until vegetables are wilted, about 5 minutes. Add ginger and garlic; cook 30 seconds.

    3. Increase heat to medium-high; add eggplant. Toss and sauté until eggplant begins to soften, about 5 minutes. Add raisins, cumin and cinnamon; stir well. Add tomatoes and hot pepper sauce; bring to a boil. Cover and reduce heat to medium-low; simmer, stirring occasionally, until eggplant is tender, about 15 minutes. If mixture becomes too thick, add hot water gradually, until sufficiently thinned.

    4. Add chick-peas and green peas; simmer, stirring occasionally, 10 minutes. Sprinkle with parsley if desired, and serve over couscous.

EACH SERVING (1 cup) PROVIDES: 1 Fat, 3 Vegetables, 2 Proteins, 1 Bread, 10 Optional Calories
PER SERVING: 377 Calories, 16 g Protein, 8 g Fat, 63 g Carbohydrate, 223 mg Sodium, 0 mg Cholesterol, 6 g Dietary Fiber

SAUTÉED ESCAROLE AND CHICK-PEAS

MAKES 4 SERVINGS

1 tablespoon + 1 teaspoon olive oil
$\frac{1}{4}$ cup chopped onion
2 garlic cloves, finely chopped
Pinch crushed red pepper flakes (optional)
8 cups chopped rinsed drained escarole
1 pound rinsed drained cooked chick-peas
Salt and freshly ground black pepper to taste
Lemon wedges to garnish (optional)

    1. In large nonstick skillet, heat oil over medium-low heat; add onion, garlic and pepper flakes. Sauté 3–4 minutes, until light gold.

    2. Add escarole; increase heat to medium. Cover and cook, stirring occasionally, until escarole is wilted, about 5–6 minutes.

    3. Uncover; add chick-peas. Increase heat to evaporate excess liquid, stirring constantly. Season with salt and pepper. Garnish with lemon wedges, if desired.

EACH SERVING (1$\frac{1}{2}$ cups) PROVIDES: 1 Fat, 4$\frac{1}{4}$ Vegetables, 2 Proteins
PER SERVING: 249 Calories, 11 g Protein, 8 g Fat, 36 g Carbohydrate, 30 mg Sodium, 0 mg Cholesterol, 6 g Dietary Fiber

TOFU PROVENÇAL

MAKES 4 SERVINGS

1 tablespoon + 1 teaspoon olive oil
1 cup thinly sliced onion
1 cup thinly sliced red bell pepper
2 garlic cloves, finely chopped
1 cup thinly sliced zucchini
2 teaspoons finely chopped fresh thyme or 1
  teaspoon dried leaves
2 cups chopped canned plum tomatoes with juice
1 pound 8 ounces firm tofu, cut into 1" cubes
Salt and freshly ground black pepper to taste
$\frac{1}{2}$ cup loosely packed fresh basil, torn into small
  pieces, or mint

1. In medium nonstick skillet, heat oil over medium-low heat; add onion. Sauté, stirring, until onion begins to brown, about 5 minutes. Add bell pepper; sauté, stirring occasionally, until bell pepper begins to soften, about 2–3 minutes. Add garlic; cook 30 seconds. Add zucchini and thyme; sauté until edges of zucchini turn golden, about 4–5 minutes.

2. Add tomatoes and juice; stir, then cover partially; cook at a steady simmer over low heat 10 minutes, stirring occasionally. Add tofu, salt and pepper; stir. Continue simmering, uncovered, 5 minutes, to heat thoroughly. Add basil; stir.

EACH SERVING (1$\frac{3}{4}$ cups) PROVIDES: 1 Fat, 2$\frac{1}{2}$ Vegetables, 3 Proteins
PER SERVING: 346 Calories, 29 g Protein, 20 g Fat, 20 g Carbohydrate, 223 mg Sodium, 0 mg Cholesterol, 2 g Dietary Fiber

TOFU-VEGETABLE STIR-FRY

Tofu, made from soybeans, is a real chameleon. With little flavor of its own, it takes on the flavors of the dish in which it is cooked. Here, Asian flavors spark the tofu to create a spicy, satisfying stir-fry.

MAKES 4 SERVINGS

2$\frac{1}{2}$ teaspoons canola oil
$\frac{1}{2}$ cup diagonally sliced carrots
2 tablespoons finely chopped fresh ginger root
4 garlic cloves, finely chopped
2 cups cut broccoli (include pared stems, cut into
  bite-size pieces)
$\frac{1}{4}$ cup low-sodium chicken broth
1 pound firm tofu, cut into small cubes
$\frac{1}{2}$ cup thinly sliced shiitake mushroom caps
1 cup julienned seeded red bell pepper
1 medium onion, cut into thin wedges
1 cup snow peas, ends trimmed
1 tablespoon + 1$\frac{1}{2}$ teaspoons soy sauce
1$\frac{1}{2}$ teaspoons dark sesame oil
Pinch crushed red pepper flakes
$\frac{1}{2}$ cup chopped scallions

1. Heat nonstick wok or large nonstick skillet over high heat. Add oil, then carrots; stir-fry 1 minute. Add ginger and garlic; stir-fry 30 seconds. Add broccoli and broth; cover. Let steam 2 minutes, then uncover and stir.

2. Add tofu, stirring 1 minute. Add mushrooms, bell pepper and onion. Stir-fry 3 minutes.

3. Add snow peas, soy sauce, sesame oil and red pepper flakes; stir-fry 1 minute. Sprinkle with scallions.

EACH SERVING (1$\frac{1}{4}$ cups) PROVIDES: 1 Fat, 3 Vegetables, 2 Proteins, 1 Optional Calorie
PER SERVING: 271 Calories, 22 g Protein, 15 g Fat, 18 g Carbohydrate, 427 mg Sodium, 0 mg Cholesterol, 4 g Dietary Fiber

MARINATED TOFU-VEGETABLE KABOBS

MAKES 4 SERVINGS

$\frac{1}{4}$ cup fresh lemon juice
2 tablespoons reduced-sodium soy sauce
1 tablespoon + 1 teaspoon dark sesame oil
1 tablespoon grated fresh ginger root
1 tablespoon finely chopped garlic
$\frac{1}{2}$ teaspoon crushed red pepper flakes or ground red pepper
1 pound firm tofu, cut into twenty-four 1" cubes
2 medium zucchini, cut into 1" cubes
1 medium red or yellow bell pepper, cut into 1" squares
1 medium onion, cut into 8 wedges, leaving root ends intact
8 small mushrooms
8 cherry tomatoes

1. To prepare marinade, in a shallow bowl, combine juice, soy sauce, oil, ginger, garlic and red pepper flakes. Add tofu, zucchini, bell pepper, onion and mushrooms. Allow to sit at room temperature at least 2 hours, turning occasionally.

2. Soak eight 12" bamboo or wooden skewers in cold water for 1 hour. Drain marinade into small bowl and reserve

3. Preheat broiler at least 15 minutes. Beginning and ending with onion, alternately thread marinated vegetables, tomatoes and tofu on skewers.

4. Broil kabobs on broiler rack, basting with marinade, about 5 minutes on each side. Vegetables should be slightly charred and tofu should be brown. Brush with marinade before serving.

EACH SERVING (2 kabobs) PROVIDES: 2$\frac{1}{4}$ Vegetables, 2 Proteins, 40 Optional Calories
PER SERVING: 251 Calories, 20 g Protein, 15 g Fat, 15 g Carbohydrate, 322 mg Sodium, 0 mg Cholesterol, 2 g Dietary Fiber

CHICK-PEAS AND PASTA

Chick-peas, also called garbanzo beans, and pasta are a classic Italian combination. You'll love the speed of this pasta dish when you want to make dinner quickly.

MAKES 4 SERVINGS

1 tablespoon + 1 teaspoon olive oil
1 medium red bell pepper, diced
1 tablespoon finely chopped garlic
1 tablespoon finely chopped rosemary
2 tablespoons chopped fresh flat-leaf parsley
Pinch crushed red pepper flakes
1 cup chopped canned plum tomatoes with $\frac{1}{2}$ cup juice
1 pound rinsed drained cooked chick-peas
Freshly ground black pepper to taste
2 cups cooked ditalini pasta
1$\frac{1}{2}$ ounces grated Parmesan cheese

1. In medium saucepan, heat oil over medium-low heat; add bell pepper, garlic, rosemary, 1 tablespoon of the parsley and the red pepper flakes. Sauté gently, stirring frequently, until garlic turns pale gold, about 5 minutes.

2. Add tomatoes and juice; increase heat to medium. Simmer, stirring frequently, 10 minutes. Add chick-peas; season with pepper. Heat thoroughly, stirring occasionally, about 5 minutes. Add pasta, cheese and remaining parsley. Mix well and serve.

EACH SERVING (1$\frac{1}{4}$ cups) PROVIDES: 1 Fat, 1 Vegetable, 2$\frac{1}{2}$ Proteins, 1 Bread
PER SERVING: 402 Calories, 19 g Protein, 11 g Fat, 58 g Carbohydrate, 355 mg Sodium, 8 mg Cholesterol, 6 g Dietary Fiber

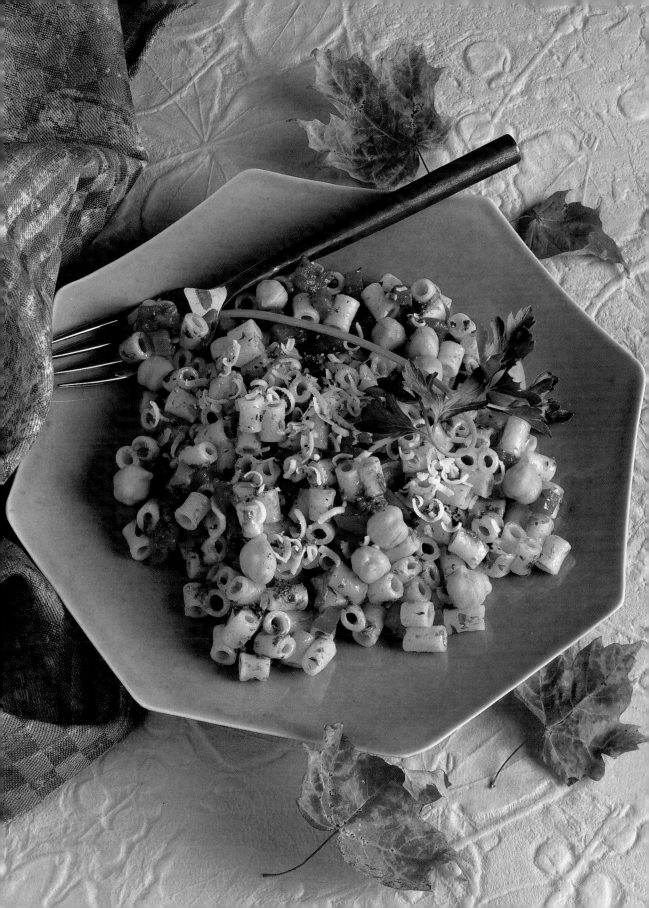

SUCCOTASH

Succotash comes from the native American word "msickquatash." Created by the Narragansett Indians, the dish originally included chicken or meat as well as vegetables. Our version is a hearty vegetarian one that goes beyond just combining corn and lima beans.

MAKES 4 SERVINGS

1 tablespoon + 1 teaspoon olive oil
1 medium red bell pepper, diced
½ cup diced zucchini
½ cup diced onion
1 garlic clove, finely chopped
1 medium tomato, seeded and diced
1 cup rinsed drained cooked green lima beans
1 cup corn kernels, fresh or frozen
2 tablespoons chopped flat-leaf parsley
1 teaspoon paprika
½ teaspoon salt
½ teaspoon black pepper
¼ teaspoon dried marjoram

1. In medium nonstick skillet, heat oil over medium heat; add bell pepper, zucchini, onion and garlic. Sauté, stirring frequently, until vegetables are wilted, about 8 minutes. Add tomato; sauté 2 minutes, stirring.

2. Add lima beans, corn, parsley, the paprika, salt, pepper and marjoram. Cover; reduce heat to medium-low. Simmer 10 minutes. Add remaining parsley and serve.

EACH SERVING (¾ cup) PROVIDES: 1 Fat, 1½ Vegetables, 1 Bread
PER SERVING: 153 Calories, 5 g Protein, 5 g Fat, 24 g Carbohydrate, 293 mg Sodium, 0 mg Cholesterol, 4 g Dietary Fiber

BEANS WITH VEGETABLES

This dish looks best when prepared with cooked dried beans. They hold their shape nicely when cooked.

MAKES 4 SERVINGS

8 broccoli spears
1 tablespoon + 1 teaspoon olive oil
1 medium red bell pepper, seeded and cut into strips
2 teaspoons finely chopped garlic
Pinch crushed red pepper flakes (optional)
2 cups cauliflower florets, cut into bite-size pieces and steamed
1 pound rinsed drained cooked cannellini (white kidney) beans*
Salt and freshly ground black pepper to taste

1. Pare broccoli stems; quarter and cut into bite-sized pieces. Cut broccoli florets into bite-sized pieces and steam until tender-crisp.

2. In a 10-inch nonstick skillet, heat oil over medium-high heat; add bell pepper. Sauté, stirring, until bell pepper begins to brown, about 4–5 minutes. Add garlic and red pepper flakes; sauté 30 seconds. Add broccoli and cauliflower; sauté until garlic is pale gold, about 2–3 minutes.

3. Add beans, tossing until heated, about 4 minutes. Season to taste with salt and pepper.

*You can substitute canned beans for the cooked dried beans.

EACH SERVING PROVIDES: 1 Fat; 2½ Vegetables, 2 Proteins
PER SERVING: 217 Calories, 12 g Protein, 5 g Fat, 33 g Carbohydrate, 22 mg Sodium, 0 mg Cholesterol, 7 g Dietary Fiber

EGYPTIAN FAVA BEAN SALAD

MAKES 4 SERVINGS

1 medium cucumber
1 pound rinsed drained cooked fava beans or red kidney beans
1 cup diced tomato
$\frac{1}{2}$ cup chopped fresh mint leaves
$\frac{1}{2}$ cup chopped fresh flat-leaf parsley
$\frac{1}{4}$ cup finely chopped red onion
$\frac{1}{4}$ cup tahini (sesame paste) mixed with 1 tablespoon cold water
$\frac{1}{4}$ cup fresh lemon juice
2 garlic cloves, finely chopped
Dash ground red pepper
Salt and freshly ground black pepper to taste

1. Pare and seed cucumber; cut cucumber lengthwise into eighths; dice.

2. In large mixing bowl, combine all ingredients. Toss well and serve at room temperature or warm slightly.

EACH SERVING (1 cup) PROVIDES: $\frac{3}{4}$ Fat, 1$\frac{1}{4}$ Vegetables, $\frac{1}{4}$ Protein, 2 Breads, 10 Optional Calories
PER SERVING: 241 Calories, 12 g Protein, 9 g Fat, 32 g Carbohydrate, 33 mg Sodium, 0 mg Cholesterol, 8 g Dietary Fiber

CRUNCHY LENTIL SALAD

MAKES 4 SERVINGS

4 cups hot cooked lentils
$\frac{1}{4}$ cup finely chopped carrot
$\frac{1}{4}$ cup finely chopped celery
1 tablespoon + 1 teaspoon extra virgin olive oil
1–2 tablespoons fresh lemon juice
1 garlic clove, finely chopped
$\frac{3}{4}$ cup plain nonfat yogurt
$\frac{1}{4}$ cup finely chopped fresh flat-leaf parsley
1 ounce coarsely chopped walnuts
Salt and freshly ground black pepper to taste
6 cups rinsed drained curly chicory

1. In large bowl, combine hot lentils, carrot, celery, olive oil, juice and garlic. Allow mixture to cool to room temperature; add yogurt, parsley, walnuts, salt and pepper. Mix thoroughly. Serve over chicory.

EACH SERVING ($\frac{3}{4}$ cup) PROVIDES: $\frac{1}{4}$ Milk, 1$\frac{1}{2}$ Fats, 3$\frac{1}{4}$ Vegetables, 1 Protein
PER SERVING: 409 Calories, 26 g Protein, 11 g Fat, 59 g Carbohydrate, 169 mg Sodium, 1 mg Cholesterol, 13 g Dietary Fiber

---

Cooking Dried Beans

◆

Buying dried beans is economical, and it's convenient to have them on hand for your favorite recipes. Beans freeze well, so cook the entire package and freeze in portion sizes for another day. Use the guidelines below to cook dried beans.

- *Pick over beans, removing any foreign particles, such as small stones. Remove any discolored, darkened or broken beans.*
- *Place in colander, rinse with cold water, then place in a large bowl.*
- *Add roughly three times as much water as beans—for example, 3 cups water to 1 cup of beans.*
- *Soak at room temperature or in the refrigerator about 24 hours.*
- *Drain and rinse beans. Place in pot and add fresh water to 2 inches above beans.*
- *Bring to a boil; reduce heat to low and simmer uncovered, stirring occasionally, until beans are tender. Depending on the beans, cooking time will be from 30 to 60 minutes.*
- *Drain beans before serving or using in a recipe.*

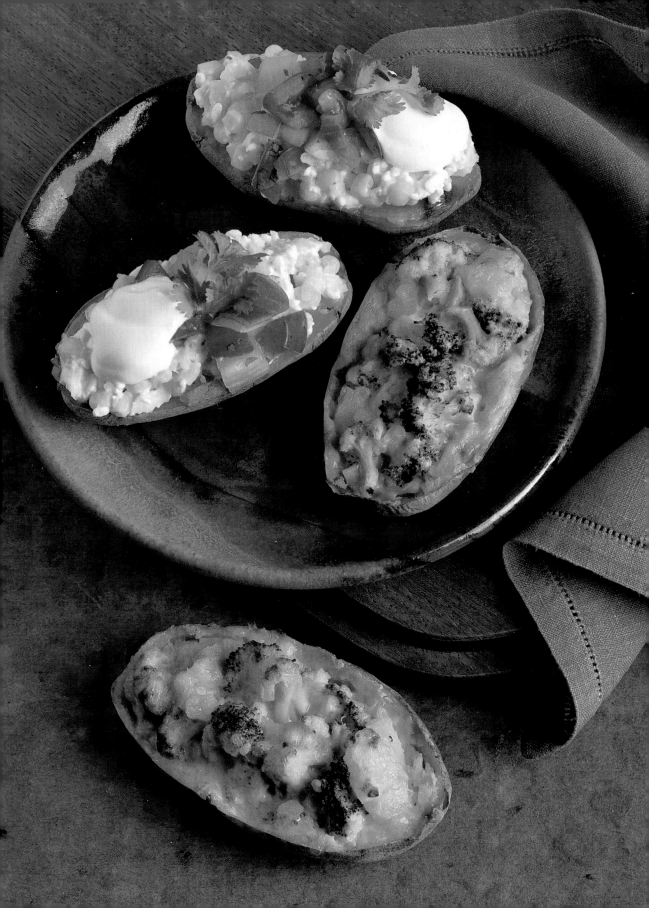

MEXICAN-STYLE BAKED POTATOES

MAKES 4 SERVINGS

Four 5-ounce russet potatoes
$2/3$ cup low-fat (1%) cottage cheese
3 ounces shredded Monterey pepperjack cheese
$1/2$ cup thawed frozen corn kernels
$1/4$ cup salsa
$1/4$ cup plain low-fat yogurt
4 sprigs fresh cilantro

1. Preheat oven to 425°F. With fork, pierce potatoes several times. Bake 1 hour or until cooked through.

2. In small bowl, stir together cottage cheese, Monterey pepperjack cheese and corn. Split hot potatoes and spoon cheese mixture into each. Top each potato with 1 tablespoon salsa, 1 tablespoon yogurt and a sprig of coriander.

EACH SERVING PROVIDES: 1$1/2$ Proteins, 1$1/4$ Breads, 10 Optional Calories
PER SERVING: 258 Calories, 14 g Protein, 8 g Fat, 34 g Carbohydrate, 410 mg Sodium, 25 mg Cholesterol, 3 g Dietary Fiber

BOILED NEW POTATOES WITH SEASONING

MAKES 4 SERVINGS

1 pound 4 ounces small new potatoes
2 garlic cloves, slivered
$1/4$ teaspoon dried rosemary leaves
$1/4$ teaspoon dried thyme leaves
$3/4$ cup low-sodium chicken broth

1. In large pot of boiling water, cook potatoes just until tender, 20–25 minutes; drain.

2. Spray large nonstick skillet with nonstick cooking spray. Add garlic, rosemary and thyme; toss. Cook over low heat, stirring constantly, 1 minute. Add potatoes and toss to coat; add broth. Increase heat to moderately high, cover and cook 2 minutes. Remove cover and continue cooking until liquid has evaporated.

EACH SERVING PROVIDES: 1 Bread, 4 Optional Calories
PER SERVING: 119 Calories, 3 g Protein, 7 g Fat, 26 g Carbohydrate, 11 mg Sodium, 0 mg Cholesterol, 2 g Dietary Fiber

TWICE-BAKED POTATOES

MAKES 4 SERVINGS

Four 5-ounce russet potatoes
3 cups chopped broccoli florets
4 ounces shredded cheddar cheese
$1/4$ cup light sour cream
$1/4$ cup skim milk
1 tablespoon + 1 teaspoon olive oil
1 teaspoon prepared mustard
$3/4$ teaspoon salt
$1/8$ teaspoon ground red pepper

1. Preheat oven to 425°F. With fork, pierce potatoes several times. Bake 1 hour or until cooked through. Reduce temperature to 375°F.

2. In large pot of boiling salted water, cook broccoli 3 minutes; drain. Rinse under cold running water; drain again.

3. Cut potatoes in half horizontally. Scoop out potato flesh, leaving $1/2$" shell intact. In medium bowl, stir together cooked potatoes, cheddar cheese, sour cream, milk, oil, mustard, salt and red pepper; fold in broccoli. Spoon mixture evenly into potato shells; place on baking sheet and bake 10 minutes or until hot and bubbly.

EACH SERVING PROVIDES: 1 Fat, 1$1/2$ Vegetables, 1$1/4$ Proteins, 1 Bread, 30 Optional Calories
PER SERVING: 375 Calories, 16 g Protein, 17 g Fat, 43 g Carbohydrate, 650 mg Sodium, 35 mg Cholesterol, 7 g Dietary Fiber

GARLIC MASHED POTATOES

Garlic and buttermilk combine to make these mashed potatoes so luscious you won't even notice they don't have a drop of fat!

MAKES 4 SERVINGS

8 garlic cloves
1 pound 4 ounces all-purpose potatoes, pared and
   thinly sliced
1 bay leaf
$\frac{1}{2}$ teaspoon salt
3 tablespoons skim buttermilk

1. Preheat oven to 375°F. Wrap garlic in foil and bake 30 minutes or until soft. When cool enough to handle, squeeze garlic from skin; set aside.

2. In large pot, combine potatoes, $1\frac{3}{4}$ cups water, bay leaf and $\frac{1}{4}$ teaspoon of the salt. Bring to a boil; reduce heat to simmer and cook 10 minutes, until potatoes are tender. Drain, reserving cooking liquid. Discard bay leaf.

3. With potato masher or beater, mash potatoes with garlic, buttermilk and remaining $\frac{1}{4}$ teaspoon salt. Thin with reserve cooking liquid as needed.

EACH SERVING PROVIDES: 1 Bread, 4 Optional Calories
PER SERVING: 99 Calories, 3 g Protein, 0 g Fat, 22 g Carbohydrate, 293 mg Sodium, 0 mg Cholesterol, 2 g Dietary Fiber

BAKED POTATOES WITH HERBED CREAM

You'll feel very self-indulgent when you put this herbed cream on your baked potato, but it's strictly on the straight and narrow!

MAKES 4 SERVINGS

Four 5-ounce russet potatoes
4 ounces Yogurt Cheese (page 359)
2 teaspoons minced chives or scallions
1 teaspoon minced fresh herbs, such as thyme, dill,
   rosemary or tarragon
1 small garlic clove, crushed
$\frac{1}{8}$ teaspoon salt
$\frac{1}{8}$ teaspoon pepper

1. Preheat oven to 425°F. With fork, pierce the potatoes several times. Bake 1 hour or until cooked through.

2. In small bowl, combine yogurt cheese, chives, herbs, garlic, salt and pepper. Split potatoes and spoon cream mixture evenly into each.

EACH SERVING PROVIDES: $\frac{1}{4}$ Milk, 1 Bread
PER SERVING: 131 Calories, 4 g Protein, 27 g Fat, 27 g Carbohydrate, 95 mg Sodium, 0 mg Cholesterol, 2 g Dietary Fiber

---

Potatoes, Please

◆

Potatoes are wonderfully satisfying—and good for you! Microwave a potato and you have the basics for a quick, delicious dinner or side dish. Try our great recipes, Mexican-Style Baked Potatoes (page 301) or Twice-Baked Potatoes (page 301).

You can also add your own potato toppings, such as salsa or nonfat yogurt with fresh herbs. Or, scoop out cooked potato and mix pulp with some tuna, shredded cheese and a dab of skim milk, then pop back in the microwave for a minute. Delicious!

To microwave a potato, scrub skin and pierce in several places to allow steam to escape. Wrap in paper towel and place in microwave oven. Microwave on High 4 to 5 minutes, turning potato over after 2 minutes, until tender. Let stand 5 minutes.

TOASTED ONION CREAM

This is a wonderful topping for baked potatoes. It's also a great dip with pita bread or cut-up vegetables.

MAKES 4 SERVINGS

2 cups finely minced yellow onion
4 ounces Yogurt Cheese (page 359)
½ teaspoon instant beef bouillon granules
   dissolved in 1 teaspoon boiling water
⅛ teaspoon black pepper

1. Spray large skillet with nonstick cooking spray. Sauté onion over medium heat about 10 minutes, stirring often, until nicely brown and caramelized. Combine with yogurt cheese, dissolved beef bouillon granules and pepper.

EACH SERVING PROVIDES: ¼ Milk, 1 Vegetable, 1 Bread, 1 Optional Calorie
PER SERVING: 163 Calories, 5 g Protein, 1 g Fat, 34 g Carbohydrate, 133 mg Sodium, 0 mg Cholesterol, 4 g Dietary Fiber

◆

LYONNAISE POTATOES

MAKES 4 SERVINGS

1 tablespoon + 1 teaspoon olive oil
1 pound 4 ounces all-purpose potatoes, boiled, peeled and sliced ¼" thick
½ teaspoon salt
¼ teaspoon dried marjoram leaves
⅛ teaspoon black pepper
1 cup thinly sliced onions
2 garlic cloves, slivered
¼ cup chicken broth

1. In large nonstick skillet, heat 1 tablespoon of the oil over moderately high heat; add potatoes. Sprinkle with salt, marjoram and pepper and cook, turning as they color, about 10 minutes.

2. Meanwhile, in separate large nonstick skillet, heat remaining teaspoon oil over medium heat; add onions. Cook 3–4 minutes. Lower heat, add garlic and cook 2 minutes. Add broth; cook 5–7 minutes longer, until soft. Transfer onions to pan with potatoes and toss together.

EACH SERVING PROVIDES: 1 Fat, ½ Vegetable, 1 Bread, 1 Optional Calorie
PER SERVING: 143 Calories, 3 g Protein, 5 g Fat, 23 g Carbohydrate, 243 mg Sodium, 0 mg Cholesterol, 2 g Dietary Fiber

◆

COLCANNON

This traditional Irish dish is particularly nice on cold evenings, when you'd like a hearty side dish with your entrée.

MAKES 6 SERVINGS

12 ounces peeled cooked all-purpose potatoes
½ cup plain nonfat yogurt
4 cups chopped green cabbage, steamed until tender
2 cups chopped leeks (white portion only), steamed until tender
3 tablespoons chopped fresh chives
¾ teaspoon salt
¼ teaspoon white pepper
Pinch ground nutmeg
2 teaspoons reduced-calorie tub margarine

1. Preheat oven to 350°F. Spray a 1½-quart casserole with nonstick cooking spray.

2. In large bowl, combine potatoes and yogurt. With mixer at low speed, beat until potatoes are chunky-smooth; stir in cabbage, leeks, chives, salt, white pepper and nutmeg, mixing well.

3. Spoon mixture into prepared casserole; dot with margarine. Bake 30 minutes, until lightly browned.

EACH SERVING PROVIDES: 2 Vegetables, ½ Bread, 15 Optional Calories
PER SERVING: 95 Calories, 3 g Protein, 1 g Fat, 19 g Carbohydrate, 320 mg Sodium, 1 mg Cholesterol, 2 g Dietary Fiber

OVEN "FRIES"

MAKES 4 SERVINGS

1 pound 4 ounces russet potatoes, pared and cut
    into 3 × $\frac{1}{2}$" strips
$\frac{3}{4}$ teaspoon salt
$\frac{1}{2}$ teaspoon granulated sugar
1 tablespoon + 1 teaspoon oil
1 teaspoon paprika

1. Preheat oven to 450°F. Spray nonstick baking sheet with nonstick cooking spray; set aside.

2. In large bowl, combine potatoes, $\frac{1}{4}$ teaspoon of the salt and the sugar; pour ice water over them to cover. Soak 15 minutes; drain well and blot dry.

3. In large bowl, toss potatoes with oil and paprika. Place in single layer on prepared baking sheet. Bake, turning potatoes over as they brown, 45 minutes, until cooked through and crisp. Sprinkle with the remaining $\frac{1}{2}$ teaspoon salt.

EACH SERVING PROVIDES: 1 Fat, 1 Bread, 2 Optional Calories
PER SERVING: 148 Calories, 3 g Protein, 5 g Fat, 24 g Carbohydrate, 420 mg Sodium, 0 mg Cholesterol, 2 g Dietary Fiber

POTATO PANCAKES

MAKES 4 SERVINGS

15 ounces pared Idaho potatoes
2 egg whites
3 tablespoons all-purpose flour
2 tablespoons minced scallion
$\frac{3}{4}$ teaspoon salt
1 tablespoon + 1 teaspoon corn or vegetable oil

1. Shred potatoes; soak in cold water for 30 minutes. Drain and blot dry.

2. Preheat oven to 375°F.

3. In medium bowl, combine potatoes, egg whites, flour, scallion and salt; mix well. Form into 12 pancakes.

4. In large nonstick skillet, heat one-third of the oil over medium heat. Cook 4 pancakes at a time, just until golden on each side, about 2 minutes; transfer to baking sheet. Continue with remaining oil and pancakes. Bake 5–7 minutes, until crisp and cooked through. Makes 12 pancakes.

EACH SERVING (3 pancakes) PROVIDES: 1 Fat, 1 Bread, 10 Optional Calories
PER SERVING: 138 Calories, 4 g Protein, 5 g Fat, 20 g Carbohydrate, 445 mg Sodium, 0 mg Cholesterol, 2 g Dietary Fiber

HASH BROWN POTATOES

MAKES 4 SERVINGS

1 teaspoon vegetable oil
1 teaspoon unsalted stick margarine
1 pound 4 ounces peeled cooked all-purpose
    potatoes, cut into $\frac{1}{2}$" cubes
1 cup minced onions
$\frac{1}{2}$ cup chicken broth
$\frac{1}{2}$ teaspoon salt
$\frac{1}{8}$ teaspoon black pepper

1. In large nonstick skillet, heat oil and margarine over medium heat; add potatoes and onions, cook 5 minutes.

2. Add broth, salt and pepper. Reduce heat and cook 15 minutes longer, patting the potato and onion mixture down and turning it over as it forms a crust.

EACH SERVING PROVIDES: $\frac{1}{2}$ Fat, $\frac{1}{2}$ Vegetable, 1 Bread, 3 Optional Calories
PER SERVING: 122 Calories, 3 g Protein, 2 g Fat, 23 g Carbohydrate, 404 mg Sodium, 0 mg Cholesterol, 2 g Dietary Fiber

Hash Brown Potatoes and scrambled eggs

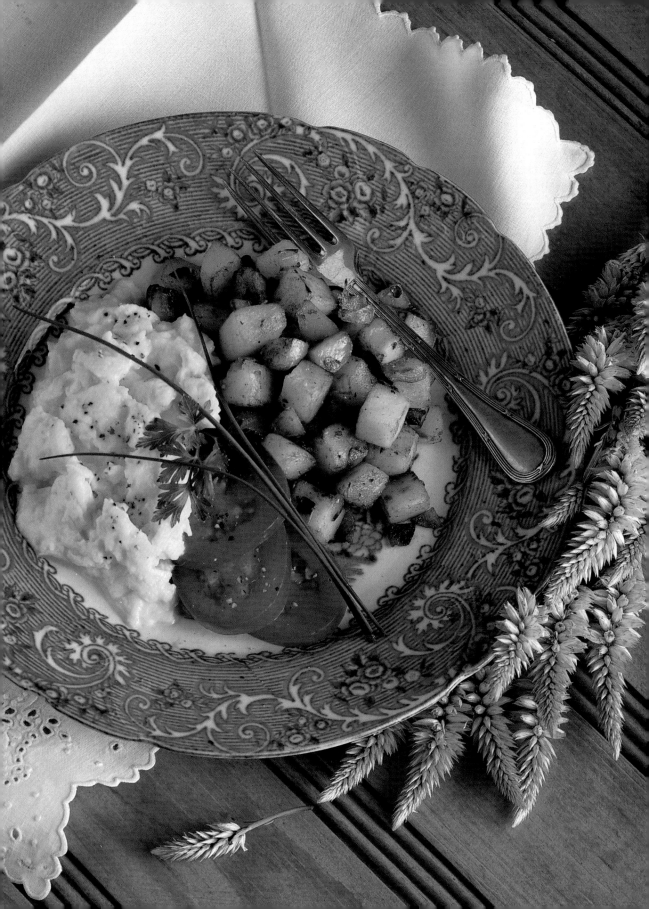

ROASTED SWEET POTATOES

MAKES 4 SERVINGS

1 tablespoon + 1 teaspoon olive oil
4 garlic cloves, unpeeled
2 sprigs fresh rosemary or $\frac{1}{2}$ teaspoon dried rosemary
1 pound pared sweet potatoes, cut into $\frac{3}{4}$" chunks
$\frac{1}{4}$ cup chicken broth
$\frac{1}{2}$ teaspoon salt

1. Preheat oven to 350°F.

2. In 9 × 9" baking pan, combine oil, garlic and rosemary. Heat in oven 7 minutes or until oil is hot; add potatoes and stir to coat. Roast 30 minutes, turning the potatoes occasionally.

3. Add broth; cook 15 minutes longer, turning the potatoes occasionally, until browned and cooked through. Sprinkle with salt and serve.

EACH SERVING PROVIDES: 1 Fat, 1 Bread, 1 Optional Calorie
PER SERVING: 165 Calories, 2 g Protein, 5 g Fat, 29 g Carbohydrate, 350 mg Sodium, 0 mg Cholesterol, 3 g Dietary Fiber

◆

SWEET POTATO CASSEROLE

Rescued from under a marshmallow topping, this sweet potato casserole is just right for holiday meals or anytime you're looking for a tantalizing side dish.

MAKES 4 SERVINGS

2 small apples, pared and thinly sliced
1 pound sweet potatoes, pared and thinly sliced
$\frac{3}{4}$ teaspoon chopped crystallized ginger
$\frac{1}{2}$ teaspoon salt
$\frac{1}{4}$ cup thawed frozen apple juice concentrate
2 tablespoons firmly packed dark brown sugar
2 teaspoons fresh lemon juice
$\frac{1}{4}$ teaspoon cinnamon
$\frac{1}{8}$ teaspoon ground cloves
2 teaspoons stick margarine, cut up

1. Preheat oven to 375°F. Spray a square baking pan with nonstick cooking spray.

2. Arrange half of the apple slices in bottom of baking pan; top with half of the sweet potato slices. Sprinkle with half the ginger and half the salt. Repeat layers, sprinkling with remaining ginger and salt.

3. In small bowl, stir together $\frac{1}{4}$ cup water, juice concentrate, brown sugar, juice, cinnamon and cloves. Pour over potato and apple layers; cover with foil and bake 45 minutes. Uncover, dot with margarine; bake 15 minutes longer, until tender, bubbly and lightly browned.

EACH SERVING PROVIDES: $\frac{1}{2}$ Fat, 1 Fruit, 1 Bread, 25 Optional Calories
PER SERVING: 225 Calories, 2 g Protein, 3 g Fat, 50 g Carbohydrate, 318 mg Sodium, 0 mg Cholesterol, 4 g Dietary Fiber

◆

MASHED SWEET POTATOES

MAKES 4 SERVINGS

1 pound sweet potatoes, pared and thinly sliced
$\frac{3}{4}$ teaspoon salt
2 teaspoons unsalted stick margarine
$\frac{1}{4}$ teaspoon ground ginger
$\frac{1}{8}$ teaspoon ground cardamom
$\frac{1}{8}$ teaspoon black pepper
$\frac{1}{8}$ teaspoon ground nutmeg

1. In medium saucepan, combine sweet potatoes, $1\frac{1}{4}$ cups water and $\frac{1}{2}$ teaspoon of the salt. Bring to a boil, cover and simmer 15–20 minutes, until tender; drain, reserving 2 tablespoons cooking liquid.

2. With a potato masher or beater, mash potatoes with reserved cooking liquid, margarine, ginger, cardamom, pepper, nutmeg and the remaining $\frac{1}{4}$ teaspoon salt.

EACH SERVING PROVIDES: $\frac{1}{2}$ Fat, 1 Bread
PER SERVING: 137 Calories, 2 g Protein, 2 g Fat, 28 g Carbohydrate, 427 mg Sodium, 0 mg Cholesterol, 3 g Dietary Fiber

*Turkey Cutlets with Cranberry Sauce (page 172),
Mashed Sweet Potatoes*

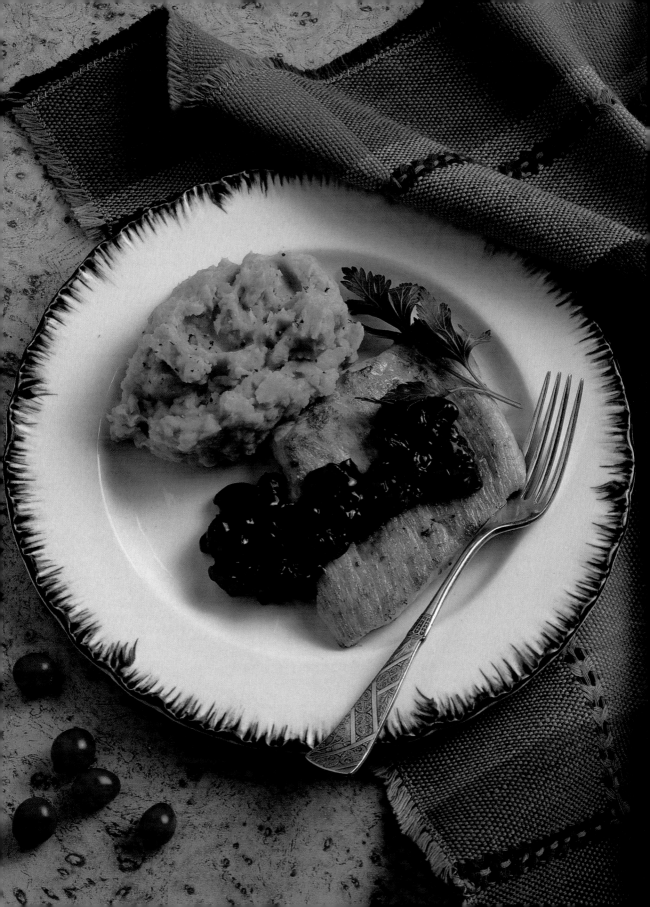

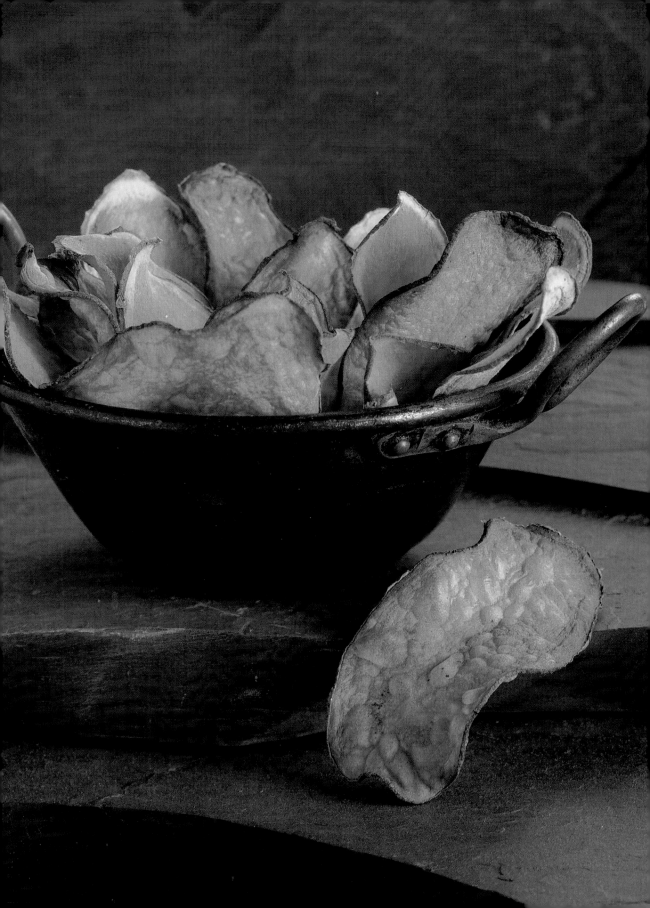

SWEET POTATO CHIPS

MAKES 4 SERVINGS

1 pound sweet potatoes, pared and sliced $\frac{1}{8}$" thick
$\frac{1}{2}$ teaspoon granulated sugar
$\frac{3}{4}$ teaspoon salt

1. In medium bowl, pour ice water over potatoes to cover; stir in sugar and $\frac{1}{4}$ teaspoon of the salt. Let stand 30 minutes.

2. Preheat oven to 350°F. Spray 2 nonstick baking sheets with nonstick cooking spray; set aside.

3. Drain potatoes, blot dry and place on prepared baking sheets in a single layer. Bake 35 to 40 minutes, turning the potato slices over frequently so that they color and crisp evenly. Sprinkle with the remaining $\frac{1}{2}$ teaspoon salt.

EACH SERVING PROVIDES: 1 Bread, 2 Optional Calories
PER SERVING: 95 Calories, 1 g Protein, 1 g Fat, 20 g Carbohydrate, 422 mg Sodium, 0 mg Cholesterol, 2 g Dietary Fiber

◆

POTATO CHIPS

MAKES 4 SERVINGS

1 pound 4 ounces russet potatoes, pared and sliced $\frac{1}{8}$" thick
$\frac{3}{4}$ teaspoon salt

1. Place potatoes in a bowl and pour ice water over to cover; stir in $\frac{1}{4}$ teaspoon of the salt and let stand 30 minutes.

2. Preheat oven to 350°F. Spray 2 nonstick baking sheets with nonstick cooking spray; set aside.

3. Drain potatoes, blot dry and place on prepared baking sheets in a single layer. Bake 45 minutes, turning the potato slices over frequently during the baking time so that they crisp evenly. Sprinkle with remaining $\frac{1}{2}$ teaspoon salt.

EACH SERVING PROVIDES: 1 Bread
PER SERVING: 107 Calories, 2 g Protein, 1 g Fat, 23 g Carbohydrate, 422 mg Sodium, 0 mg Cholesterol, 2 g Dietary Fiber

POTATO AND BEAN SALAD WITH WALNUT VINAIGRETTE

MAKES 4 SERVINGS

1 pound 1 ounce cooked small new or red bliss potatoes
1$\frac{1}{4}$ cups green beans
2 tablespoons + 2 teaspoons balsamic vinegar
$\frac{1}{2}$ fluid ounce (1 tablespoon) dry white wine
1 teaspoon Dijon mustard
Salt and freshly ground black pepper to taste
2 teaspoons extra virgin olive oil
2 teaspoons canola oil or other vegetable oil
$\frac{1}{4}$ cup finely chopped shallots or scallions
1 ounce walnuts, finely chopped
4 ounces rinsed drained cooked kidney beans (room temperature)

1. Cool potatoes to room temperature; cut into halves or quarters. Trim green beans; steam until tender-crisp. Cut into 1" pieces.

2. To prepare vinaigrette, in small bowl, whisk together vinegar, wine, mustard, salt and pepper. Add olive oil and canola oil, a little at a time, whisking constantly. Mix in shallots and walnuts.

3. In large bowl, combine potatoes, green beans and kidney beans; pour dressing over and toss thoroughly. Allow to stand at room temperature about 1 hour. Toss again and serve.

EACH SERVING PROVIDES: 1$\frac{1}{2}$ Fats, $\frac{3}{4}$ Vegetable, $\frac{3}{4}$ Protein, 1 Bread, 3 Optional Calories
PER SERVING: 261 Calories, 7 g Protein, 10 g Fat, 38 g Carbohydrate, 54 mg Sodium, 0 mg Cholesterol, 5 g Dietary Fiber

GREEN BEAN AND POTATO SALAD

MAKES 4 SERVINGS

3 tablespoons wine vinegar
1 tablespoon Dijon mustard
$\frac{1}{2}$ teaspoon freshly ground black pepper
$\frac{1}{4}$ teaspoon salt
1 tablespoon + 1 teaspoon olive oil
3 cups green beans, cut into 2" pieces and steamed
1 pound boiled or steamed potatoes, cut into $\frac{1}{4}$"
  slices
$\frac{1}{2}$ cup chopped red onion
$\frac{1}{2}$ cup chopped fresh dill

1. To prepare vinaigrette, whisk together vinegar, mustard, pepper and salt; then whisk in oil.

2. Place green beans, potatoes and onion in a medium mixing bowl. Add vinaigrette and dill; toss thoroughly. Serve warm or at room temperature.

EACH SERVING (1$\frac{1}{2}$ cups) PROVIDES: 1 Fat, 1$\frac{3}{4}$ Vegetables, 1 Bread
PER SERVING: 206 Calories, 5 g Protein, 5 g Fat, 38 g Carbohydrate, 267 mg Sodium, 0 mg Cholesterol, 4 g Dietary Fiber

BAKED POTATOES WITH SOUR CREAM

MAKES 4 SERVINGS

Four 5-ounce russet potatoes
$\frac{1}{4}$ cup nonfat sour cream
3 tablespoons thinly sliced chives
$\frac{3}{4}$ teaspoon salt
$\frac{1}{8}$ teaspoon black pepper
$\frac{1}{8}$ teaspoon ground nutmeg

1. Preheat oven to 425°F. With fork, pierce potatoes several times. Bake 1 hour or until cooked through.

2. In small bowl, whisk together sour cream, chives, salt, pepper and nutmeg. Split potatoes and spoon $\frac{1}{4}$ of cream mixture into each.

EACH SERVING PROVIDES: 1 Bread, 10 Optional Calories
PER SERVING: 126 Calories, 4 g Protein, 0 g Fat, 27 g Carbohydrate, 433 mg Sodium, 0 mg Cholesterol, 2 g Dietary Fiber

Lemon–Poppy Seed Crisps, Coconut-Macadamia Kisses
(page 331), Apple-Oatmeal Cookies (page 330)

CHAPTER TWELVE

DESSERTS

CHOCOLATE LAYER CAKE

MAKES 12 SERVINGS

1 cup + 2 tablespoons all-purpose flour
$\frac{1}{3}$ cup unsweetened cocoa powder
1 teaspoon espresso powder or instant coffee
   granules
1 teaspoon baking powder
1 teaspoon baking soda
$\frac{1}{4}$ teaspoon salt
$\frac{1}{3}$ cup + 2 teaspoons granulated sugar
2 tablespoons + 2 teaspoons reduced-calorie tub
   margarine
1 large egg
1 teaspoon vanilla extract
1 cup skim buttermilk
$\frac{1}{2}$ cup reduced-calorie apricot spread (16 calories
   per 2 teaspoons)
1 tablespoon confectioners' sugar

1. Preheat oven to 350°F. Spray two 8" square baking pans with nonstick cooking spray.

2. In small bowl, combine flour, cocoa powder, espresso powder, baking powder, baking soda and salt; set aside.

3. In medium bowl, with mixer on high speed, cream sugar and margarine; add egg and vanilla extract, beating until smooth. Gradually beat in flour mixture alternately with buttermilk, until batter is smooth.

4. Evenly divide batter between prepared pans; bake 10 minutes, until toothpick inserted in center comes out clean. Transfer pans to rack; let cool. Insert sharp knife around edges of each pan; remove cakes from pans. Transfer 1 cake to serving platter flat side up; set aside.

5. Meanwhile, in small saucepan, heat fruit spread over low heat about 2–3 minutes, until melted. Brush $\frac{1}{4}$ cup of the melted spread on top of cake on serving platter. Brush the remaining fruit spread on flat underside of remaining cake; arrange on top of cake on serving platter, fruit-spread sides together.

6. Evenly sprinkle top of cake with confectioners' sugar. Cut into 12 equal pieces.

EACH SERVING PROVIDES: $\frac{1}{4}$ Fat, $\frac{1}{2}$ Bread, 65 Optional Calories
PER SERVING: 119 Calories, 3 g Protein, 3 g Fat, 22 g Carbohydrate, 243 mg Sodium, 19 mg Cholesterol, 1 g Dietary Fiber

◆

UPSIDE-DOWN BLUEBERRY-CORNMEAL CAKE

MAKES 12 SERVINGS

$1\frac{1}{2}$ cups fresh or thawed frozen blueberries
$\frac{1}{2}$ cup minus 1 tablespoon granulated sugar
1 teaspoon cornstarch
3 ounces uncooked yellow cornmeal
$\frac{1}{3}$ cup + 2 teaspoons all-purpose flour
1 teaspoon baking powder
$\frac{1}{4}$ teaspoon salt
$\frac{1}{4}$ cup reduced-calorie tub margarine
1 large egg
$1\frac{1}{2}$ teaspoons lemon zest
$\frac{1}{4}$ cup skim milk

1. Preheat oven to 375°F. Spray an 8" square baking pan with nonstick cooking spray.

2. In small saucepan bring blueberries, 1 tablespoon of the sugar and the cornstarch to a boil; cook, stirring frequently, about 2–3 minutes, until thickened. Pour berry mixture into prepared baking pan.

3. In small bowl, combine cornmeal, flour, baking powder and salt; set aside.

4. In medium bowl, with mixer on high speed, cream the remaining $\frac{1}{3}$ cup + 2 teaspoons sugar and the margarine; add egg and lemon zest and beat until smooth. Gradually add cornmeal mixture alternately with milk, beating until batter is smooth.

5. Evenly scrape batter over berry mixture. Bake 20–25 minutes, until toothpick inserted in center comes out clean. Transfer to rack for 5 minutes; invert onto serving platter.

EACH SERVING PROVIDES: $\frac{1}{2}$ Fat, $\frac{1}{2}$ Bread, 45 Optional Calories
PER SERVING: 105 Calories, 2 g Protein, 3 g Fat, 19 g Carbohydrate, 132 mg Sodium, 18 mg Cholesterol, 1 g Dietary Fiber

Chocolate Layer Cake

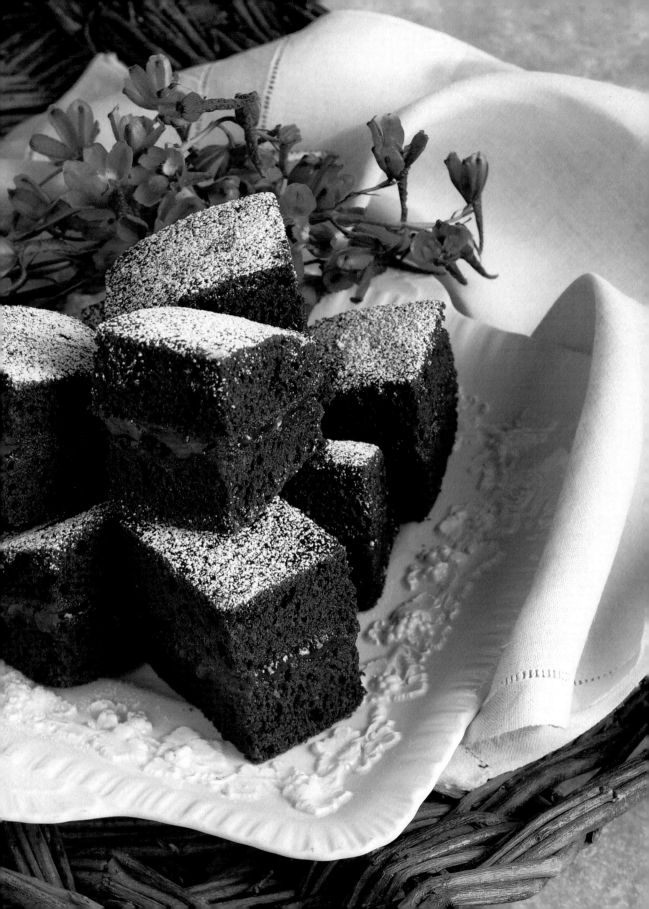

VANILLA LAYER CAKE WITH CHOCOLATE-GINGER FROSTING

MAKES 12 SERVINGS

1 cup + 2 tablespoons cake flour
1 teaspoon baking soda
$\frac{1}{4}$ teaspoon salt
$\frac{1}{3}$ cup + 2 teaspoons granulated sugar
2 tablespoons + 2 teaspoons reduced-calorie tub margarine
1 large egg
$2\frac{1}{2}$ teaspoons vanilla extract
$\frac{1}{2}$ cup skim milk
$1\frac{1}{4}$ cups part-skim ricotta cheese
$\frac{1}{4}$ cup unsweetened cocoa powder
$\frac{1}{4}$ cup firmly packed dark brown sugar
2 teaspoons unsalted butter, softened
$\frac{3}{4}$ teaspoons ground ginger

1. Preheat oven to 350°F. Spray two 8" round cake pans with nonstick cooking spray.

2. To prepare cake, in small bowl, combine cake flour, baking soda and salt; set aside.

3. In medium bowl with mixer on high speed, cream sugar and margarine; add egg and 2 teaspoons of the vanilla extract, beating until smooth. Gradually beat in flour mixture, alternately with milk, until batter is smooth.

4. Evenly divide batter between prepared pans; bake 15–20 minutes, until toothpick inserted in center comes out clean. Let cakes cool in pans 5 minutes; remove cakes from pans and set on racks to cool. Transfer 1 cake to serving platter; set aside.

5. Meanwhile, to prepare frosting, in food processor or blender, combine ricotta cheese, cocoa powder, brown sugar, butter, ginger and remaining $\frac{1}{2}$ teaspoon vanilla extract; process until smooth.

6. Spread thin layer of frosting over cake on serving platter; top with remaining cake. Spread remaining frosting over top and sides of entire cake. Cut into 12 equal pieces.

EACH SERVING PROVIDES: $\frac{1}{4}$ Fat, $\frac{1}{2}$ Protein, $\frac{1}{2}$ Bread, 55 Optional Calories
PER SERVING: 149 Calories, 5 g Protein, 5 g Fat, 22 g Carbohydrate, 220 mg Sodium, 28 mg Cholesterol, 1 g Dietary Fiber

---

Just Desserts

◆

Be sure to get your just desserts, and follow these tips to bake the best cakes and cookies!

- *Cakes and cookies bake best in shiny aluminum, tin or stainless steel pans for the most even distribution of heat. Check for smooth seams to make cleaning easier.*
- *Use a cold baking sheet for each batch of cookies; when spooned onto a warm sheet, batter will begin to spread and melt before baking.*
- *Cookies are done when they have a little brown border and an imprint remains when gently touched in the center. Adjust baking time if the first batch comes out over- or underdone.*
- *As a general rule, batter should fill a tin by no more than two thirds. During baking, the mixture will then rise just to or slightly above the rim. If you use a larger tin than called for, the cake will end up flat; if you use a smaller tin than called for, there's a possibility that the batter will overflow, causing a cracked or wrinkled surface—and a messy oven.*
- *Because heat rises, oven temperatures are not uniform throughout. For best results, place baking pans in the center of the oven, and do not place one pan directly over another. If necessary, stagger pans on the same rack so they don't touch each other or the sides of the oven. If baking two sheets of cookies or two cake pans simultaneously, reverse top and bottom pans halfway through baking time for more even baking and browning.*

CARAMEL CAKE WITH BOURBON-PEAR SAUCE

MAKES 12 SERVINGS

½ cup granulated sugar
2¼ cups all-purpose flour
1 teaspoon baking powder
1 teaspoon baking soda
¼ teaspoon salt
¼ cup reduced-calorie tub margarine
¾ cup skim buttermilk, at room temperature
½ cup firmly packed dark brown sugar
½ cup egg substitute, at room temperature
½ teaspoon vanilla extract
3 large Bosc pears, pared and cut into ½" cubes
2 teaspoons bourbon

1. To prepare caramel syrup, in small saucepan, combine granulated sugar and 1 tablespoon water. Cook over low heat, washing down sides of pan with a brush dipped in cold water and keeping sugar moving, 6–7 minutes, until amber colored. Remove from heat; carefully stir in ½ cup boiling water. Cook, stirring constantly, until sugar dissolves. Let cool.

2. Preheat oven to 350°F. Spray a 9" round cake pan with nonstick cooking spray.

3. In medium bowl, combine flour, baking powder, baking soda and salt; set aside.

4. In large bowl, with mixer on high speed, beat margarine until creamy; add buttermilk, brown sugar, egg substitute, ¼ cup of the prepared caramel syrup and the vanilla extract, mixing until well blended. Gradually add flour mixture, stirring to mix well (do not overmix).

5. Scrape batter into prepared pan. Bake 25–30 minutes, until toothpick inserted in center comes out clean. Let cake cool in pan 5 minutes; remove cake from pan and set on rack to cool.

6. Meanwhile, in medium saucepan, combine the remaining caramel syrup and the pears; bring to a boil. Reduce heat to low; simmer, covered, 15 minutes. Remove from heat. With fork or potato masher, lightly mash pear mixture until it resembles a chunky sauce; stir in bourbon. Pour pear mixture into medium serving bowl; let cool slightly.

7. To serve, cut cake into 12 equal pieces; top each piece with an equal amount of pear sauce.

EACH SERVING PROVIDES: ½ Fat, ½ Fruit, 1 Bread, 80 Optional Calories
PER SERVING: 228 Calories, 4 g Protein, 3 g Fat, 48 g Carbohydrate, 261 mg Sodium, 1 mg Cholesterol, 3 g Dietary Fiber

FROSTED CARROT CAKE

We've recreated the ever-popular carrot cake, down to the cream cheese frosting, in a newer, lighter version for your whole family to enjoy.

MAKES 8 SERVINGS

¾ cup all-purpose flour
½ cup uncooked yellow cornmeal
1½ teaspoons double-acting baking powder
½ teaspoon ground cinnamon
¼ teaspoon salt
¼ teaspoon ground ginger
½ cup thawed frozen apple juice concentrate
1 large egg
¼ cup skim milk
2 tablespoons + 2 teaspoons vegetable oil
2 tablespoons firmly packed dark brown sugar
1 cup shredded carrots
½ cup golden raisins
½ cup light cream cheese
1 tablespoon honey

1. Preheat oven to 375°F. Spray a 9" Bundt pan with nonstick cooking spray.

2. In medium bowl, combine flour, cornmeal, baking powder, cinnamon, salt and ginger; set aside.

3. In medium bowl, beat together apple juice concentrate, egg, milk, oil and brown sugar; stir in carrots and raisins. Gradually add flour mixture, stirring just until combined.

4. Scrape batter evenly into prepared pan. Bake 35–40 minutes, until toothpick inserted in center comes out clean. Transfer pan to rack; let cool completely.

5. Meanwhile, to prepare frosting, in food processor or blender, combine cream cheese and honey; process until smooth. Invert cake onto serving platter; spread cream cheese mixture evenly over top and sides. Cut cake into 8 equal pieces.

EACH SERVING PROVIDES: 1 Fat, 1 Fruit, ¼ Vegetable, 1 Bread, 60 Optional Calories
PER SERVING: 243 Calories, 5 g Protein, 8 g Fat, 39 g Carbohydrate, 263 mg Sodium, 34 mg Cholesterol, 2 g Dietary Fiber

COFFEE CHIFFON CAKE

MAKES 12 SERVINGS

2¼ cups sifted cake flour
1½ cups granulated sugar
1 tablespoon baking powder
1 teaspoon salt
¾ cup strong black coffee
6 eggs, separated, at room temperature
¼ cup vegetable oil
1 teaspoon vanilla extract
2 egg whites, at room temperature
1 tablespoon confectioners sugar

1. Preheat oven to 325°F.

2. In large bowl, sift together flour, ¾ cup of the sugar, the baking powder and salt; add coffee, egg yolks, oil and vanilla extract, stirring until smooth.

3. In separate large bowl, with mixer on medium speed, beat all 8 egg whites until foamy; gradually beat in the remaining ¾ cup sugar, beating until egg whites are stiff but not dry. Stir one-fourth of the whites into the batter. Fold the remaining whites into the batter.

4. Scrape batter into an ungreased 10" tube pan; smooth top with a spatula. Bake 1 hour, or until a cake tester inserted in center comes out clean. Invert cake onto rack; let cool completely. Sprinkle with confectioners sugar; transfer to serving platter. Cut into 12 equal pieces.

EACH SERVING PROVIDES: 1 Fat, ½ Protein, 1 Bread, 95 Optional Calories
PER SERVING: 247 Calories, 5 g Protein, 7 g Fat, 40 g Carbohydrate, 347 mg Sodium, 106 mg Cholesterol, 0 g Dietary Fiber

BRANDIED FRUIT CAKE

MAKES 12 SERVINGS

1¼ cups all-purpose flour
1 cup whole-wheat flour
1 teaspoon baking powder
1 teaspoon baking soda
¼ teaspoon salt
¼ cup reduced-calorie tub margarine
½ cup firmly packed dark brown sugar
1 tablespoon grated fresh ginger
1 teaspoon cinnamon
½ teaspoon ground nutmeg
¼ teaspoon ground cloves
1 cup skim buttermilk
½ cup egg substitute
1 teaspoon grated orange zest
1 teaspoon grated lemon zest
1 teaspoon vanilla extract
12 dried apricot halves
½ cup golden raisins
6 large pitted prunes, chopped
6 dried dates, pitted and chopped
3 tablespoons brandy, bourbon or rum

1. Preheat oven to 350°F. Spray a 9" Bundt pan with nonstick cooking spray.

2. In medium bowl, sift together all-purpose flour, whole-wheat flour, baking powder, baking soda and salt; set aside.

3. In large bowl, with mixer on high speed, beat margarine until creamy; add brown sugar, ginger, cinnamon, nutmeg and cloves, beating until fluffy. Add buttermilk, egg substitute, orange zest, lemon zest and vanilla extract; mix until well blended.

4. Gradually stir flour mixture into egg mixture, mixing just until combined. Gently stir in apricots, raisins, prunes, dates and brandy.

5. Scrape batter into prepared pan. Bake 35–40 minutes, until toothpick inserted in center comes out clean. Let cake cool in pan 5 minutes. Remove cake from pan; set on rack to cool. Transfer to serving platter; cut into 12 equal pieces.

EACH SERVING PROVIDES: ½ Fat, 1 Fruit, 1 Bread, 60 Optional Calories
PER SERVING: 212 Calories, 5 g Protein, 3 g Fat, 42 g Carbohydrate, 268 mg Sodium, 1 mg Cholesterol, 3 g Dietary Fiber

VARIATION

Omit brandy, bourbon or rum from recipe, and decrease Optional Calories to 50.

◆

SPICED FIG CAKE

Dense and fruity, you'll find this reminiscent of holiday fruitcakes from the past.

MAKES 8 SERVINGS

8 large dried figs, coarsely chopped
⅓ cup reduced-calorie tub margarine
¼ cup firmly packed dark brown sugar
2 large eggs, lightly beaten
¾ cup all-purpose flour
¾ teaspoon ground ginger
½ teaspoon cinnamon
½ teaspoon black pepper
½ teaspoon baking powder
⅛ teaspoon ground cloves
⅛ teaspoon salt

1. Preheat oven to 350°F. Spray an 8" square baking pan with nonstick cooking spray.

2. In medium saucepan, combine figs, margarine, brown sugar and 2 tablespoons water; bring to a boil. Reduce heat to low; simmer, covered, 5 minutes. Set aside; let cool. Stir in beaten eggs.

3. In medium bowl, combine flour, ginger, cinnamon, pepper, baking powder, cloves and salt. Add fig mixture; stir just until combined. Pour into prepared baking pan; bake about 20 minutes, until toothpick inserted in center comes out clean.

EACH SERVING PROVIDES: 1 Fat, 1 Fruit, ¼ Protein, ½ Bread, 25 Optional Calories
PER SERVING: 164 Calories, 3 g Protein, 6 g Fat, 27 g Carbohydrate, 157 mg Sodium, 53 mg Cholesterol, 0 g Dietary Fiber

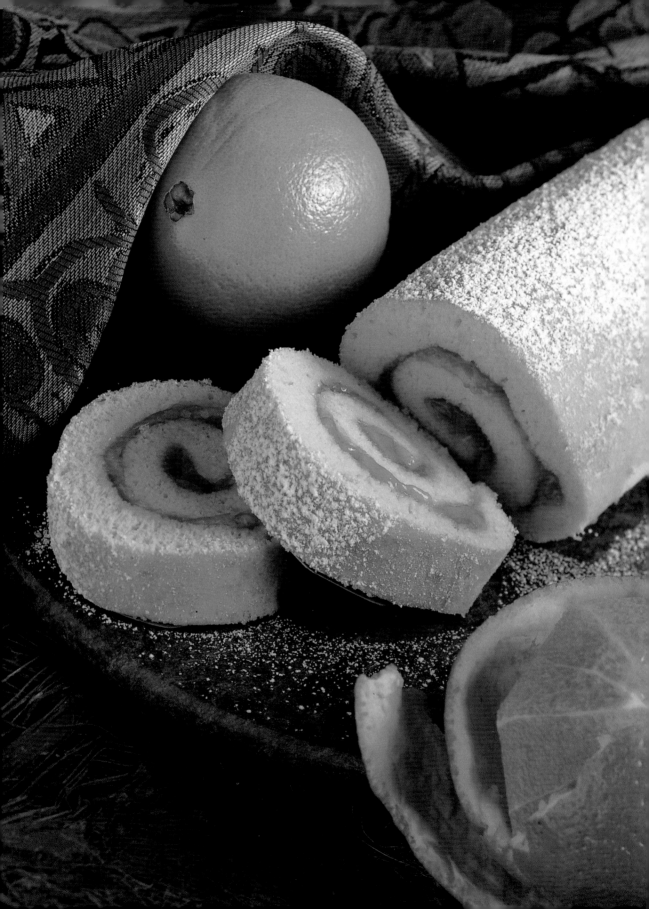

ROLLED ORANGE SPONGE CAKE

MAKES 10 SERVINGS

2 tablespoons confectioners sugar
4 large eggs, separated
3 egg whites, at room temperature
$\frac{3}{4}$ cup granulated sugar
2 tablespoons finely grated orange zest
1 tablespoon fresh lemon juice
$\frac{1}{8}$ teaspoon salt
1 cup minus 1 tablespoon sifted cake flour
$\frac{1}{2}$ cup + 2 tablespoons orange spreadable fruit

1. Preheat oven to 350°F. Line a 15$\frac{1}{2}$ × 10 $\frac{1}{2}$ × 1" jelly-roll pan with wax paper. Dust clean dish towel with 1 tablespoon of the confectioners sugar; set aside.

2. In medium bowl, with mixer on medium speed, beat all 7 egg whites until soft peaks form; set aside.

3. In large bowl, with whisk, beat egg yolks until thick; gradually beat in granulated sugar, beating until thick and light. Add orange zest, juice and salt; beat to combine. Gradually stir in cake flour, mixing well. Stir one-fourth of the beaten egg whites into batter; fold in remaining whites. Evenly spread batter into prepared pan. Bake 12–15 minutes, until golden (top should spring back when touched lightly with finger).

4. To remove cake from pan, insert a thin knife around edge of pan; invert cake onto prepared dish towel. Peel paper off cake. Starting at narrow end, roll cake up with towel. Transfer rolled cake to rack; let cool.

5. Unroll cake, removing towel. Evenly spread spreadable fruit over cake; reroll. Arrange cake, seam-side down, on serving platter. Sprinkle with the remaining 1 tablespoon confectioners sugar.

EACH SERVING PROVIDES: 1 Fruit, $\frac{1}{2}$ Protein, $\frac{1}{2}$ Bread, 65 Optional Calories
PER SERVING: 175 Calories, 4 g Protein, 2 g Fat, 35 g Carbohydrate, 70 mg Sodium, 85 mg Cholesterol, 0 g Dietary Fiber

BANANA CUPCAKES

MAKES 12 SERVINGS

2$\frac{1}{4}$ cups all-purpose flour
1 teaspoon baking powder
$\frac{1}{2}$ teaspoon baking soda
$\frac{1}{8}$ teaspoon salt
4 ripe medium bananas, cut into chunks
1 cup skim buttermilk
$\frac{1}{2}$ cup reduced-calorie tub margarine
$\frac{1}{2}$ cup minus 1 tablespoon firmly packed light brown sugar
1 large egg, at room temperature
$\frac{1}{2}$ cup dried currants
1$\frac{1}{4}$ cups part-skim ricotta cheese
2 tablespoons unsweetened cocoa powder
1 tablespoon rum

1. Preheat oven to 350°F. Line 12 muffin cups with double papers.

2. In medium bowl, sift together flour, baking powder, baking soda and salt; set aside.

3. In large bowl, with mixer on medium speed, combine bananas, buttermilk, margarine, $\frac{1}{4}$ cup of the brown sugar and the egg; beat to mix well.

4. Stir in flour mixture; mix just until blended. Add currants; stir to mix well.

5. Fill each muffin cup with an equal amount of batter. Bake 35–40 minutes, until a toothpick inserted in center comes out clean. Transfer pan to rack; let cool completely.

6. Meanwhile, to prepare frosting, in food processor or blender combine ricotta cheese, remaining 3 tablespoons brown sugar, the cocoa and rum; process until smooth. Evenly spread frosting on cooled cupcakes.

EACH SERVING PROVIDES: 1 Fat, 1 Fruit, $\frac{1}{2}$ Protein, 1 Bread, 40 Optional Calories
PER SERVING: 254 Calories, 7 g Protein, 7 g Fat, 42 g Carbohydrate, 253 mg Sodium, 26 mg Cholesterol, 2 g Dietary Fiber

LEMON ANGEL FOOD CAKE WITH BERRY TOPPING

MAKES 12 SERVINGS

1½ cups granulated sugar
1 cup + 2 tablespoons sifted cake flour
¼ teaspoon salt
12 egg whites, at room temperature
1¼ teaspoons cream of tartar
1 tablespoon + 1 teaspoon grated lemon zest
1 teaspoon vanilla extract
2¼ cups raspberries
2¼ cups sliced strawberries
2 tablespoons raspberry liqueur

1. Preheat oven to 375°F. Onto sheet of wax paper sift together ¾ cup of the sugar, the cake flour and salt; set aside.

2. In large bowl, with mixer on low speed, beat egg whites 1–2 minutes, or until small bubbles appear and surface is frothy. Sprinkle cream of tartar over whites; with mixer at medium speed, add the remaining ¾ cup of sugar in a slow, steady stream, beating until all the sugar has been added. Stop beating; scrape around sides and bottom of bowl with a spatula. Add 1 tablespoon of the lemon zest and vanilla extract; continue beating until whites are stiff but not dry.

3. Sift one-third of the flour mixture over top of beaten egg whites; with rubber spatula, quickly fold into whites, scraping sides and bottom of bowl. Repeat procedure 2 more times, using half of the remaining flour mixture each time, making sure all of the flour mixture is blended into whites.

4. Scrape batter into an ungreased 9" or 10" tube pan; with spatula, smooth surface. Bake on oven rack set in lower third of the oven 25–30 minutes, or until a cake tester inserted in center comes out clean.

5. To remove cake from pan, insert a thin knife around edge of pan; invert onto serving platter. Let cool completely.

6. Meanwhile, in large bowl, combine raspberries, strawberries, liqueur and the remaining 1 teaspoon lemon zest; let stand 30 minutes.

7. To serve, cut cake into 12 equal pieces; top each piece with an equal amount of berry sauce.

EACH SERVING PROVIDES: ½ Fruit, ¼ Protein, ½ Bread, 105 Optional Calories
PER SERVING: 175 Calories, 5 g Protein, 0 g Fat, 38 g Carbohydrate, 101 mg Sodium, 0 mg Cholesterol, 2 g Dietary Fiber

---

Baking Tips

◆

Baking is a pleasure with these no-fail baking tips.

- *Always follow directions to preheat the oven when called for.*
- *When several dry ingredients such as baking powder, salt and spices are added together, premeasure them into a small cup. For a clean-up short-cut, use 3-ounce paper cups and toss them away once you have added the ingredients.*
- *Do the same for larger quantities like flour mixtures: Sift them onto a sheet of wax paper or a paper plate and then use the paper or the plate to hold the spatula after you've scraped the mixing bowl. That way, you'll have no extra bowls to wash and your counter will stay clean as well.*
- *If your stationary mixer head lifts up or your mixer is handheld, at the end of the mixing process, lift beaters slowly at the lowest setting, allowing the batter to spin off the mixing blades into the bowl.*
- *Most baked goods freeze well. Use moisture- and vapor-proof wrapping; press out all air and seal. Label with the name, date, and portion size. Use within 2 to 3 months.*

MOCHA-CINNAMON ANGEL FOOD CAKE

MAKES 12 SERVINGS

1½ cups granulated sugar
½ cup + 1 tablespoon sifted cake flour
½ cup unsweetened cocoa powder
1 teaspoon cinnamon
1 teaspoon espresso powder or instant coffee
  granules
¼ teaspoon salt
12 egg whites, at room temperature
1¼ teaspoons cream of tartar
2 teaspoons vanilla extract
1 tablespoon confectioners sugar

1. Preheat oven to 375°F. Onto sheet of wax paper, sift together ¾ cup of the sugar, the cake flour, cocoa powder, cinnamon, espresso powder and salt; set aside.

2. In medium bowl, with mixer at low speed, beat egg whites 1–2 minutes, or until frothy and small bubbles appear; sprinkle cream of tartar over whites. With mixer at medium speed, add remaining ¾ cup sugar in a slow, steady stream, beating until all of the sugar has been added. Stop beating; scrape around sides and bottom of bowl with spatula. Add vanilla extract; continue beating on medium speed until egg whites are stiff but not dry.

3. Sift one-third of the flour mixture over beaten egg whites; with rubber spatula, quickly fold into whites, scraping sides and bottom of bowl. Repeat procedure 2 more times using one-half of the remaining flour mixture each time, making sure all flour is blended into whites.

4. Scrape batter into an ungreased 9" or 10" tube pan; with a spatula, smooth surface. Bake on oven rack set in lower third of the oven 25–30 minutes, or until a cake tester inserted in the center comes out clean.

5. To remove cake from pan, insert a thin knife around edge of pan; invert cake onto serving platter. Let cool completely. Dust with confectioners sugar.

EACH SERVING PROVIDES: ¼ Protein, ¼ Bread, 110 Optional Calories
PER SERVING: 144 Calories, 5 g Protein, 1 g Fat, 32 g Carbohydrate, 101 mg Sodium, 0 mg Cholesterol, 1 g Dietary Fiber

VARIATION

Omit confectioners sugar from recipe; decrease Optional Calories to 105.

CHEESECAKE

MAKES 16 SERVINGS

12 graham crackers (2½" squares) made into
  crumbs
2 cups light cream cheese
1 cup nonfat sour cream
½ cup granulated sugar
2 teaspoons vanilla extract
2 large eggs
2 teaspoons grated lemon zest

1. Preheat oven to 325°F. Wrap outside of a 10" springform pan with heavy-duty aluminum foil. Spray sides and bottom with nonstick cooking spray. Sprinkle graham cracker crumbs evenly over bottom and ¾ of the way up sides.

2. In large bowl, with electric mixer, beat cream cheese, sour cream, sugar and vanilla extract until smooth. Add eggs, one at a time, beating at low speed until blended. Stir in lemon zest.

3. Pour batter into prepared pan. Set springform pan into large roasting pan. Pour boiling water into roasting pan to come halfway up sides of springform pan. Bake 30–35 minutes, or until almost completely set. Turn off oven, place a wooden spoon in door to keep open and leave cake in oven for 30 minutes. Remove to a cooling rack and run a thin knife around outer edge to release cake. Let cool completely and then refrigerate. With a thin sharp knife, cut into 16 even slices.

EACH SERVING PROVIDES: ¼ Bread, 100 Optional Calories
PER SERVING: 128 Calories, 5 g Protein, 6 g Fat, 14 g Carbohydrate, 210 mg Sodium, 42 mg Cholesterol, 0 g Dietary Fiber

PUMPKIN CHEESECAKE

An amazingly rich-tasting cheesecake, just right to serve as the finale to a holiday meal.

MAKES 6 SERVINGS

9 graham crackers (2½" squares), made into
  crumbs
1 cup low-fat (1%) cottage cheese
¾ cup part-skim ricotta cheese
¾ cup egg substitute
½ cup granulated sugar
1 teaspoon ground ginger
1 teaspoon vanilla extract
½ teaspoon ground nutmeg
½ teaspoon cinnamon
⅛ teaspoon salt
1½ cups pumpkin purée

1. Preheat oven to 350°F. Spray a 9" glass pie plate with nonstick cooking spray. Sprinkle graham cracker crumbs over bottom of pie plate; set aside.

2. In food processor or blender, combine cottage cheese and ricotta cheese; process 1 minute, until smooth. Transfer cheese mixture to large bowl. Add egg substitute, sugar, ginger, vanilla extract, nutmeg, cinnamon and salt; stir to mix well. Reserve ¼ cup of cheese mixture; set aside.

3. Add pumpkin to cheese mixture in large bowl; stir until blended. Scrape batter into prepared pie plate. Drizzle the reserved cheese mixture in 3 concentric circles over the pumpkin batter. With knife, lightly draw the batter from the center toward the outer edge; starting about 2 inches from line, lightly draw the knife from the outer edge toward to center. Repeat pattern around the pie, alternating directions, until a spiderweb pattern is formed.

5. Bake 45–50 minutes, until knife inserted in center comes out clean. Cool completely on rack. Cover and refrigerate until ready to serve.

EACH SERVING PROVIDES: ⅛ Vegetable, 1½ Proteins, ½ Bread, 60 Optional Calories
PER SERVING: 218 Calories, 12 g Protein, 4 g Fat, 33 g Carbohydrate, 344 mg Sodium, 11 mg Cholesterol, 1 g Dietary Fiber

DOUBLE APPLE STRUDEL

Like grandmother's, but better! Keep phyllo dough covered with a slightly damp towel while you work, as it dries out quickly.

MAKES 12 SERVINGS

3 small apples, pared, cored and diced
$4\frac{1}{2}$ ounces dried apple slices, coarsely chopped
$\frac{1}{3}$ cup + 2 teaspoons dark raisins
$\frac{1}{3}$ cup granulated sugar
2 tablespoons cornstarch
$\frac{1}{2}$ teaspoon cinnamon
1 teaspoon vanilla extract
3 ounces walnuts
1 ounce gingersnap cookies
$\frac{1}{4}$ cup reduced-calorie tub margarine, melted
12 sheets thawed frozen phyllo dough (12 × 17" each)*

1. To prepare filling, in large nonstick skillet, combine apples, dried apples, $\frac{1}{2}$ cup water, the raisins, sugar, cornstarch and cinnamon. Cook, covered, over medium heat, stirring occasionally, 10 minutes, until apples are very tender and mixture has thickened. Stir in vanilla; let cool completely.

2. In food processor, combine walnuts and gingersnaps; process to form crumbs; set aside. Reserve 2 teaspoons of the margarine; set aside. Place dry towels on work surface.

3. To assemble strudel, place sheet of dough on dry towel, keeping remaining phyllo sheets covered with a damp towel; lightly brush with some of the margarine. Top with 1 sheet of dough; lightly brush with some more of the margarine and sprinkle with 1 tablespoon of the crumb mixture. Repeat procedure, using all of the dough, crumb mixture and margarine, ending with dough.

4. Preheat oven to 375°F. Spray jelly-roll pan with nonstick cooking spray.

5. Spoon apple filling over dough, leaving a 2" border. Using towel, starting at wide end, roll strudel, jelly-roll style, enclosing filling. Transfer, seam-side down, to prepared pan; brush top with reserved 2 teaspoons margarine. Make 12 shallow cuts through top layers of phyllo dough (do not cut into filling).

6. Bake 40–45 minutes, until golden. Let cool 10 minutes; cut at scored sections.

*Phyllo dough must be thawed in refrigerator at least 8 hours or overnight.

EACH SERVING PROVIDES: 1 Fat, 1 Fruit, $\frac{1}{4}$ Protein, $\frac{1}{2}$ Bread, 50 Optional Calories
PER SERVING: 210 Calories, 3 g Protein, 8 g Fat, 34 g Carbohydrate, 154 mg Sodium, 0 mg Cholesterol, 1 g Dietary Fiber

◆

APPLE COBBLER

MAKES 4 SERVINGS

$\frac{3}{4}$ cup buttermilk baking mix
$\frac{1}{4}$ cup buttermilk
2 tablespoons granulated sugar
$\frac{1}{2}$ teaspoon ground cardamom
4 apples
1 tablespoon fresh lemon juice

1. Preheat oven to 350°F. Spray a 1-quart baking dish with nonstick cooking spray.

2. In small bowl, combine baking mix, buttermilk, 1 tablespoon of the sugar and the cardamom; stir until smooth. Set aside.

3. In medium saucepan combine apples, the remaining 1 tablespoon sugar and the lemon juice; bring to a boil. Reduce heat to low; cook, stirring constantly, 5 minutes, until fruit is soft. Pour into prepared baking dish.

4. With spoon, evenly drop batter over fruit. Bake 20–25 minutes, until browned. Let cool.

EACH SERVING ($\frac{1}{4}$ of cobbler) PROVIDES: 1 Fruit, 1 Bread, 50 Optional Calories
PER SERVING: 191 Calories, 3 g Protein, 4 g Fat (1 g unsaturated), 38 g Carbohydrate, 304 mg Sodium, 1 mg Cholesterol, 3 g Dietary Fiber

FRESH FRUIT AND HONEY NAPOLEON

Light and flaky phyllo dough stands in for puff paste in this elegant dessert with a hint of honey.

MAKES 6 SERVINGS

2 tablespoons reduced-calorie tub margarine, melted
2 tablespoons honey
6 sheets thawed frozen phyllo dough (12 × 17" each)*
1 medium papaya, pared, seeded and cut into $\frac{1}{2}$" chunks
$\frac{3}{4}$ cup blueberries
1 tablespoon fresh lemon juice
$\frac{3}{4}$ cup whipped topping
1 tablespoon confectioners sugar

1. Preheat oven to 375°F. Spray large baking sheet with nonstick cooking spray. In small bowl, combine margarine and honey; set aside.

2. To assemble layers, keeping phyllo sheets covered with a damp towel, layer 1 sheet of dough at a time, brushing each sheet with 2 teaspoons of the margarine mixture, using all of the dough and margarine mixture.

3. Cut dough crosswise into three 5½"-wide strips; cut dough lengthwise into six 2" strips, forming eighteen rectangular pieces. Bake 8–10 minutes, until browned and crisp. Transfer pan to rack; let cool.

4. Meanwhile, in medium bowl combine papaya, blueberries and juice.

5. To serve, on each of six serving plates, place 1 piece of baked phyllo dough; top each with 1 tablespoon whipped topping and 1 tablespoon of the fruit mixture. Repeat procedure using all of the baked phyllo dough, equal amounts of the remaining whipped topping and fruit mixture, ending with baked phyllo dough. Evenly dust each with confectioners sugar. Serve immediately.

*Phyllo dough must be thawed in the refrigerator for at least 8 hours.

EACH SERVING PROVIDES: ½ Fat, ½ Fruit, ½ Bread, 65 Optional Calories
PER SERVING: 150 Calories, 2 g Protein, 5 g Fat, 26 g Carbohydrate, 138 mg Sodium, 1 mg Cholesterol, 1 g Dietary Fiber

CHOCOLATE-APRICOT BARS

MAKES 12 SERVINGS

$1\frac{1}{2}$ cups all-purpose flour
3 ounces uncooked quick oats
$\frac{1}{4}$ cup firmly packed light brown sugar
Pinch salt
$\frac{1}{2}$ cup reduced-calorie tub margarine, well chilled
$\frac{3}{4}$ cup apricot spreadable fruit
2 ounces semisweet chocolate chips*

1. Preheat oven to 350°F. Spray a 9" baking pan with nonstick cooking spray.

2. In medium bowl, combine flour, oats, brown sugar and salt. With pastry blender or 2 knives, cut in margarine and 2 tablespoons water until mixture is a crumbly dough. Press dough into prepared pan; bake 25–35 minutes, until golden.

3. Evenly top bar mixture with spreadable fruit; bake 15 minutes. Let cool.

4. Meanwhile, in double boiler over simmering water, melt chocolate chips; remove from heat, stirring until smooth. With spatula, scrape the chocolate into a paper cone or small pastry bag. Evenly drizzle cooled apricot bars with the melted chocolate. Let cool completely. Cut into 12 equal bars.

*Chocolate can be melted in a microwave oven. In a 1-quart glass bowl, microwave chocolate chips on High 1½ minutes, stirring halfway through cooking.

EACH SERVING PROVIDES: 1 Fat, 1 Fruit, 1 Bread, 40 Optional Calories
PER SERVING: 199 Calories, 3 g Protein, 6 g Fat, 35 g Carbohydrate, 87 mg Sodium, 0 mg Cholesterol, 1 g Dietary Fiber

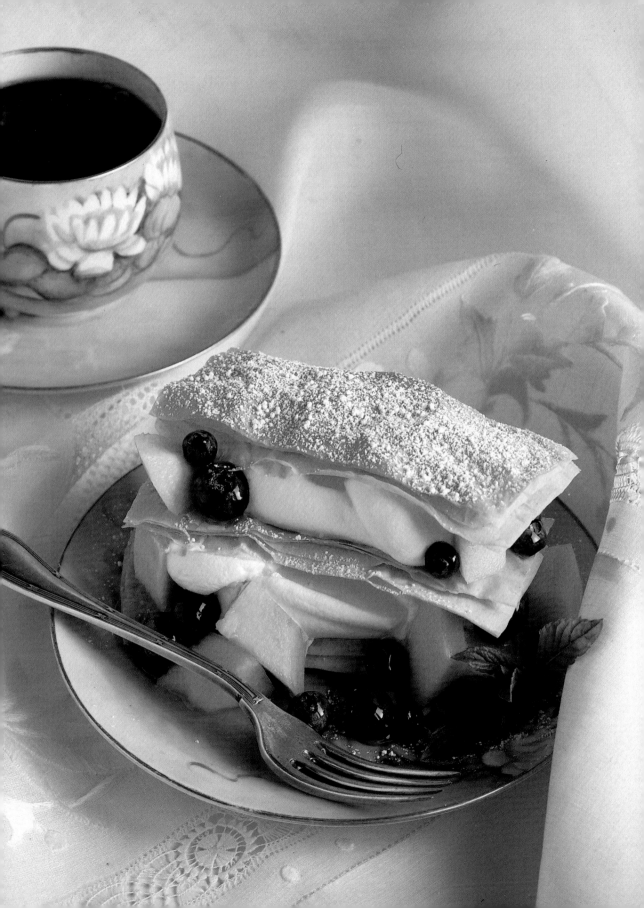

NECTARINE-CHERRY TART

MAKES 12 SERVINGS

$\frac{1}{4}$ cup reduced-calorie tub margarine
2 tablespoons granulated sugar
1 large egg
1 cup + 2 tablespoons all-purpose flour
6 small nectarines, pared, pitted and sliced
12 ounces cherries, pitted
$\frac{1}{4}$ cup thawed frozen orange juice concentrate
1 teaspoon grated orange zest
2 teaspoons cornstarch, dissolved in 2 tablespoons
   cold water

1. To prepare tart shell, in food processor, combine margarine and sugar; pulse until well blended. Add egg; pulse to blend. Add flour; pulse several times until mixture forms soft dough.

2. Press dough evenly over bottom and up sides of a 14 × 5 × 1" tart pan with removable bottom; with fork, prick dough. Line shell with foil; fill with dried beans or pie weights. Heat oven to 350°F. Bake 10 minutes; remove weights and foil. Bake shell 10–12 minutes longer, until golden. Cook on rack.

3. To prepare filling, in large saucepan, combine nectarines, cherries, juice concentrate and zest; bring to a boil. Reduce heat to low; simmer 5 minutes, until fruit is soft. With slotted spoon, transfer fruit to bowl; let cool. Reserve fruit juice.

4. Stir dissolved cornstarch into fruit juice; cook, stirring constantly, about 1 minute, until thickened. Evenly pour juice filling over tart shell; arrange fruit over filling. Let cool 10 minutes; remove tart from pan. Cut into 12 equal wedges.

EACH SERVING PROVIDES: $\frac{1}{2}$ Fat, 1 Fruit, $\frac{1}{2}$ Bread, 15 Optional Calories
PER SERVING: 129 Calories, 3 g Protein, 3 g Fat, 24 g Carbohydrate, 42 mg Sodium, 18 mg Cholesterol, 2 g Dietary Fiber

STRAWBERRY PIE WITH RICE CRUST

The unusual rice crust gives this pie its fresh new taste appeal; and, unlike the usual pastry shell, this crust is low in fat!

MAKES 6 SERVINGS

6 ounces uncooked brown rice
2 eggs, lightly beaten
1 tablespoon granulated sugar
6 cups strawberries, sliced
2 tablespoons cornstarch
1 tablespoon fresh lemon juice
Granulated sugar substitute to equal 8 teaspoons
   sugar
2–3 drops red food coloring (optional)

1. To prepare crust, spray an 8" pie plate with nonstick cooking spray. In medium saucepan, bring $2\frac{1}{2}$ cups water to a boil; add rice. Reduce heat to low; simmer, covered, 50 minutes, or until rice is tender. Remove from heat.

2. Preheat oven to 400°F. Add eggs and sugar to rice mixture; stir to mix well. Spoon rice mixture into prepared pie plate. With rubber spatula, press rice mixture evenly on bottom and up the sides of plate.

3. Bake 10–15 minutes, or until firm and slightly golden; let cool completely.

4. To prepare filling, in food processor, combine $1\frac{1}{2}$ cups of the strawberries, the cornstarch and juice; purée until smooth.

5. In small saucepan, bring strawberry purée to a boil; reduce heat to low. Cook, stirring frequently, 3 minutes, or until purée is thickened. Remove from heat; stir in sweetener and food coloring, if using. Let cool.

6. Meanwhile, arrange the remaining strawberry slices over rice crust; spoon cooled purée over berries. Refrigerate, covered, until firm.

EACH SERVING PROVIDES: 1 Fruit, $\frac{1}{4}$ Protein, 1 Bread, 25 Optional Calories
PER SERVING: 198 Calories, 6 g Protein, 3 g Fat, 38 g Carbohydrate, 25 mg Sodium, 71 mg Cholesterol, 5 g Dietary Fiber

Banana "Cream" Pie

An old-fashioned favorite with a new profile: in a near-perfect disguise, a nonfat yogurt base with a deceptively rich taste replaces the traditional "cream" filling.

Makes 8 Servings

12 graham crackers (2½" squares), made into crumbs
1 tablespoon + 1 teaspoon margarine
4 medium bananas, cut into thin diagonal slices
2 tablespoons fresh lime juice
1 envelope unflavored gelatin
⅓ cup granulated sugar
1½ cups plain nonfat yogurt
1 teaspoon vanilla extract
Grated lime zest

1. Preheat oven to 350°F. Spray a 9" pie plate with nonstick cooking spray.

2. In medium bowl, with fork, combine graham cracker crumbs and margarine. Press into bottom and up sides of pie plate. Bake 3–5 minutes, until firm; let cool.

3. In medium bowl, toss banana slices with juice; reserve 1 cup. Arrange remaining banana slices over graham cracker crust.

4. In small saucepan, sprinkle gelatin over ½ cup cold water; let stand 2 minutes. Add sugar; cook over medium-high heat, stirring constantly, 2–3 minutes, until mixture boils and gelatin and sugar are dissolved. Remove from heat.

5. With whisk, add yogurt and vanilla extract to gelatin mixture; pour over bananas in pie plate. Decoratively arrange reserved banana slices on top of pie; evenly sprinkle with lime zest. Refrigerate, covered with plastic wrap, until well chilled.

EACH SERVING PROVIDES: ¼ Milk, ½ Fat, 1 Fruit, ½ Bread, 30 Optional Calories
PER SERVING: 175 Calories, 4 g Protein, 3 g Fat, 33 g Carbohydrate, 120 mg Sodium, 1 mg Cholesterol, 1 g Dietary Fiber

Buttermilk Pie

Makes 12 Servings

¼ cup reduced-calorie tub margarine, cold
¾ cup + 2 tablespoons granulated sugar
4 large eggs
1⅓ cups minus 1 teaspoon all-purpose flour
2 cups low-fat (1.5%) buttermilk, at room temperature
¼ cup reduced-calorie tub margarine, melted, at room temperature
¼ cup fresh lemon juice
1 tablespoon grated lemon zest
Pinch salt

1. Preheat oven to 350°F.

2. To prepare pie crust, in food processor, combine cold margarine and 2 tablespoons of the sugar; pulse until well blended. Add 1 of the eggs; pulse to blend. Add 1 cup + 2 tablespoons of the flour and pulse several times, until mixture forms soft dough.

3. Press dough evenly over bottom and up sides of 10" pie plate; with fork, prick dough. Line crust with foil; fill with dried beans or pie weights. Bake 10 minutes; remove weights and foil. Bake 10–12 minutes longer, until golden; cool on rack. Increase oven temperature to 425°F.

4. To prepare filling, combine the remaining ¾ cup sugar and the remaining 3 tablespoons flour. With whisk, beat in the remaining 3 eggs, the buttermilk, melted margarine, lemon juice, zest and salt. Pour into pie crust.

5. Bake 10 minutes; cover crust edges with foil. Reduce heat to 350°F; bake 30 minutes longer, until knife inserted in center comes out clean. Let cool. Serve slightly warm or at room temperature.

EACH SERVING PROVIDES: 1 Fat, ¼ Protein, ½ Bread, 80 Optional Calories
PER SERVING: 187 Calories, 5 g Protein, 6 g Fat, 28 g Carbohydrate, 148 mg Sodium, 73 mg Cholesterol, 0 g Dietary Fiber

RASPBERRY BROWNIES

Chocolate can be melted in a microwave oven. In a 1-quart glass bowl, microwave chocolate chips on High power 1½ minutes, stirring halfway through cooking.

MAKES 8 SERVINGS

3 ounces semisweet chocolate, coarsely chopped, or semisweet chocolate chips
4 large eggs, at room temperature
½ cup granulated sugar
1 teaspoon vanilla extract
¼ teaspoon salt
½ cup reduced-calorie tub margarine, melted, at room temperature
¾ cup all-purpose flour
½ cup raspberry spreadable fruit

1. Preheat oven to 350°F. Spray an 8" square baking pan with nonstick cooking spray.

2. In double boiler over simmering water, melt chocolate; remove from heat, stirring until smooth. Set aside; let cool to room temperature.

3. In large bowl, with mixer at high speed, beat eggs and sugar 7 minutes, until pale yellow and tripled in volume; beat in vanilla extract and salt. Add margarine; stir to mix well. Stir in flour, mixing well.

4. Pour half of mixture into medium bowl. Stir melted chocolate into one portion of the batter and the spreadable fruit into the other portion. Scrape chocolate batter into prepared pan, reserving ½ cup. Scrape raspberry batter over the chocolate batter; scatter spoonfuls of the reserved chocolate batter over the raspberry batter, using all of the chocolate batter. With knife, cut through batter to create a marbled effect.

5. Bake 20–25 minutes, until a toothpick inserted in center comes out almost clean. Transfer pan to rack; let cool completely. Cut into 16 equal squares.

EACH SERVING PROVIDES: 1½ Fats, 1 Fruit, ½ Protein, ½ Bread, 100 Optional Calories
PER SERVING: 274 Calories, 5 g Protein, 12 g Fat, 39 g Carbohydrate, 211 mg Sodium, 106 mg Cholesterol, 0 g Dietary Fiber

TRIPLE-GINGER GINGERBREAD

Crystallized ginger is the surprise ingredient in this ginger trio; serve gingerbread warm with a cup of herbal tea.

MAKES 12 SERVINGS

1¼ cups all-purpose flour
1 cup whole-wheat flour
1 teaspoon baking powder
1 teaspoon baking soda
¼ teaspoon salt
¼ cup reduced-calorie tub margarine
½ cup firmly packed dark brown sugar
1 tablespoon grated fresh ginger root
2 teaspoons ground ginger
¼ teaspoon ground cloves
1 cup skim buttermilk
½ cup egg substitute
2 tablespoons crystallized ginger, chopped
1 teaspoon vanilla extract
⅓ cup + 2 teaspoons golden raisins

1. Preheat oven to 350°F. Spray a 9" square baking pan with nonstick cooking spray.

2. In medium bowl, combine all-purpose flour, whole-wheat flour, baking powder, baking soda and salt; set aside.

3. In large bowl, with mixer on high speed, beat margarine until creamy; add brown sugar, fresh ginger, ground ginger and cloves, beating until fluffy. Stir in buttermilk, egg substitute, crystallized ginger and vanilla extract; add flour mixture and mix until well blended. Fold in raisins.

4. Scrape batter into prepared pan. Bake 25–30 minutes, until toothpick inserted in center comes out clean. Transfer pan to rack; let cool completely. Cut into 12 equal pieces.

EACH SERVING PROVIDES: ½ Fat, 1 Bread, 55 Optional Calories
PER SERVING: 171 Calories, 4 g Protein, 3 g Fat, 34 g Carbohydrate, 269 mg Sodium, 1 mg Cholesterol, 2 g Dietary Fiber

DOUBLE GINGERBREAD

MAKES 12 SERVINGS

2 cups all-purpose flour
2 tablespoons + 2 teaspoons dark brown sugar
2 tablespoons crystallized ginger, minced
2 teaspoons ground ginger
2 teaspoons baking soda
½ teaspoon salt
⅓ cup molasses or maple syrup
1 egg, beaten
1 cup boiling apple cider

1. Preheat oven to 350°F. Spray an 8" square pan with nonstick cooking spray.

2. In large bowl, combine flour, brown sugar, crystallized ginger, ground ginger, baking soda and salt. In small bowl, whisk together molasses and egg. Gradually beat in boiling cider.

3. Add cider mixture to flour mixture, and stir just until flour disappears; do not overblend. Pour into prepared pan, and bake 20–25 minutes, or until cake tester comes out clean. Cool on rack 10 minutes and remove from pan. Cut into 12 equal pieces. Serve warm, or at room temperature.

EACH SERVING PROVIDES: ¼ Fruit, ¾ Bread, 65 Optional Calories
PER SERVING: 140 Calories, 3 g Protein, 1 g Fat, 30 g Carbohydrate, 314 mg Sodium, 18 mg Cholesterol, 1 g Dietary Fiber

PEACH BARS

MAKES 24 SERVINGS

2¼ cups all-purpose flour, sifted
½ teaspoon baking powder
¼ teaspoon salt
1 cup firmly packed light brown sugar
1 cup reduced-calorie tub margarine, at room temperature
1 large egg, at room temperature
1 teaspoon almond extract
⅓ cup + 2 teaspoons peach spreadable fruit

1. Preheat oven to 350°F. Spray a 9" square baking pan with nonstick cooking spray.

2. In medium bowl, combine flour, baking powder and salt; set aside.

3. In large bowl, with mixer at medium-high speed, cream brown sugar and margarine until light and fluffy; beat in egg and almond extract. With mixer on low speed, gradually beat in flour mixture, beating until blended. With spatula, evenly and smoothly spread bar mixture into prepared pan; evenly top with spreadable fruit.

4. Bake 25–30 minutes, until lightly browned and mixture begins to shrink from sides of pan. Transfer pan to rack; let cool completely. Cut into 24 equal bars.

EACH SERVING PROVIDES: 1 Fat, ¼ Fruit, ½ Bread, 35 Optional Calories
PER SERVING: 125 Calories, 1 g Protein, 4 g Fat, 21 g Carbohydrate, 112 mg Sodium, 9 mg Cholesterol, 0 g Dietary Fiber

APPLE-OATMEAL COOKIES

MAKES 12 SERVINGS

4½ ounces uncooked quick oats, toasted until
   lightly browned
½ cup + 1 tablespoon all-purpose flour
½ teaspoon cinnamon
¼ teaspoon baking soda
¼ teaspoon salt
¼ cup firmly packed light brown sugar
¼ cup reduced-calorie tub margarine
1 medium Golden Delicious apple (6 ounces),
   pared and coarsely grated
1 large egg
½ teaspoon vanilla extract
⅓ cup + 2 teaspoons dark raisins

1. Preheat oven to 350° F. Spray 2 baking sheets with nonstick cooking spray.

2. In large bowl, combine oats, flour, cinnamon, baking soda and salt; set aside.

3. In medium bowl, with mixer on high speed, cream brown sugar and margarine until light and fluffy; add apple, egg and vanilla extract, and beat until well blended. Add oat mixture; stir to mix well. Add raisins; stir until combined.

4. Drop dough by tablespoonfuls onto prepared sheets forming 24 equal cookies and leaving 2 inches between each. Flatten each cookie with spatula.

5. Bake in center of middle oven rack 12–15 minutes, until lightly browned. Transfer to cooling rack; let cool completely. Store in air-tight container.

EACH SERVING (2 cookies) PROVIDES: ½ Fat, ¼ Fruit, ¾ Bread, 30 Optional Calories
PER SERVING: 125 Calories, 3 g Protein, 3 g Fat, 22 g Carbohydrate, 116 mg Sodium, 18 mg Cholesterol, 1 g Dietary Fiber

PEANUT BUTTER COOKIES

MAKES 12 SERVINGS

1 cup + 2 tablespoons all-purpose flour
½ teaspoon baking soda
½ teaspoon salt
¼ cup reduced-calorie tub margarine
¼ cup natural chunky-style peanut butter (no
   sugar or salt added)
⅓ cup + 2 teaspoons firmly packed dark brown
   sugar
1 large egg
½ teaspoon vanilla extract
2 ounces peanut butter morsels

1. Preheat oven to 350°F. Spray 2 baking sheets with nonstick cooking spray.

2. In medium bowl, combine flour, baking soda and salt; set aside.

3. In separate medium bowl, with mixer on high speed, cream margarine and peanut butter. Gradually beat in brown sugar; add egg and vanilla extract, beating until light and fluffy. With mixer on low speed, gradually beat in flour mixture, beating until blended. Stir in peanut butter morsels.

4. Drop dough by generous tablespoonfuls onto prepared baking sheets, forming 12 cookies on each sheet and leaving about 2 inches between each cookie. With tines of fork, slightly press each cookie to flatten, then press down in opposite direction, creating a checkerboard pattern.

5. Bake on center oven rack 12–15 minutes, until browned on bottom. Transfer to cooling rack; let cool completely. Store in air-tight container.

EACH SERVING (2 cookies) PROVIDES: 1 Fat, ¼ Protein, ½ Bread, 55 Optional Calories
PER SERVING: 152 Calories, 4 g Protein, 7 g Fat, 19 g Carbohydrate, 219 mg Sodium, 18 mg Cholesterol, 0 g Dietary Fiber

LEMON–POPPY SEED CRISPS

MAKES 8 SERVINGS

$\frac{3}{4}$ cup all-purpose flour
1 tablespoon poppy seeds
$\frac{1}{4}$ cup granulated sugar
2 tablespoons + 2 teaspoons reduced-calorie tub margarine
1 teaspoon grated lemon zest
Pinch salt

1. Preheat oven to 350°F. Spray baking sheet with nonstick cooking spray.
2. In small bowl, combine flour and poppy seeds; set aside.
3. In large bowl, with mixer at medium-high speed, beat sugar, margarine, lemon zest and salt until light and fluffy. With mixer on low speed, beat in flour mixture just until combined. Gather dough into a ball; wrap half in plastic wrap and refrigerate.
4. Roll remaining dough between 2 sheets of wax paper, forming a 7" circle. With a fluted pastry wheel or pizza cutter, cut into 16 equal wedges. With spatula, transfer wedges to prepared baking sheet.
5. Bake 10–12 minutes, just until golden. Transfer crisps to rack; let cool. Repeat procedure using remaining dough.

EACH SERVING (4 crisps) PROVIDES: $\frac{1}{2}$ Fat, $\frac{1}{2}$ Bread, 30 Optional Calories
PER SERVING: 90 Calories, 1 g Protein, 3 g Fat, 15 g Carbohydrate, 54 mg Sodium, 0 mg Cholesterol, 0 g Dietary Fiber

COCONUT-MACADAMIA KISSES

Light, sweet, studded with the rich taste of macadamia nuts, these kisses are a very special treat. They will keep well, stored in an airtight container.

MAKES 18 SERVINGS

3 large egg whites, at room temperature
Pinch salt
$\frac{1}{2}$ cup granulated sugar
$\frac{1}{4}$ cup shredded coconut
1 teaspoon coconut extract
$1\frac{1}{2}$ ounces macadamia nuts (18 nuts), halved

1. Preheat oven to 250°F. Line baking sheet with parchment paper or foil.
2. In medium bowl, with mixer on medium speed, combine egg whites and salt; beat until foamy. Gradually beat in sugar, beating until shiny and stiff peaks form when beater is lifted. Fold in coconut and coconut extract.
3. Into pastry bag fitted with large star tip, spoon meringue mixture. Pipe 36 equal rosettes on prepared baking sheet. Arrange half of a macadamia nut in center of each rosette.
4. Bake 40 minutes, until edges begin to dry and kisses are lightly browned. Turn oven off; let kisses dry in oven, about 3 hours or overnight, until crisp. Peel paper (or foil) from kisses. Store in air-tight container.

EACH SERVING (2 kisses) PROVIDES: $\frac{1}{4}$ Fat, 30 Optional Calories
PER SERVING: 46 Calories, 1 g Protein, 2 g Fat, 6 g Carbohydrate, 19 mg Sodium, 0 mg Cholesterol, 0 g Dietary Fiber

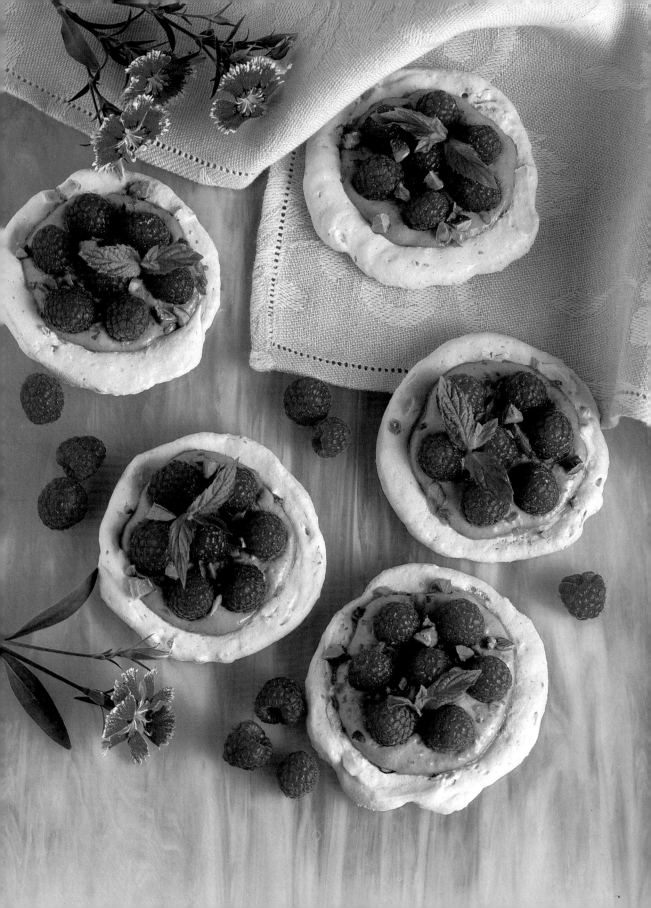

TOASTED ALMOND MERINGUES WITH RASPBERRY FILLING

MAKES 6 SERVINGS

3 large egg whites, at room temperature
$\frac{1}{8}$ teaspoon salt
$\frac{1}{2}$ cup + 1 tablespoon superfine sugar*
$1\frac{1}{2}$ ounces almonds, toasted and finely chopped
$2\frac{1}{4}$ cups raspberries
$\frac{3}{4}$ cup + 2 tablespoons part-skim ricotta cheese
2 tablespoons light cream cheese
1 teaspoon grated lemon zest

1. Preheat oven to 200°F. Line large baking sheet with parchment paper; draw six $3\frac{1}{2}$" circles on paper.

2. In large bowl, with mixer on high speed, beat egg whites and salt until foamy. Beat in $\frac{1}{2}$ cup of the sugar, 1 tablespoon at a time, until stiff peaks form. Gently fold in 1 ounce of the almonds.

3. Spoon meringue into pastry bag fitted with a No. 6 round tip; fill circles on parchment paper with meringue. With back of a spoon, push meringue up, forming a slightly higher edge on each circle. Bake 2 hours. Turn oven off; cool meringues in oven 1 hour.

4. Meanwhile, in blender or food processor, combine 1 cup of the raspberries, the ricotta cheese, cream cheese, the remaining tablespoon of sugar and the lemon zest; process until smooth.

5. To serve, on each of 6 plates, place 1 meringue. Fill each with an equal amount of the berry mixture, top with remaining $1\frac{1}{4}$ cups raspberries and sprinkle with remaining $\frac{1}{2}$ ounce almonds.

*If superfine sugar is not available, process granulated sugar in blender until superfine.

EACH SERVING PROVIDES: $\frac{1}{2}$ Fat, $\frac{1}{2}$ Fruit, 1 Protein, 80 Optional Calories
PER SERVING: 205 Calories, 8 g Protein, 8 g Fat, 28 g Carbohydrate, 146 mg Sodium, 14 mg Cholesterol, 3 g Dietary Fiber

CHOCOLATE-ORANGE PUDDING

MAKES 4 SERVINGS

1 envelope unflavored gelatin
1 cup low-fat (1%) milk
$\frac{1}{3}$ cup firmly packed dark brown sugar
$\frac{3}{4}$ cup part-skim ricotta cheese
$\frac{1}{4}$ cup unsweetened cocoa powder
1 tablespoon + 1 teaspoon orange liqueur
1 teaspoon vanilla extract

1. In small saucepan, sprinkle gelatin over milk; let stand 1 minute, until softened. Stir in brown sugar; cook over medium-low heat, stirring constantly, about 2 minutes, until gelatin is completely dissolved (do not boil).

2. In blender, combine ricotta cheese, cocoa powder, orange liqueur and vanilla extract; process on medium speed, about 1 minute, until puréed, scraping down sides of container as necessary.

3. Reduce speed to low; gradually add milk mixture; process until combined. Evenly pour pudding into each of four 6-ounce custard cups. Cover with plastic wrap; refrigerate until set, at least 2 hours.

EACH SERVING PROVIDES: $\frac{1}{4}$ Milk, $\frac{3}{4}$ Protein, 90 Optional Calories
PER SERVING: 193 Calories, 10 g Protein, 5 g Fat, 28 g Carbohydrate, 100 mg Sodium, 17 mg Cholesterol, 2 g Dietary Fiber

Toasted Almond Meringues with Raspberry Filling

TOASTED COCONUT CUSTARD

MAKES 4 SERVINGS

1 cup low-fat (1%) milk
1/3 cup instant nonfat dry milk powder
2 tablespoons granulated sugar
1 teaspoon coconut extract
2 large eggs
1/2 teaspoon vanilla extract
1 tablespoon + 1 teaspoon shredded sweetened coconut, toasted until golden

1. Preheat oven to 350°F. Spray four 6-ounce custard cups with nonstick cooking spray.

2. In medium saucepan, combine milk, milk powder, sugar and coconut extract. Cook over medium-high heat, stirring frequently, 3–4 minutes, until mixture boils and sugar is dissolved.

3. In medium bowl, with whisk, beat eggs until light; gradually whisk in hot milk mixture and vanilla extract. Fill each prepared custard cup with one-fourth of the custard mixture; sprinkle each with 1 teaspoon coconut.

4. Arrange cups in medium shallow pan; pour hot water (not boiling) halfway up side of pan. Bake 20–25 minutes, until custards are set, or a knife inserted in center comes out clean. Cover and refrigerate until chilled.

EACH SERVING PROVIDES: 1/2 Milk, 1/2 Protein, 30 Optional Calories
PER SERVING: 121 Calories, 7 g Protein, 4 g Fat, 14 g Carbohydrate, 97 mg Sodium, 110 mg Cholesterol, 0 g Dietary Fiber

CAPPUCCINO CUSTARD

MAKES 4 SERVINGS

1 cup low-fat (1%) milk
1/3 cup instant nonfat dry milk powder
1 tablespoon + 1 1/2 teaspoons instant espresso powder
1 tablespoon granulated sugar
2 large eggs
1 teaspoon vanilla extract
1/8 teaspoon cinnamon

1. Preheat oven to 325°F. Spray four 6-ounce custard cups with nonstick cooking spray.

2. In medium saucepan, combine milk, milk powder, espresso powder and sugar. Cook over medium-high heat, stirring frequently, 3–4 minutes, until mixture boils and sugar is dissolved; remove from heat.

3. In medium bowl, with whisk, beat eggs until light; gradually whisk in hot milk mixture and vanilla extract. Fill each prepared custard cup with one-fourth of the custard mixture; evenly sprinkle each with cinnamon.

4. Arrange cups in medium shallow baking pan; pour hot water (not boiling) halfway up pan. Bake 20–25 minutes, until custard is set, or a knife inserted in center comes out clean. Cover and refrigerate until chilled.

EACH SERVING PROVIDES: 1/2 Milk, 1/2 Protein, 10 Optional Calories
PER SERVING: 105 Calories, 7 g Protein, 4 g Fat, 10 g Carbohydrate, 93 mg Sodium, 110 mg Cholesterol, 0 g Dietary Fiber

BREAD PUDDING WITH ANISE

MAKES 4 SERVINGS

4 slices 2-day-old white bread
2 tablespoons + 2 teaspoons reduced-calorie tub
  margarine
⅓ cup + 2 teaspoons golden raisins
2 cups low-fat (1%) milk
2 eggs
3 tablespoons honey
½ teaspoon anise seeds, lightly crushed with a
  rolling pin
½ teaspoon vanilla extract
Pinch salt

1. Spray a 1½-quart casserole with nonstick cooking spray.

2. Evenly spread both sides of each slice of bread with an equal amount of margarine; cut each into quarters. Arrange 2 quartered slices in bottom of the prepared casserole; sprinkle with 3 tablespoons of the raisins. Repeat procedure with remaining 2 bread slices and the remaining 3 tablespoons of raisins; set aside.

3. In small bowl, whisk together milk, eggs, honey, anise seeds, vanilla extract and salt; pour over bread mixture. Let stand at room temperature 1 hour.

4. Preheat oven to 350°F.

5. Set casserole in a large shallow baking pan; pour hot water (not boiling) halfway up baking pan. Bake 1 hour, or until a knife inserted in center comes out clean. Let cool slightly and serve.

EACH SERVING PROVIDES: ½ Milk, 1 Fat, ¾ Fruit, ½ Protein, 1 Bread, 45 Optional Calories
PER SERVING: 283 Calories, 10 g Protein, 9 g Fat, 43 g Carbohydrate, 336 mg Sodium, 111 mg Cholesterol, 1 g Dietary Fiber

RICE PUDDING WITH GOLDEN RAISINS

Short-grain rice, the kind used to make risotto, is the key to the creaminess of this pudding with a homey, old-fashioned taste.

MAKES 4 SERVINGS

2 cups skim milk
¼ cup granulated sugar
4 ounces uncooked arborio or other short-grain
  rice
2 large eggs
¼ cup golden raisins
1 teaspoon vanilla extract
Pinch cinnamon
1 tablespoon + 1 teaspoon reduced-calorie tub
  margarine

1. In small saucepan, bring 1 cup of the milk, the sugar and 2 tablespoons water to a boil; stir in rice. Reduce heat to low; simmer 30 minutes, stirring occasionally.

2. Preheat oven to 325°F. Spray a 1½-quart baking dish with nonstick cooking spray.

3. In small bowl, combine the remaining 1 cup milk, the eggs, raisins, vanilla extract and cinnamon. Stir cooked rice into milk mixture. Pour into the prepared baking dish; dot with margarine. Bake 25 minutes, stirring twice during baking.

EACH SERVING PROVIDES: ½ Milk, ½ Fat, ½ Fruit, ½ Protein, 1 Bread, 45 Optional Calories
PER SERVING: 280 Calories, 9 g Protein, 5 g Fat, 49 g Carbohydrate, 133 mg Sodium, 109 mg Cholesterol, 0 g Dietary Fiber

Maple Tapioca with Dried Cranberries

Makes 4 Servings

2 cups low-fat (1%) milk
$\frac{1}{2}$ cup dried cranberries
$\frac{1}{3}$ cup maple syrup
3 tablespoons uncooked quick-cooking tapioca
$\frac{1}{8}$ teaspoon salt
1 large egg white
$\frac{1}{4}$ teaspoon vanilla extract

1. In medium saucepan, combine milk, cranberries, maple syrup, tapioca and salt; let stand 5 minutes.

2. Meanwhile, in bowl of electric mixer, beat egg white until stiff peaks form; set aside.

3. Bring milk mixture to a boil. Reduce heat to low; cook, stirring constantly, 15–20 minutes, until tapioca is tender and clear. Stir in beaten egg white and vanilla extract.

4. Scrape tapioca into medium serving bowl; let cool. Serve warm or chilled.

EACH SERVING PROVIDES: $\frac{1}{2}$ Milk, 1 Fruit, 110 Optional Calories
PER SERVING: 193 Calories, 5 g Protein, 1 g Fat, 42 g Carbohydrate, 181 mg Sodium, 5 mg Cholesterol, 0 g Dietary Fiber

Baked Plums

Makes 4 Servings

4 large plums, pitted and sliced
2 tablespoons firmly packed dark brown sugar
$\frac{1}{2}$ teaspoon cinnamon
2 tablespoons + 2 teaspoons reduced-calorie tub margarine

1. Preheat oven to 450°F. Spray an 8" or 9" pie plate with nonstick cooking spray.

2. Arrange plum slices in prepared pie plate; evenly sprinkle with brown sugar and cinnamon. Dot with margarine.

3. Bake 15 minutes, until plums are soft and margarine is bubbling.

EACH SERVING PROVIDES: 1 Fat, 1 Fruit, 25 Optional Calories
PER SERVING: 119 Calories, 1 g Protein, 5 g Fat, 21 g Carbohydrate, 76 mg Sodium, 0 mg Cholesterol, 2 g Dietary Fiber

◆

Broiled Pecan Pineapple

Makes 4 Servings

12 ounces pineapple, pared and cut into $\frac{1}{2}$" chunks
14 pecan halves, coarsely chopped
2 tablespoons firmly packed light brown sugar

1. Preheat broiler. Line bottom of shallow baking pan with foil.

2. Arrange pineapple chunks on prepared pan; top with pecans. Sprinkle brown sugar over pineapple and pecans.

3. Broil 6" from heat, 2–3 minutes, until sugar has melted and nuts are lightly browned. Serve warm.

EACH SERVING PROVIDES: 1 Fat, $\frac{1}{2}$ Fruit, 25 Optional Calories
PER SERVING: 115 Calories, 1 g Protein, 5 g Fat, 19 g Carbohydrate, 4 mg Sodium, 0 mg Cholesterol, 1 g Dietary Fiber

PEACH SOUFFLÉ

MAKES 4 SERVINGS

¼ cup + 1 tablespoon granulated sugar
2 medium peaches, pared, pitted and sliced
1½ teaspoons fresh lemon juice
4 large eggs, separated, at room temperature
2 large egg whites, at room temperature
¼ cup confectioners sugar (reserve 1 tablespoon)

1. Preheat oven to 450°F. Spray a 6-cup soufflé dish with nonstick cooking spray; coat bottom and sides of dish with 2 tablespoons of the granulated sugar and refrigerate.

2. In blender or food processor, combine the remaining 3 tablespoons of the granulated sugar, the peach slices and lemon juice; purée until smooth. Add egg yolks and process until well blended; transfer to large bowl.

3. In medium bowl, with mixer on medium speed, beat all 6 egg whites until stiff peaks form. Sprinkle confectioners sugar over egg whites; continue beating until stiff peaks form again. Stir one-fourth of the beaten egg whites into peach mixture; fold in remaining whites.

4. Scrape batter into prepared dish; set in small roasting pan. Pour hot water (not boiling) halfway up side of roasting pan. Bake 10 minutes. Evenly sprinkle with reserved tablespoon confectioners sugar; serve immediately.

EACH SERVING PROVIDES: ½ Fruit, 1 Protein, 110 Optional Calories
PER SERVING: 202 Calories, 8 g Protein, 5 g Fat, 31 g Carbohydrate, 91 mg Sodium, 213 mg Cholesterol, 1 g Dietary Fiber

NECTARINE SOUFFLÉ

Substitute 2 small nectarines for the peaches; proceed according to directions.

WATERMELON SORBET

MAKES 4 SERVINGS

4 cups pitted watermelon chunks
¼ cup superfine sugar*
2 tablespoons fresh lime juice

1. In processor, combine watermelon, sugar and lime juice; purée until smooth.

2. Pour watermelon mixture into a 2-quart freezer-safe container with tight-fitting cover; place in freezer, covered, 4–6 hours, until mixture resembles set gelatin.

3. In food processor, in 2 separate batches, purée set watermelon mixture; return to same container. Freeze, covered, overnight.

4. To serve, let stand at room temperature 5 minutes; evenly spoon into 4 dessert dishes.

*If superfine sugar is not available, process granulated sugar in blender until superfine.

EACH SERVING PROVIDES: 1 Fruit, 45 Optional Calories
PER SERVING: 102 Calories, 1 g Protein, 1 g Fat, 25 g Carbohydrate, 3 mg Sodium, 0 mg Cholesterol, 1 g Dietary Fiber

---

Get the Brown Out

◆

Do you like to serve cut-up fresh fruit, but hate the fact that it turns brown? Then you'll love this tip for keeping apple slices fresh-looking and pretty. It also works well on other fruit that tends to darken when exposed to air.

- *Wash apples. Halve, then cut into quarters. Remove the section of core from each quarter; slice fruit.*
- *Dip fruit into a bowl of lemon juice. You can also use a bowl of ascorbic-acid color keeper.*
- *Drain fruit on paper towel after dipping.*

BLUEBERRY SHERBET

MAKES 8 SERVINGS

3 cups thawed frozen blueberries
½ cup granulated sugar
1 tablespoon fresh lime juice
1 envelope unflavored gelatin
2 cups low-fat (1.5%) buttermilk

1. In large saucepan, combine blueberries, sugar and juice; sprinkle with gelatin. Let stand 2 minutes. Simmer over medium-low heat, stirring constantly, about 3 minutes, until sugar and gelatin are completely dissolved. Remove from heat; stir in buttermilk.

2. Pour berry mixture into a 2½-quart freezer-safe container with tight-fitting cover; place in freezer, covered, 4–6 hours, until mixture resembles set gelatin.

3. In food processor, in 2 separate batches, purée set berry mixture; return to same container. Freeze, covered, overnight.

4. To serve, let stand at room temperature 5 minutes; evenly spoon into 8 dessert dishes.

EACH SERVING PROVIDES: ¼ Milk, ½ Fruit, 45 Optional Calories
PER SERVING: 114 Calories, 3 g Protein, 1 g Fat, 23 g Carbohydrate, 69 mg Sodium, 4 mg Cholesterol, 1 g Dietary Fiber

PINK GRAPEFRUIT AND RASPBERRY GRANITA

MAKES 6 SERVINGS

1½ cups fresh or drained thawed frozen raspberries
2 cups pink grapefruit juice
½ cup superfine sugar*

1. Set fine sieve over a 2-quart freezer-safe container with tight-fitting cover; press raspberries through sieve. Discard seeds.

2. Add grapefruit juice and sugar to container; stir to mix well. Freeze, covered, stirring with a fork every half hour, about 6 hours, until frozen.

* If superfine sugar is not available, process granulated sugar in blender until superfine.

EACH SERVING PROVIDES: 1 Fruit, 60 Optional Calories
PER SERVING: 112 Calories, 1 g Protein, 0 g Fat, 28 g Carbohydrate, 1 mg Sodium, 0 mg Cholesterol, 1 g Dietary Fiber

FROZEN MANGO-LIME MOUSSE

The tropical flavors of mango and lime make this the perfect choice to follow a spicy Mexican or Caribbean entrée.

MAKES 4 SERVINGS

2 medium mangoes (10 ounces each), pared, pitted and cut into ½" cubes
½ cup part-skim ricotta cheese
¼ cup granulated sugar
2 tablespoons fresh lime juice
1 teaspoon grated lime zest
1 envelope unflavored gelatin
1 cup low-fat (1%) milk

1. In food processor or blender, combine mangoes, ricotta cheese, sugar, juice and the zest.

2. Meanwhile, sprinkle gelatin over ¼ cup cold water; let stand 2 minutes, until softened. Pour into food processor.

3. In small saucepan, bring milk to a boil. Pour into food processor; purée until smooth.

4. Into each of four 8-ounce freezer-safe dishes pour one-fourth of the mango mixture; cover with plastic wrap. Freeze about 2 hours, until set.

EACH SERVING PROVIDES: ¼ Milk, 1¼ Fruits, ½ Protein, 45 Optional Calories
PER SERVING: 189 Calories, 8 g Protein, 3 g Fat, 35 g Carbohydrate, 75 mg Sodium, 12 mg Cholesterol, 1 g Dietary Fiber

SPICED BERRY MOLD

In this buffet showpiece, the berries are suspended in shimmering jelled cranberry juice and look like little jewels.

MAKES 8 SERVINGS

2 cups cranberry juice cocktail
$\frac{1}{4}$ cup granulated sugar
2 envelopes unflavored gelatin
2 cinnamon sticks
$\frac{1}{4}$ teaspoon ground cloves
$\frac{3}{4}$ cup blueberries
$\frac{3}{4}$ cup raspberries

1. In medium saucepan, combine juice, sugar, gelatin, cinnamon sticks and cloves; bring to a boil. Reduce heat to low; cook, stirring constantly, until gelatin is dissolved. Let cool 3–7 minutes, until slightly jelled; remove and discard cinnamon sticks. Stir in blueberries and raspberries.

2. Into a 1-quart ungreased mold, pour berry mixture; cover with plastic wrap. Chill until firm.

EACH SERVING PROVIDES: 1 Fruit, 25 Optional Calories
PER SERVING: 80 Calories, 2 g Protein, 0 g Fat, 19 g Carbohydrate, 6 mg Sodium, 0 mg Cholesterol, 1 g Dietary Fiber

---

Sectioning Grapefruit and Oranges

◆

Here's the easy way to section your fresh grapefruit and oranges.

- *Begin by cutting off the peel and the white membrane, using a very sharp utility knife or a serrated knife for peeling citrus fruits.*
- *Remove the sections by cutting into the center of the fruit between one section and the membrane. Then turn the knife and slide it down the other side of the section, next to the membrane.*
- *Remove any seeds. Allow the grapefruit or orange sections to fall into a bowl along with any juice.*

MINTED GRAPEFRUIT AND ORANGES

MAKES 4 SERVINGS

$\frac{1}{2}$ cup chopped fresh mint
2 tablespoons granulated sugar
1 medium grapefruit
2 small oranges
Mint leaves, optional

1. To prepare mint syrup, in small saucepan, combine chopped mint, $\frac{1}{4}$ cup water and the sugar; bring to a boil. Reduce heat to low; simmer 3 minutes. Remove from heat; let cool 10 minutes.

2. Meanwhile, remove skin and membranes from grapefruit. Over small bowl, with a paring knife, cut grapefruit into sections. Remove skin and membranes from oranges; cut each crosswise into 4 equal slices. Combine with grapefruit sections.

3. Strain cooled mint syrup over fruit, squeezing any juice from the mint leaves into bowl. Refrigerate, covered with plastic wrap, until well chilled. To serve, garnish with whole mint leaves, if desired.

EACH SERVING PROVIDES: 1 Fruit, 25 Optional Calories
PER SERVING: 73 Calories, 1 g Protein, 0 g Fat, 18 g Carbohydrate, 0 mg Sodium, 0 mg Cholesterol, 2 g Dietary Fiber

BLACK AND WHITE STRAWBERRIES

You've probably seen chocolate-dipped fruit in elegant restaurants. Our version uses semisweet and white chocolate for a dramatic presentation.

MAKES 4 SERVINGS

$1\frac{1}{2}$ ounces semisweet chocolate chips
$1\frac{1}{2}$ teaspoons framboise or raspberry liqueur
$\frac{1}{2}$ ounce white chocolate, chopped, or white chocolate chips
2 cups strawberries, with hulls attached (about 16 berries)

1. Line an 18" baking sheet with wax paper.

2. In small microwavable bowl, combine semisweet chocolate chips, framboise and $1\frac{1}{2}$ teaspoons water; microwave on High power $1\frac{1}{2}$ minutes, stirring twice during cooking time.

3. Holding 1 berry by the hull, dip berry halfway into the melted chocolate; set on wax paper. Repeat procedure with remaining berries and chocolate.

4. In small microwavable bowl, melt white chocolate in microwave on High power 1 minute, stirring once during cooking time.

5. With tines of a fork, drizzle white chocolate over strawberries. Refrigerate until chocolate has hardened. Serve chilled.

EACH SERVING (4 strawberries) PROVIDES: $\frac{1}{2}$ Fruit, 80 Optional Calories
PER SERVING: 97 Calories, 1 g Protein, 4 g Fat, 15 g Carbohydrate, 4 mg Sodium, 0 mg Cholesterol, 2 g Dietary Fiber

ALMOND-FUDGE TRUFFLES

Make these at holiday time and pack them in a pretty tin with the recipe attached for a wonderful, personal gift.

MAKES 24 SERVINGS

$\frac{1}{2}$ cup + 2 tablespoons unsweetened cocoa powder
1 cup sifted confectioners sugar
$\frac{1}{2}$ cup light cream cheese, at room temperature
$\frac{1}{2}$ teaspoon almond extract

1. On sheet of wax paper, reserve 2 tablespoons cocoa powder; set aside.

2. In food processor or with mixer on high speed, combine confectioners sugar, the remaining $\frac{1}{2}$ cup cocoa powder, the cream cheese and almond extract; process until well blended.

3. Drop cream cheese mixture by rounded teaspoonfuls in the reserved cocoa powder, making 24 portions; roll into balls and refrigerate.

EACH SERVING (1 piece) PROVIDES: 45 Optional Calories
PER SERVING: 45 Calories, 1 g Protein, 1 g Fat, 6 g Carbohydrate, 27 mg Sodium, 2 mg Cholesterol, 1 g Dietary Fiber

Cheese Soufflé (page 354)

CHAPTER THIRTEEN

BASIC TECHNIQUES AND RECIPES

BÉCHAMEL SAUCE

Béchamel sauce is very nice served over vegetables,
poached fish or poached chicken.

MAKES 4 SERVINGS

1 tablespoon + 1 teaspoon reduced-calorie tub
  margarine
$\frac{1}{4}$ cup all-purpose flour
3 cups low-fat (1%) milk
2 whole cloves
1 small bay leaf
3 peppercorns
$\frac{1}{4}$ teaspoon salt
Pinch nutmeg

In medium saucepan over medium-low heat,
melt margarine; whisk flour into margarine. Gradually add milk, whisking constantly, until smooth.
Add cloves and bay leaf to milk mixture. Stir in
peppercorns, salt and nutmeg. Simmer gently over
low heat, whisking frequently, 10 minutes. Strain.

EACH SERVING (3 fluid ounces) PROVIDES: $\frac{3}{4}$ Milk, $\frac{1}{2}$ Fat, $\frac{1}{4}$ Bread, 10
Optional Calories
PER SERVING: 123 Calories, 7 g Protein, 4 g Fat, 15 g Carbo-
hydrate, 263 mg Sodium, 7 mg Cholesterol, 0 g Dietary Fiber

MORNAY SAUCE

With its cheese flavor, Mornay sauce adds a hearty
touch to vegetables or fish.

MAKES 8 SERVINGS

3 cups low-fat (1%) milk
$\frac{1}{4}$ cup all-purpose flour
1 small onion, peeled
3 whole cloves
1 bay leaf
3 peppercorns
$\frac{1}{4}$ teaspoon salt
$\frac{1}{8}$ teaspoon ground nutmeg
2 slices low-fat processed Swiss cheese (2 ounces),
  cut in small pieces
$\frac{3}{4}$ ounce Parmesan cheese, grated
Pinch ground red pepper

1. In medium saucepan over low heat, whisk
milk into flour. Stud onion with cloves and bay
leaf and add to milk mixture. Stir in peppercorns,
salt and nutmeg. Simmer gently 10 minutes.
Strain.

2. Return to heat; stir in cheeses and ground
red pepper. Cook just until cheeses are melted.

EACH SERVING ($\frac{3}{4}$ cup) PROVIDES: $\frac{1}{4}$ Milk, $\frac{1}{4}$ Protein, 25 Optional
Calories
PER SERVING: 85 Calories, 6 g Protein, 3 g Fat, 8 g Carbohydrate,
172 mg Sodium, 10 mg Cholesterol, 0 g Dietary Fiber

HERBED CHEESE SAUCE

For those occasions when the broccoli or cauliflower needs a little embellishing, stir up this tasty cheese sauce.

MAKES 4 SERVINGS

1 cup low-fat (1%) milk
1 tablespoon all-purpose flour
3 ounces reduced-fat cheddar cheese, grated
1 tablespoon Parmesan cheese, grated
1 tablespoon chopped fresh basil
1 teaspoon chopped fresh tarragon
1 teaspoon chopped fresh thyme
$\frac{3}{4}$ teaspoon prepared mustard
$\frac{1}{4}$ teaspoon freshly ground black pepper
Pinch ground nutmeg

1. In small saucepan, heat $\frac{2}{3}$ cup of the milk over medium heat. Set aside; keep warm.

2. In medium saucepan, whisk together the remaining $\frac{1}{3}$ cup of milk and the flour until smooth. Cook over medium heat, stirring constantly; bring to a boil. Boil, stirring constantly, 5 minutes, until very thick.

3. Gradually whisk in warm milk, cheddar cheese, Parmesan cheese, basil, tarragon, thyme, mustard, pepper and nutmeg. Cook over low heat, stirring constantly, until cheeses are melted.

EACH SERVING (¼ cup) PROVIDES: ¼ Milk, 1 Protein, 15 Optional Calories
PER SERVING: 108 Calories, 9 g Protein, 5 g Fat, 6 g Carbohydrate, 216 mg Sodium, 18 mg Cholesterol, 0 g Dietary Fiber

MUSHROOM SAUCE

Perfect for chicken, this sauce is also excellent served over pasta.

MAKES 4 SERVINGS

2 teaspoons unsalted margarine
2 tablespoons minced shallots
1 garlic clove, minced
4 cups thinly sliced mushrooms
$\frac{1}{2}$ teaspoon rubbed sage
$\frac{1}{4}$ teaspoon salt
$\frac{1}{8}$ teaspoon black pepper
2 tablespoons brandy
1 tablespoon + $1\frac{1}{2}$ teaspoons all-purpose flour
1 cup evaporated skimmed milk
2 tablespoons nonfat sour cream

1. In large nonstick skillet, heat margarine; add shallots. Sauté until soft, about 2 minutes. Add garlic; cook 1 minute longer. Stir in mushrooms, sage, salt and pepper; cook, stirring frequently, until mushrooms are tender, about 6 minutes.

2. Increase heat to high; cook until almost all liquid has evaporated, about 3 minutes. Add brandy; cook 1 minute. Stir in flour; cook, stirring constantly, until smooth. Add evaporated milk; simmer 7 minutes. Stir in sour cream.

EACH SERVING (½ cup) PROVIDES: ½ Milk, ½ Fat, 2 Vegetables, 35 Optional Calories
PER SERVING: 123 Calories, 7 g Protein, 2 g Fat, 14 g Carbohydrate, 217 mg Sodium, 3 mg Cholesterol, 1 g Dietary Fiber

MUSTARD SAUCE

MAKES 8 SERVINGS

$\frac{1}{3}$ cup grainy mustard
$\frac{1}{3}$ cup low-fat (1.5%) buttermilk
1 tablespoon minced shallots
1 tablespoon light sour cream
2 teaspoons tomato paste
1 tablespoon rinsed capers

In small bowl, stir together mustard, buttermilk, shallots, sour cream and tomato paste; fold in capers.

EACH SERVING (1$\frac{3}{4}$ tablespoons) PROVIDES: 5 Optional Calories
PER SERVING: 20 Calories, 1 g Protein, 1 g Fat, 2 g Carbohydrate, 148 mg Sodium, 1 mg Cholesterol, 0 g Dietary Fiber

HORSERADISH SAUCE

With a nip of horseradish, this sauce is very good with hamburgers or grilled meat.

MAKES 8 SERVINGS

$\frac{1}{2}$ cup drained prepared horseradish
$\frac{1}{2}$ cup plain nonfat yogurt
$\frac{1}{3}$ cup nonfat sour cream
2 teaspoons whole-grain mustard
1 teaspoon granulated sugar
$\frac{1}{2}$ teaspoon Worcestershire sauce
$\frac{1}{8}$ teaspoon black pepper
2 tablespoons chopped parsley

In medium bowl, whisk together horseradish, yogurt, sour cream, mustard, sugar, Worcestershire sauce and pepper. Stir in parsley just before serving.

EACH SERVING (1$\frac{1}{2}$ tablespoons) PROVIDES: 15 Optional Calories
PER SERVING: 35 Calories, 2 g Protein, 2 g Fat, 4 g Carbohydrate, 41 mg Sodium, 4 mg Cholesterol, 0 g Dietary Fiber

LEMON-DILL SAUCE

MAKES 8 SERVINGS

$\frac{1}{3}$ cup fresh lemon juice
2 teaspoons cornstarch
$\frac{1}{2}$ teaspoon granulated sugar
$\frac{1}{4}$ teaspoon dried thyme leaves
$\frac{1}{4}$ teaspoon salt
1 tablespoon + 1 teaspoon snipped fresh dill
1 tablespoon + 1 teaspoon unsalted margarine
1 tablespoon chopped parsley
$\frac{1}{4}$ teaspoon grated lemon zest

In medium stainless steel saucepan, whisk lemon juice into cornstarch; add $\frac{1}{3}$ cup + 1 tablespoon water, the sugar, thyme and salt and bring to a boil. Boil, stirring constantly, 2 minutes. Remove from heat; stir in dill, margarine, parsley and lemon zest.

EACH SERVING (2 tablespoons) PROVIDES: $\frac{1}{2}$ Fat, 3 Optional Calories
PER SERVING: 23 Calories, 0 g Protein, 2 g Fat, 2 g Carbohydrate, 68 mg Sodium, 0 mg Cholesterol, 0 g Dietary Fiber

MINT SAUCE

MAKES 4 SERVINGS

1 cup lightly packed fresh mint, finely chopped
$\frac{1}{2}$ cup white wine vinegar
2 teaspoons granulated sugar

1. In medium stainless steel bowl, add mint; set aside.

2. In small stainless steel saucepan, bring vinegar and sugar to a boil. Cook, stirring constantly, 1–2 minutes, until sugar dissolves; pour vinegar mixture over the mint. Let steep for at least one hour before serving. Pour into jar with tight-fitting cover; refrigerate up to 1 week.

EACH SERVING (2 tablespoons) PROVIDES: 8 Optional Calories
PER SERVING: 15 Calories, 0 g Protein, 0 g Fat, 4 g Carbohydrate, 0 mg Sodium, 0 mg Cholesterol, 0 g Dietary Fiber

PEANUT SAUCE

This Indonesian-inspired sauce adds excitement to chicken and is also a tempting dipping sauce for grilled vegetables.

MAKES 8 SERVINGS

2 tablespoons + 2 teaspoons creamy peanut butter
2 garlic cloves, crushed
2 tablespoons soy sauce
1 tablespoon + 1 teaspoon granulated sugar
1 tablespoon water
$1\frac{1}{4}$ teaspoons rice wine vinegar
1 tablespoon chopped fresh cilantro or $\frac{1}{2}$ teaspoon dried coriander

In small food processor or blender, combine peanut butter and garlic; purée until smooth. Add remaining ingredients and purée until well combined.

EACH SERVING (1 tablespoon) PROVIDES: $\frac{1}{2}$ Fat, $\frac{1}{4}$ Protein, 8 Optional Calories
PER SERVING: 43 Calories, 2 g Protein, 3 g Fat, 4 g Carbohydrate, 283 mg Sodium, 0 mg Cholesterol, 0 g Dietary Fiber

SALSA

MAKES 4 SERVINGS

3 cups chopped seeded plum tomatoes
3 tablespoons shredded fresh basil
3 tablespoons chopped fresh cilantro
1 tablespoon minced green bell pepper
2 teaspoons minced scallion
2 garlic cloves, minced
$\frac{1}{2}$ teaspoon coarse (kosher) salt
1 tablespoon red wine vinegar

1. In medium bowl, combine tomatoes, basil, cilantro, bell pepper, scallion, garlic and salt; toss well. Let stand 30 minutes; drain off any liquid that accumulates.

2. Sprinkle vinegar over tomato mixture; toss again.

EACH SERVING PROVIDES: $1\frac{1}{2}$ Vegetables
PER SERVING: 34 Calories, 1 g Protein, 0 g Fat, 8 g Carbohydrate, 196 mg Sodium, 0 mg Cholesterol, 2 g Dietary Fiber

TOMATO SAUCE

MAKES 4 SERVINGS

2 teaspoons olive oil
$\frac{1}{2}$ cup minced onion
$\frac{1}{4}$ cup minced carrot
2 garlic cloves, minced
$3\frac{1}{2}$ cups canned crushed tomatoes
3 tablespoons fresh orange juice
2 teaspoons honey
1 cinnamon stick, split lengthwise
$\frac{1}{4}$ teaspoon salt

In large nonstick skillet, heat oil over low heat; add onion. Cook until onion is soft, about 7 minutes. Add carrot and garlic; cook 5 minutes. Stir in tomatoes, orange juice, honey, cinnamon stick and salt; cook 20 minutes. Remove cinnamon stick before serving.

EACH SERVING ($\frac{3}{4}$ cup) PROVIDES: $\frac{1}{2}$ Fat, 2 Vegetables, 15 Optional Calories
PER SERVING: 91 Calories, 2 g Protein, 3 g Fat, 16 g Carbohydrate, 481 mg Sodium, 0 mg Cholesterol, 2 g Dietary Fiber

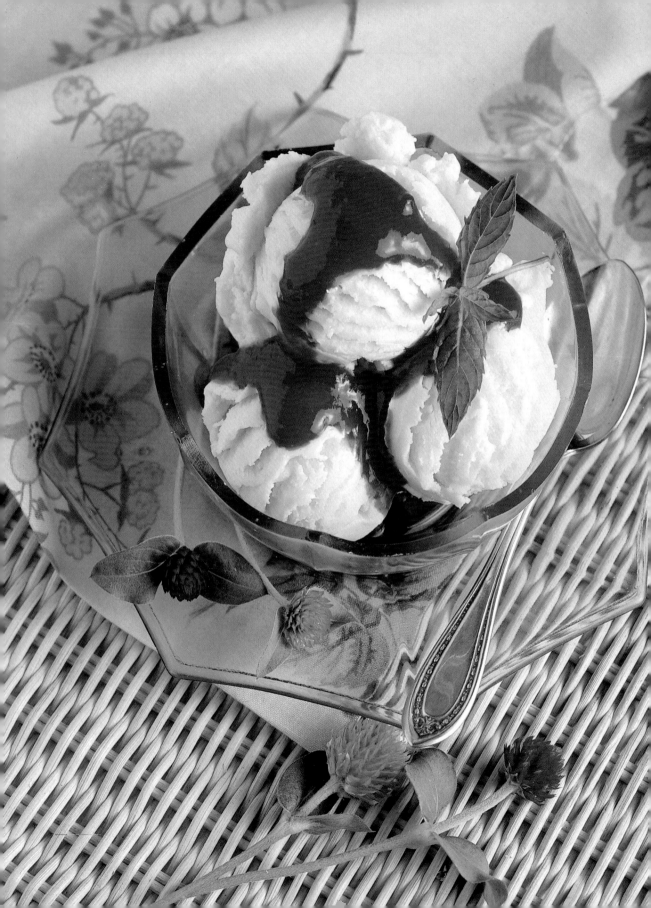

RASPBERRY SAUCE

This is delightful on frozen yogurt or sorbet, and you can create a wide range of flavor combinations, such as chocolate frozen yogurt and raspberry sauce or peach sorbet and raspberry sauce.

MAKES 8 SERVINGS

1½ cups fresh or thawed frozen raspberries
¼ cup raspberry spreadable fruit
1 tablespoon honey
¾ teaspoon vanilla extract
⅛ teaspoon ground allspice

In food processor or blender, purée raspberries. Push puréed raspberries through strainer; discard seeds. Return purée to food processor; add spreadable fruit, honey, vanilla extract and allspice; purée until smooth.

EACH SERVING (1 tablespoon) PROVIDES: ¾ Fruit, 10 Optional Calories
PER SERVING: 42 Calories, 0 g Protein, 0 g Fat, 10 g Carbohydrate, 0 mg Sodium, 0 mg Cholesterol, 1 g Dietary Fiber

CRANBERRY SAUCE

MAKES 16 SERVINGS

3 cups cranberries
1 small navel orange, cut into ¼" pieces
⅔ cup firmly packed dark brown sugar
½ cup orange juice
1 cinnamon stick, split lengthwise
¼ teaspoon ground cloves

In medium saucepan, combine cranberries, orange pieces, brown sugar, juice, cinnamon stick and cloves; bring to a boil. Reduce heat to low; simmer 30 minutes, or until all berries have popped and sauce is syrupy.

EACH SERVING (3 tablespoons) PROVIDES: ¼ Fruit, 35 Optional Calories
PER SERVING: 52 Calories, 0 g Protein, 0 g Fat, 13 g Carbohydrate, 4 mg Sodium, 0 mg Cholesterol, 0 g Dietary Fiber

CHOCOLATE SAUCE

MAKES 4 SERVINGS

3 tablespoons unsweetened cocoa powder
½ cup evaporated skimmed milk
⅓ cup granulated sugar
1 tablespoon + 1 teaspoon light corn syrup
¾ teaspoon vanilla extract

In medium heavy-bottomed saucepan, whisk ¼ cup water and cocoa powder until dissolved. Whisk in evaporated milk, sugar, corn syrup and vanilla; bring to a boil. Lower heat to a simmer and cook, stirring constantly, 6–8 minutes, until thick. Serve warm or at room temperature.

EACH SERVING (3 tablespoons) PROVIDES: ¼ Milk, 85 Optional Calories
PER SERVING: 120 Calories, 3 g Protein, 1 g Fat, 28 g Carbohydrate, 46 mg Sodium, 1 mg Cholesterol, 1 g Dietary Fiber

SWEET LEMON SAUCE

MAKES 8 SERVINGS

¼ cup + 2 tablespoons granulated sugar
1 tablespoon cornstarch
⅓ cup fresh lemon juice
½ teaspoon grated lemon zest
1 tablespoon + 1 teaspoon unsalted margarine
  (optional)

In medium heavy-bottomed saucepan, stir together sugar and cornstarch; whisk in ½ cup water and the juice. Bring to a boil and boil 2 minutes. Place over hot water bath 15 minutes. Remove from heat and stir in lemon zest; swirl in margarine, if using.

EACH SERVING (2 tablespoons with margarine) PROVIDES: ½ Fat, 40 Optional Calories
EACH SERVING (2 tablespoons without margarine) PROVIDES: 40 Optional Calories
PER SERVING (with margarine): 60 Calories, 0 g Protein, 2 g Fat, 11 g Carbohydrate, 23 mg Sodium, 0 mg Cholesterol, 0 g Dietary Fiber
PER SERVING (without margarine) PROVIDES: 43 Calories, 0 g Protein, 0 g Fat, 11 g Carbohydrate, 0 mg Sodium, 0 mg Cholesterol, 0 g Dietary Fiber

PEPPER AND APPLE CHUTNEY

MAKES 8 SERVINGS

2 cups diced red bell peppers
1 cup diced onions
$\frac{1}{4}$ cup granulated sugar
2 tablespoons dark raisins
3 garlic cloves, slivered
1 teaspoon yellow mustard seeds
$\frac{3}{4}$ teaspoon ground ginger
$\frac{1}{2}$ teaspoon salt
$\frac{2}{3}$ cup apple cider vinegar
$\frac{1}{4}$ cup thawed frozen apple juice concentrate
1 small Granny Smith apple, pared, cored and cut into $\frac{1}{2}$" chunks

1. In medium stainless steel saucepan, combine bell peppers, onions, sugar, raisins, garlic, mustard seeds, ginger and salt; stir well to combine. Stir in vinegar and apple juice concentrate. Bring to a boil; cover and simmer 35 minutes.

2. Stir in apple; cook, uncovered, 7–10 minutes longer, until apple is tender and chutney has thickened.

EACH SERVING (3 tablespoons) PROVIDES: $\frac{1}{2}$ Fruit, $\frac{3}{4}$ Vegetable, 25 Optional Calories
PER SERVING: 74 Calories, 1 g Protein, 0 g Fat, 19 g Carbohydrate, 141 mg Sodium, 0 mg Cholesterol, 1 g Dietary Fiber

PESTO

MAKES 6 SERVINGS

$2\frac{1}{2}$ cups packed thoroughly washed and dried basil leaves
2 garlic cloves, crushed
2 tablespoons + 2 teaspoons pine nuts
1 tablespoon + 1 teaspoon olive oil
$\frac{1}{4}$ teaspoon salt
$3\frac{3}{4}$ ounces grated Parmesan cheese

In food processor or blender, combine basil, garlic, $\frac{1}{2}$ cup water, the pine nuts, oil and salt; purée until smooth. Add Parmesan cheese and purée 30 seconds.

EACH SERVING (2 tablespoons) PROVIDES: 1 Fat, 1 Protein
PER SERVING: 144 Calories, 9 g Protein, 11 g Fat, 5 g Carbohydrate, 422 mg Sodium, 14 mg Cholesterol, 0 g Dietary Fiber

---

Microwave Cooking Tips

◆

Your microwave can be a great help in the kitchen, slashing prep time as well as cleanup time. You'll find these tips helpful and easy!

- *For greater volume when whipping egg whites, place them in a glass measuring cup; microwave 8–10 seconds for 2 whites, 10–12 seconds for 3 whites.*
- *For maximum juice from a lemon or lime, microwave 1 minute before squeezing.*
- *Melt 2 tablespoons margarine in 20–30 seconds.*
- *One-half cup skim milk can be warmed in 30–45 seconds, scalded in 45–60 seconds.*
- *Plump dried fruits by sprinkling with a teaspoon of water; microwave for 15–45 seconds.*
- *Soften lumpy sugar in a microwavable dish or container with a slice of apple or bread; microwave 15 seconds.*

VEGETABLE STOCK

MAKES 8 SERVINGS

2 cups chopped onions
1½ cups sliced leeks (white part only)
1 cup chopped carrots
1 cup chopped celery
1 cup chopped parsnips
6 large dried mushrooms
12 sprigs flat-leaf parsley
6 fresh sprigs dill
12 black peppercorns
1½ teaspoons salt or to taste

1. In large stockpot sprayed with nonstick cooking spray, add onions, leeks, carrots, celery and parsnips; cook, stirring, until vegetables are soft, about 10 minutes. Add 9 cups water, the mushrooms, parsley, dill, peppercorns and salt. Bring to a boil. Reduce heat so liquid bubbles gently. Simmer, partially covered, 2 hours.

2. Line a colander with a double layer of cheesecloth; place over large bowl. Strain stock through colander, pressing vegetables with a wooden spoon to extract juices. Discard remaining solids; cool and use immediately, or place in 1-cup freezer containers and freeze for later use.

EACH SERVING (1 cup) PROVIDES: 20 Optional Calories
PER SERVING: 17 Calories, 1 g Protein, 0 g Fat, 4 g Carbohydrate, 423 mg Sodium, 0 mg Cholesterol, 1 g Dietary Fiber

BEEF STOCK

MAKES 8 SERVINGS

4 pounds meaty beef neck bones or beef soup bones
1 large onion, root ends trimmed, unpeeled, cut into chunks
2 medium carrots, washed, untrimmed, cut into 1" pieces
1 large celery stalk with leaves, cut into 1" pieces
1 large leek, trimmed and washed, cut into 1" pieces
1 small purple turnip, washed and cut into chunks
8 sprigs flat-leaf parsley
2 sprigs fresh thyme
1 bay leaf
12 black peppercorns
1½ teaspoons salt or to taste

1. Preheat oven to 400°F.

2. In a shallow roasting pan, roast bones, turning occasionally with tongs, until they begin to brown, about 30 minutes.

3. Lift bones with tongs into a large stockpot. Add 12 cups water and the remaining ingredients; bring to a boil. Reduce heat so liquid bubbles gently. Simmer, partially covered, 2 hours, skimming foam and fat occasionally.

4. Line a colander with a double layer of cheesecloth; place over large bowl. Strain stock through colander, pressing remaining solids with a wooden spoon to extract juices; discard solids. Cool stock. Refrigerate until fat rises to surface; remove. Or, place stock into 1-cup freezer containers and freeze; remove fat when ready to use.

EACH SERVING (1 cup) PROVIDES: 20 Optional Calories
PER SERVING: 19 Calories, 1 g Protein, 0 g Fat, 3 g Carbohydrate, 427 mg Sodium, 0 mg Cholesterol, 0 g Dietary Fiber

CHICKEN STOCK

MAKES 8 SERVINGS

4 pounds chicken wings, backs, or a mixture of
   wings, backs and giblets (no liver)
1 large onion, quartered
2 medium carrots, washed and trimmed, cut in 1"
   pieces
2 large celery stalks with leaves, cut in 1" pieces
1 large leek, washed and trimmed, cut in 1" pieces
2 fresh thyme sprigs
8 flat-leaf parsley sprigs
12 black peppercorns
$1\frac{1}{2}$ teaspoons salt or to taste

1. In large stockpot, place chicken and 12
cups water; bring to a boil. Skim off foam that col-
lects on surface. Add onion, carrots, celery, leek,
thyme, parsley, peppercorns and salt. Reduce heat
so liquid bubbles gently. Simmer, partially covered, 2 hours, skimming foam and fat occasionally.

2. Line a colander with a double layer of
cheesecloth; place over large bowl. Strain stock
through colander, pressing remaining solids with a
wooden spoon; discard solids. Cool stock. Refrigerate until fat rises to surface; remove. Or, place
stock into 1-cup freezer containers and freeze;
remove fat when ready to use.

EACH SERVING (1 cup) PROVIDES: 20 Optional Calories
PER SERVING: 23 Calories, 1 g Protein, 1 g Fat, 3 g Carbohydrate,
446 mg Sodium, 0 mg Cholesterol, 0 g Dietary Fiber

RED WINE MARINADE

*This is a good marinade for beef, lamb or pork. Cool
the marinade and then add the meat; marinate in the
refrigerator several hours or overnight.*

MAKES 4 SERVINGS

$\frac{1}{2}$ cup thinly sliced onion
$\frac{1}{2}$ cup thinly sliced carrot
2 garlic cloves, thinly sliced
1 cup dry red wine
2 sprigs fresh thyme or $\frac{1}{2}$ teaspoon dried
1 bay leaf
$\frac{1}{4}$ teaspoon juniper berries, lightly crushed
6 peppercorns

Spray medium stainless steel saucepan with
nonstick cooking spray; add onion, carrot and garlic. Sauté 5 minutes. Add wine, thyme, bay leaf,
juniper berries and peppercorns; bring to a boil.
Boil 7–8 minutes or until slightly reduced. Strain
and discard solids.

EACH SERVING ($2\frac{1}{2}$ tablespoons) PROVIDES: 50 Optional Calories
PER SERVING: 60 Calories, 1 g Protein, 0 g Fat, 5 g Carbohydrate,
9 mg Sodium, 0 mg Cholesterol, 1 g Dietary Fiber

TERIYAKI MARINADE

A great marinade for pork, beef, chicken or fish. It also doubles as a tempting dipping sauce!

MAKES 6 SERVINGS

$\frac{1}{4}$ cup reduced-sodium soy sauce
3 tablespoons light corn syrup
3 tablespoons fresh orange juice
1 tablespoon firmly packed dark brown sugar
1 garlic clove, crushed
$\frac{1}{2}$ teaspoon ground ginger

In small jar with tight-fitting lid, combine all ingredients; shake until well combined.

EACH SERVING (2 tablespoons) PROVIDES: 35 Optional Calories
PER SERVING: 49 Calories, 1 g Protein, 0 g Fat, 12 g Carbohydrate, 413 mg Sodium, 0 mg Cholesterol, 0 g Dietary Fiber

TOMATO MARINADE

You'll love this spicy marinade for fish or chicken. Makes enough for four chicken breast halves or four fish fillets.

MAKES 4 SERVINGS

1 cup mixed vegetable juice
1 tablespoon minced scallion
1 garlic clove, crushed
1 teaspoon lime juice
$\frac{1}{4}$ teaspoon ground coriander (optional)
$\frac{1}{4}$ teaspoon ground cumin
Pinch ground red pepper

In small jar with tight-fitting lid, combine all ingredients; shake until well combined.

EACH SERVING PROVIDES: $\frac{1}{2}$ Vegetable
PER SERVING: 14 Calories, 0 g Protein, 0 g Fat, 3 g Carbohydrate, 222 mg Sodium, 0 mg Cholesterol, 0 g Dietary Fiber

YOGURT MARINADE

Use this marinade for chicken, beef, lamb or fish. Makes enough for four chicken breast halves or four fish fillets.

MAKES 4 SERVINGS

$\frac{1}{2}$ cup coarsely chopped onion
4 garlic cloves, crushed
2 tablespoons chopped fresh ginger root
1 tablespoon fresh lemon juice
1 cup plain low-fat yogurt
$\frac{1}{2}$ teaspoon salt
$\frac{1}{2}$ teaspoon ground coriander
$\frac{1}{2}$ teaspoon ground cumin
$\frac{1}{4}$ teaspoon black pepper
$\frac{1}{4}$ teaspoon cinnamon
$\frac{1}{8}$ teaspoon ground cardamom
$\frac{1}{8}$ teaspoon ground cloves

In food processor or blender, combine onion, garlic, ginger and juice; purée to a paste. Add yogurt, salt, coriander, cumin, pepper, cinnamon, cardamom and cloves; purée until well combined.

EACH SERVING ($\frac{1}{2}$ cup) PROVIDES: $\frac{1}{4}$ Vegetable, 25 Optional Calories
PER SERVING: 53 Calories, 4 g Protein, 1 g Fat, 8 g Carbohydrate, 315 mg Sodium, 3 mg Cholesterol, 0 g Dietary Fiber

HERB MARINADE

This recipe may be doubled.

MAKES 6 SERVINGS

2 tablespoons Dijon mustard
1 tablespoon + 1 teaspoon chopped fresh
  rosemary
2 teaspoons chopped fresh oregano
2 teaspoons minced shallots
$1\frac{1}{2}$ teaspoons red wine vinegar
2 garlic cloves, minced

In small jar with tight-fitting lid, combine all ingredients; add 1 tablespoon water and shake well. Rub on chicken or lamb and marinate one hour or up to overnight.

PER SERVING: 5 Calories, 0 g Protein, 0 g Fat, 1 g Carbohydrate, 166 mg Sodium, 0 mg Cholesterol, 0 g Dietary Fiber

DRY RUB MARINADE

MAKES 3 SERVINGS

$1\frac{1}{2}$ teaspoons coarse (kosher) salt
1 bay leaf, crumbled
$\frac{1}{2}$ teaspoon rubbed sage
$\frac{1}{2}$ teaspoon granulated sugar
$\frac{1}{8}$ teaspoon ground allspice
$\frac{1}{8}$ teaspoon ground ginger
$\frac{1}{8}$ teaspoon cinnamon

In small bowl, combine all ingredients. To use: rub onto meat (pork roast, thin chops or cutlets, flank steak, roast beef, steak or lamb) 2 hours before cooking, using about 1 teaspoon per 12 ounces uncooked meat.

1 TEASPOON PROVIDES: 3 Optional Calories
PER SERVING: 5 Calories, 0 g Protein, 0 g Fat, 0 g Carbohydrate, 736 mg Sodium, 0 mg Cholesterol, 0 g Dietary Fiber

HERBED VINEGAR

MAKES 1 QUART

1 quart distilled white vinegar
$\frac{1}{4}$ cup packed washed and dried basil leaves
8 fresh rosemary sprigs
8 fresh thyme sprigs
3 strips orange zest, cut into $3 \times \frac{1}{2}$" pieces
8 peppercorns
5 allspice berries
1 cinnamon stick, split lengthwise

In medium stainless steel saucepan, bring vinegar to a boil. Add basil, rosemary, thyme, zest, peppercorns, allspice and cinnamon stick; boil 1 minute. Transfer to sterilized 1-quart jar or bottle. Store in a cool, dark place and allow flavors to mellow for 2 weeks before using. Use in reasonable amounts.

PER QUART: 3 Calories, 0 g Protein, 0 g Fat, 1 g Carbohydrate, 0 mg Sodium, 0 mg Cholesterol, 0 g Dietary Fiber

OMELET

MAKES 1 SERVING

1 egg
2 egg whites
¼ teaspoon salt
1 teaspoon vegetable oil

1. In small bowl, whisk together egg, egg whites, 1 tablespoon water and the salt.

2. Preheat broiler; place broiler rack 4 inches from heat.

3. In 6-inch flameproof nonstick skillet, heat oil over medium-high heat. Pour in egg mixture, pulling the sides of the omelet in towards the center as the edges cook. When the bottom is set, run the pan under the broiler for 30 seconds to cook the top. Fold in half and turn out onto serving plate.

EACH SERVING PROVIDES: 1 Fat, 1 Protein, 40 Optional Calories
PER SERVING: 148 Calories, 13 g Protein, 10 g Fat, 1 g Carbohydrate, 713 mg Sodium, 213 mg Cholesterol, 0 g Dietary Fiber

◆

SWEET PUFFY OMELET

A sweet version of the basic omelet, this makes a nice brunch dish.

MAKES 1 SERVING

1 large egg, separated
⅛ teaspoon salt
2 egg whites
1 tablespoon raspberry spreadable fruit, melted
½ teaspoon confectioners sugar

1. Preheat oven to 400°F. Spray small ovenproof nonstick skillet or a 6" cake pan with nonstick cooking spray.

2. In medium bowl, whisk together egg yolk, 1 tablespoon water and the salt.

3. In clean medium bowl, with clean whisk, beat egg whites until stiff but not dry; fold into yolk mixture. With rubber spatula or back of large spoon, spread mixture evenly over bottom of prepared skillet.

4. Bake 10 minutes, or until toothpick inserted in center comes out dry.

5. With spatula, carefully loosen edges; turn omelet out onto a warm plate. Gently fold in half; top with melted fruit spread. Dust top of omelet with confectioners sugar.

EACH SERVING PROVIDES: 1 Fruit, 1 Protein, 50 Optional Calories
PER SERVING: 162 Calories, 13 g Protein, 6 g Fat, 13 g Carbohydrate, 449 mg Sodium, 213 mg Cholesterol, 0 g Dietary Fiber

◆

FRITTATA

MAKES 4 SERVINGS

3 large eggs
3 egg whites
2 tablespoons grated Parmesan cheese
½ teaspoon salt
2 teaspoons olive oil

1. In medium bowl, whisk together eggs, egg whites, 2 tablespoons water, 1 tablespoon of the Parmesan cheese and the salt.

2. Preheat broiler with rack set 6" from heat.

3. In large flameproof nonstick skillet, heat oil over low heat. Add egg mixture and cook without stirring for 10–12 minutes, until bottom is set and top is slightly loose. Sprinkle top with remaining 1 tablespoon Parmesan cheese.

4. Place pan under broiler until top is just set, about 1 minute. Invert onto a serving platter and cut into 4 wedges.

EACH SERVING PROVIDES: ½ Fat, 1 Protein, 15 Optional Calories
PER SERVING: 100 Calories, 8 g Protein, 7 g Fat, 1 g Carbohydrate, 408 mg Sodium, 161 mg Cholesterol, 0 g Dietary Fiber

CHEESE SOUFFLÉ

MAKES 4 SERVINGS

1 cup low-fat (1%) milk
3 tablespoons all-purpose flour
8 slices (6.4 ounces) low-fat processed cheddar
   cheese, diced
$\frac{1}{2}$ teaspoon salt
$\frac{1}{8}$ teaspoon ground red pepper
2 eggs, separated
2 egg whites

1. In medium heavy-bottomed saucepan, whisk milk into flour; cook over low heat until thickened and no longer floury, about 5 minutes. Stir in cheese, $\frac{1}{4}$ teaspoon of the salt and the ground red pepper.

2. Preheat oven to 350°F.

3. In small bowl, stir small amount of the cheese mixture into the egg yolks, then stir egg yolk mixture into cheese mixture.

4. In separate large bowl, beat all 4 egg whites until foamy; beat in remaining $\frac{1}{4}$ teaspoon salt and beat until peaks are stiff but not dry. Stir $\frac{1}{4}$ of the egg-white mixture into the cheese mixture; gently fold in remaining whites. Scrape into a 3-quart ungreased soufflé dish. Bake 35 minutes or until puffed high and cooked through. Serve immediately.

EACH SERVING PROVIDES: $\frac{1}{4}$ Milk, 1$\frac{1}{2}$ Proteins, $\frac{1}{4}$ Bread, 10 Optional Calories
PER SERVING: 228 Calories, 19 g Protein, 11 g Fat, 9 g Carbo-hydrate, 663 mg Sodium, 139 mg Cholesterol, 0 g Dietary Fiber

SPINACH AND CHEESE QUICHE

MAKES 12 SERVINGS

Plain Pie Crust, prebaked (see page 356)
1$\frac{1}{2}$ cups evaporated skimmed milk
$\frac{1}{3}$ cup low-fat cottage cheese
1$\frac{1}{2}$ ounces Parmesan cheese, grated
2 eggs
3 egg whites
$\frac{1}{2}$ teaspoon salt
$\frac{1}{4}$ teaspoon black pepper
1 package (10 ounces) thawed and squeezed dry
   frozen chopped spinach (2 cups)

1. Preheat oven to 425°F. In medium bowl, whisk together evaporated milk, cottage cheese, Parmesan cheese, eggs, egg whites, salt and pepper. Spread spinach evenly in bottom of pie shell.

2. Place pie plate on jelly-roll pan; pour filling on top of spinach. Bake 15 minutes. Reduce temperature to 350°F and bake 20 minutes longer, until filling is set. Cool 10 minutes before serving.

EACH SERVING PROVIDES: $\frac{1}{4}$ Milk, $\frac{1}{2}$ Fat, $\frac{1}{4}$ Vegetable, $\frac{1}{2}$ Protein, $\frac{1}{2}$ Bread, 15 Optional Calories
PER SERVING: 126 Calories, 8 g Protein, 5 g Fat, 13 g Carbo-hydrate, 394 mg Sodium, 44 mg Cholesterol, 1 g Dietary Fiber

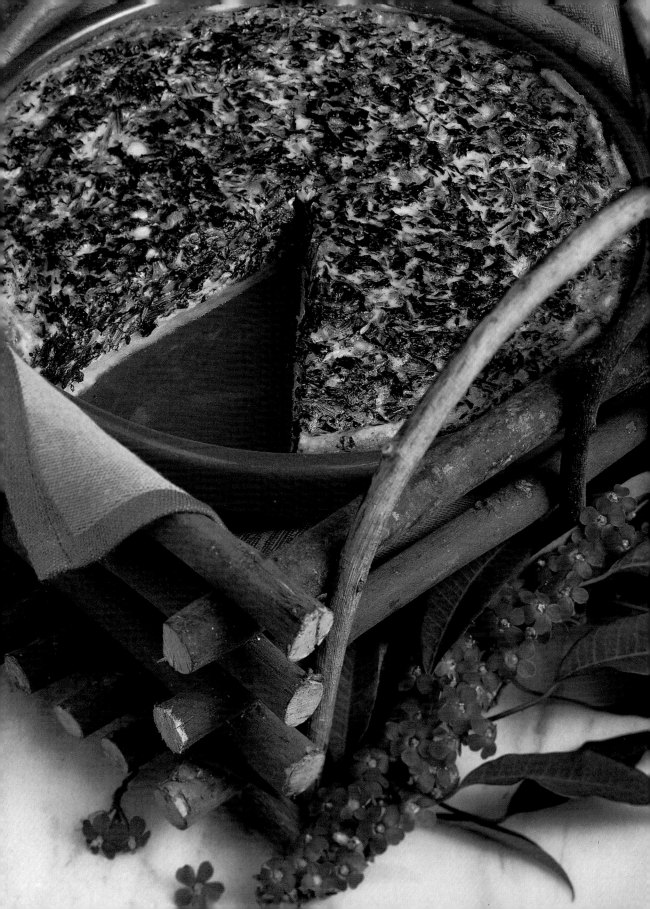

PLAIN PIE CRUST

*The secret of good pastry? Keep it cold, work quickly,
and let it rest to relax the gluten before rolling it out.
For best results, make the crust about
24 hours before you'd like to bake it.*

MAKES 8 SERVINGS

1 cup + 2 tablespoons all-purpose flour
1 teaspoon granulated sugar
$\frac{1}{4}$ teaspoon baking powder
$\frac{1}{8}$ teaspoon salt
2 tablespoons + 2 teaspoons unsalted margarine,
   well chilled, diced
$\frac{1}{3}$ cup lowfat (1%) cottage cheese
$\frac{1}{4}$ cup plain low-fat yogurt

1. In large bowl, combine 1 cup of the flour,
the sugar, baking powder and salt. With pastry
blender or two knives, cut in margarine until mixture resembles coarse crumbs. Stir in cottage
cheese and yogurt until mixture forms soft ball.
Gather dough into a ball; wrap in plastic wrap.
Refrigerate several hours or overnight.

2. Sprinkle work surface with the remaining
flour; roll dough into a 13" circle. Fit dough into a
9" pie plate, pressing to form a stand-up rim; flute
rim, if desired. Chill. Prick bottom with fork.

FOR PREBAKED CRUST:

3. Preheat oven to 400ºF. Line crust with foil;
fill with dried beans or pie weights. Bake 10 minutes, until crust is set; remove foil and beans; bake
5 to 8 minutes longer or until golden. Cool crust
on rack.

EACH SERVING PROVIDES: 1 Fat, $\frac{3}{4}$ Bread, 15 Optional Calories
PER SERVING: 111 Calories, 3 g Protein, 4 g Fat, 15 g Carbohydrate, 93 mg Sodium, 1 mg Cholesterol, 0 g Dietary Fiber

TART CRUST

MAKES 8 SERVINGS

1 cup + 2 tablespoons all-purpose flour, chilled
2 tablespoons granulated sugar
$\frac{1}{2}$ teaspoon salt
2 tablespoons + 2 teaspoons unsalted margarine,
   well chilled, diced
$\frac{1}{4}$ cup plain low-fat yogurt
1 egg yolk

1. In large bowl, combine 1 cup of the flour,
the sugar and salt. With pastry blender or two
knives, cut in margarine until mixture resembles
coarse crumbs. Stir in yogurt and egg yolk; gather
dough into ball; wrap in plastic wrap. Refrigerate
several hours or overnight.

2. Sprinkle work surface with the remaining
2 tablespoons flour; roll dough into a 13" circle.
Fit dough into a 9" tart pan, pressing dough to fit
into sides of pan and rolling dough over to form a
stand-up rim. Chill. Prick bottom with fork.

FOR PREBAKED CRUST:

3. Preheat oven to 400ºF. Line crust with foil;
fill with dried beans or pie weights. Bake 15 minutes, until crust is set; remove foil and beans and
bake 5 to 8 minutes longer, or until golden. Cool
crust on rack.

EACH SERVING PROVIDES: 1 Fat, $\frac{3}{4}$ Bread, 15 Optional Calories
PER SERVING: 114 Calories, 3 g Protein, 5 g Fat, 15 g Carbohydrate, 74 mg Sodium, 27 mg Cholesterol, 0 g Dietary Fiber

CRUMB CRUST

MAKES 8 SERVINGS

¾ cup honey graham cracker crumbs
¾ cup fine plain dried bread crumbs
1½ teaspoons granulated sugar
¼ teaspoon cinnamon
⅛ teaspoon ground cloves
1 tablespoon + 1 teaspoon unsalted stick
   margarine, frozen
2 tablespoons apple juice

1. Preheat oven to 375°F. Spray a 9" spring-form pan with nonstick cooking spray.

2. In medium bowl, combine graham cracker crumbs, bread crumbs, sugar, cinnamon and cloves; with two forks, cut in margarine until mixture resembles cornmeal.

3. Add apple juice; stir until crumb mixture is thoroughly moistened. Press mixture onto bottom and up sides of prepared pan. Bake 15 minutes, or until golden. Let cool slightly before filling.

EACH SERVING PROVIDES: ½ Fat, 1 Bread, 5 Optional Calories
PER SERVING: 96 Calories, 2 g Protein, 3 g Fat, 15 g Carbohydrate, 138 mg Sodium, 0 mg Cholesterol, 1 g Dietary Fiber

CROUTONS

You can either use your own day-old bread or buy it from a local bakery at a reduced price. You can also freeze leftover bread until you have enough to make croutons.

MAKES 8 SERVINGS

8 ounces day-old bread, cubed
1 tablespoon salt-free seasoning blend
2 teaspoons garlic powder

1. Preheat oven to 300°F.

2. On baking sheet, arrange bread cubes in a single layer, keeping the cubes close together; evenly sprinkle with seasoning blend and garlic powder.

3. Bake 30–40 minutes, until golden brown and thoroughly dried. Store 1-ounce portions in sealable plastic bags for up to one week, or freeze.

EACH SERVING (1 ounce) PROVIDES: 1 Bread
PER SERVING: 83 Calories, 3 g Protein, 1 g Fat, 15 g Carbohydrate, 154 mg Sodium, 0 mg Cholesterol, 1 g Dietary Fiber

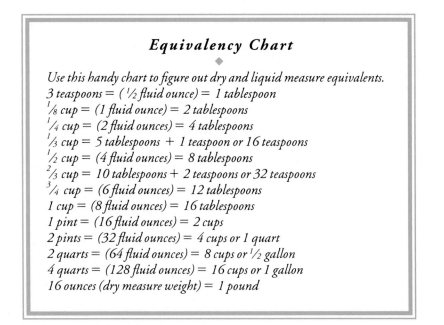

Equivalency Chart

◆

Use this handy chart to figure out dry and liquid measure equivalents.
3 teaspoons = (½ fluid ounce) = 1 tablespoon
⅛ cup = (1 fluid ounce) = 2 tablespoons
¼ cup = (2 fluid ounces) = 4 tablespoons
⅓ cup = 5 tablespoons + 1 teaspoon or 16 teaspoons
½ cup = (4 fluid ounces) = 8 tablespoons
⅔ cup = 10 tablespoons + 2 teaspoons or 32 teaspoons
¾ cup = (6 fluid ounces) = 12 tablespoons
1 cup = (8 fluid ounces) = 16 tablespoons
1 pint = (16 fluid ounces) = 2 cups
2 pints = (32 fluid ounces) = 4 cups or 1 quart
2 quarts = (64 fluid ounces) = 8 cups or ½ gallon
4 quarts = (128 fluid ounces) = 16 cups or 1 gallon
16 ounces (dry measure weight) = 1 pound

MAPLE SPICE GRANOLA

MAKES 10 SERVINGS

15 ounces rolled oats
$\frac{1}{3}$ cup instant nonfat dry milk powder
1 teaspoon cinnamon
$\frac{1}{2}$ teaspoon ground ginger
$\frac{1}{4}$ teaspoon ground cloves
$\frac{1}{4}$ teaspoon ground nutmeg
1 cup apple cider
$\frac{1}{3}$ cup maple syrup
1 teaspoon vanilla extract
$\frac{1}{2}$ teaspoon natural maple extract
$\frac{1}{4}$ cup raisins, chopped
12 dried apricot halves, finely diced

1. Preheat oven to 300°F. Divide oats between two large roasting pans or jelly-roll pans. Shake pans to spread evenly. Bake for 20 minutes, stirring once with spatula.

2. Pour oats into large bowl; add milk powder and spices and stir to combine thoroughly.

3. In small saucepan, heat cider to boiling. Add maple syrup, vanilla and maple extract and stir until dissolved and smooth. Add cider mixture to oats mixture and toss to combine.

4. Spray the roasting or jell-roll pans with nonstick cooking spray. Divide oats mixture between the two pans, spreading evenly, and bake 15–20 minutes until evenly toasted, stirring occasionally.

5. Add raisins and apricots and stir gently to combine. Cool mixture completely in pans; break up any large chunks. Transfer to airtight canister or sealable plastic bags.

EACH SERVING PROVIDES: $\frac{1}{2}$ Fruit, 2 Breads, 40 Optional Calories
PER SERVING: 236 Calories, 8 g Protein, 3 g Fat, 46 g Carbohydrate, 17 mg Sodium, 0 mg Cholesterol, 5 g Dietary Fiber

TROPICAL FRUIT AND NUT GRANOLA

For an interesting change of flavor, substitute 4$\frac{1}{2}$ ounces each of oat, rye and wheat flakes for the rolled oats.

MAKES 12 SERVINGS

13 $\frac{1}{2}$ ounces rolled oats
$\frac{1}{3}$ cup instant nonfat dry milk powder
$\frac{2}{3}$ cup pineapple juice
$\frac{1}{3}$ cup honey
2 teaspoons almond extract
1 teaspoon vanilla extract
1 teaspoon coconut extract
1 ounce sliced almonds
$\frac{1}{2}$ cup flaked coconut
1$\frac{1}{2}$ ounces dried pineapple, diced
1$\frac{1}{2}$ ounces dried dates, chopped

1. Preheat oven to 300°F. Divide oats between two large roasting pans or jelly-roll pans. Shake pans to spread evenly. Bake for 20 minutes, stirring once with spatula.

2. Pour oats into large bowl; add milk powder and stir to combine thoroughly.

3. In small saucepan, heat pineapple juice and $\frac{1}{3}$ cup water to boiling. Add honey and almond, vanilla and coconut extract and stir until dissolved and smooth. Add pineapple juice mixture to oats mixture and toss to combine.

4. Spray the roasting or jell-roll pans with nonstick cooking spray. Divide mixture between the two pans, spreading evenly; bake 15 minutes until evenly toasted, stirring once. Add almonds and coconut and bake 5–10 minutes longer, stirring occasionally.

5. Add pineapple and dates; stir gently to combine. Cool mixture completely in pans; break up any large chunks. Transfer to airtight canister or sealable plastic bags.

EACH SERVING PROVIDES: $\frac{1}{2}$ Fruit, 1$\frac{1}{2}$ Breads, 55 Optional Calories
PER SERVING: 228 Calories, 7 g Protein, 5 g Fat, 40 g Carbohydrate, 24 mg Sodium, 0 mg Cholesterol, 4 g Dietary Fiber

CRÊPES

Crêpes can be either sweet or savory. For sweet, sprinkle finished crêpes with confectioners sugar, or fill with your favorite spreadable fruit. For a savory crêpe, fill with minced cooked chicken and vegetables.

MAKES 4 SERVINGS

¾ cup skim milk
½ cup all-purpose flour
1 egg
1 egg white
2 teaspoons vegetable oil
¼ teaspoon salt

1. In food processor or blender, combine milk, flour, egg, egg white, oil and salt; blend until smooth and creamy. Let stand 30 minutes.

2. Spray a 6" nonstick skillet with nonstick cooking spray; set over medium-high heat. Pour a scant 3 tablespoons of batter into pan, swirling to coat bottom. Cook 30 seconds or until lightly browned; turn crêpe over and cook 10 seconds longer. Transfer to a plate. Repeat with remaining batter to make 11 more crêpes.

EACH SERVING (3 crêpes) PROVIDES: ½ Fat, ¼ Protein, ½ Bread, 35 Optional Calories
PER SERVING: 123 Calories, 6 g Protein, 5 g Fat, 14 g Carbohydrate, 189 mg Sodium, 54 mg Cholesterol, 0 g Dietary Fiber

YOGURT CHEESE

This cheese is extraordinarily versatile; you'll find it used in recipes in this book, too.

MAKES 4 SERVINGS

3 cups plain nonfat yogurt

Spoon yogurt into a coffee filter or cheese-cloth-lined sieve; place over bowl. Refrigerate, covered with plastic wrap, 24 hours. Discard liquid.

EACH SERVING (¼ cup + 2 tablespoons) PROVIDES: 1 Milk
PER SERVING: 60 Calories, 7 g Protein, 0 g Fat, 6 g Carbohydrate, 60 mg Sodium, 0 mg Cholesterol, 0 g Dietary Fiber

---

Nuts

◆

Shelled nuts should be stored in the freezer or refrigerator to preserve freshness. Because their oil content is high, nuts can turn rancid under less-than-ideal storage conditions.

A time-saving preparation tip is to weigh out nuts in 1-ounce amounts and put each ounce in an individual zip-closure sandwich bag. Label with name, amount and date before storing. Bring to room temperature before adding to recipe.

Nuts are one ingredient that are best processed by hand; a blender or food processor tends to pulverize them and release their oils, causing them to clump. By hand-chopping or grinding, you have more control over the texture. Another time-saving preparation tip is to put nuts in a plastic bag; press out air and seal tightly. Then pound with a mallet until the desired texture is achieved.

HOLIDAY MENUS

HOLIDAY MENUS

◆

Holidays and special occasions can be challenging, but the good news is that you can plan meals that are healthful, creative and delicious while following a sensible, healthy food plan! You can still serve traditional meals that showcase your favorite holiday foods and not feel the least deprived.

And, even better, no one will think they are eating "diet" food. In fact, you'll probably find that friends and family enjoy these sensible recipes as much as, if not more than, your original holiday menu.

While you'll love to serve these menus on the specific holiday designated, feel free to use them anytime you'd like to entertain. Our Fourth of July bash would also be great for a barbecue with the neighbors; Easter dinner could be served at a dinner party anytime in the spring; our Mother's Day Brunch would be welcome whenever you're entertaining a large group.

The menus are planned to give you a balanced meal—you'll find complete Weight Watchers Selection Information for each menu, so you'll know exactly how to record your meal. And each individual recipe has Weight Watchers Selection Information, as well as nutrition information. You'll find this useful when you'd like to bring a dish to a holiday meal held at someone else's home. Volunteer to bring Pumpkin-Ricotta Cheesecake (page 403) to Thanksgiving Dinner, or Roasted Vegetable-Pasta Salad (page 388) to a picnic, and it will be much easier to follow your food plan.

Each menu has its own shopping list and preparation schedule to help you plan your holiday meals. At right is a list of staple items that most people have on hand; these staple items have not been included in the shopping lists.

STAPLE ITEMS

♦

BAKING NEEDS

Baking powder
Baking soda
Cornstarch
Cream of tartar
Flour—all-purpose and whole-wheat
Nonfat dry milk powder
Sugar—brown, confectioners and granulated
Unflavored gelatin
Unsweetened cocoa powder
Vanilla extract

CONDIMENTS

Barbecue sauce
Chili sauce
Hot pepper sauce
Ketchup
Lemon and lime juice
Mustard—prepared and Dijon
Red and white wine
Soy sauce—regular or reduced-sodium
Teriyaki sauce—regular or reduced-sodium
Vinegars—red wine and white
Worcestershire sauce—regular or low-sodium

HERBS, SPICES AND SEASONINGS

Allspice, Basil leaves, Bay leaves, Black peppercorns, Chili powder, Cinnamon, Cloves, Dry
mustard, Garlic powder, Ginger, Ground red
pepper, Nutmeg, Oregano, Paprika, Parsley,
Pepper, Rosemary, Sage, Salt, Savory, Sesame
seeds, Tarragon, Thyme

REFRIGERATOR STAPLES

Eggs
Margarine—regular and reduced-calorie tub
Parmesan cheese
Plain nonfat yogurt
Reduced-calorie mayonnaise
Skim milk
Yeast

PANTRY STAPLES

Coffee and tea
Dried bread crumbs
Evaporated skimmed milk
Gravy flavoring
Honey
Low-sodium broths
Oils—vegetable and olive
Peanut butter
Reduced-calorie pancake syrup
Reduced-calorie whole-wheat and white bread
Rice—short- and long-grain

VALENTINE'S DAY DESSERTS FOR CHOCOLATE LOVERS

---

*Healthy eating is still possible—and quite luscious—on Valentine's Day!
Make any of these enticing chocolate desserts and you can indulge your passion for chocolate, as well as show you care about your loved ones' health.*

◆ MENU ◆

Chocolate Banana Pâté

Chocolate Mousse Pie

Chocolate-Walnut Baklava

Chocolate-Banana Pâté

Bananas
Whipped topping
Fresh or frozen raspberries
Pineapple juice

Chocolate Mousse Pie

Whipped topping
Rum extract

Chocolate-Walnut Baklava

Walnuts
Dark raisins
Semisweet chocolate
Unsalted reduced-calorie tub margarine
Phyllo dough

PREP SCHEDULE

◆ Chocolate-Banana Pâté can be made ahead. Or, if you like, prepare raspberry sauce before making pâté and store in the refrigerator.

◆ Make Chocolate Mousse Pie either the day before serving or early in the morning, so it has time to chill.

◆ Make Chocolate-Walnut Baklava the day before serving or early in the morning, so it has time to cool.

CHOCOLATE BANANA PÂTÉ

MAKES 8 SERVINGS

1 envelope unflavored gelatin
$\frac{1}{4}$ cup unsweetened cocoa powder
$\frac{1}{4}$ cup granulated sugar
1 tablespoon honey
2 very ripe medium bananas
$\frac{3}{4}$ cup plain nonfat yogurt
2 teaspoons vanilla extract
1 cup whipped topping
$2\frac{1}{4}$ cups fresh or thawed frozen raspberries
1 tablespoon cornstarch
$\frac{1}{3}$ cup pineapple juice

1. Line an 8" loaf pan with aluminum foil; set aside.

2. In small saucepan, sprinkle gelatin over $\frac{1}{2}$ cup cold water; let stand 2 minutes. Stir in cocoa, 2 tablespoons of the sugar and the honey; cook, stirring constantly, 4–5 minutes, until gelatin is dissolved. Remove from heat; let cool.

3. In medium bowl, mash bananas until very smooth. Stir in yogurt, gelatin mixture and vanilla; gently fold in whipped topping. Spoon into prepared pan and freeze until firm, about 8 hours.

4. Meanwhile, in small saucepan, combine raspberries and the remaining 2 tablespoons sugar; bring to a boil, stirring to crush berries. In small bowl, dissolve cornstarch in pineapple juice. Add to saucepan; stir to mix well. Cook 30–40 seconds, until thick. Strain through a fine mesh sieve; cool completely.

5. To serve, remove pâté from pan; peel off foil. Cut into $\frac{1}{2}$"-thick slices; serve with raspberry sauce.

EACH SERVING PROVIDES: 1 Fruit, 80 Optional Calories
PER SERVING: 136 Calories, 3 g Protein, 3 g Fat, 20 mg Sodium, 0 mg Cholesterol

CHOCOLATE MOUSSE PIE

MAKES 8 SERVINGS

$1\frac{1}{2}$ cups all-purpose flour
$\frac{1}{4}$ teaspoon salt
$\frac{1}{8}$ teaspoon baking powder
$\frac{1}{2}$ cup reduced-calorie tub margarine
1 teaspoon unflavored gelatin
2 tablespoons boiling water
$\frac{1}{3}$ cup granulated sugar
$\frac{1}{3}$ cup unsweetened cocoa powder
1 cup evaporated skimmed milk, well chilled
$1\frac{1}{2}$ teaspoons vanilla extract
1 cup whipped topping
1 tablespoon confectioners sugar
$\frac{1}{2}$ teaspoon rum extract
Unsweetened cocoa powder to garnish (optional)

1. To prepare pie crust, in medium bowl, stir together $1\frac{1}{3}$ cups of the flour, the salt and the baking powder. With 2 knives or pastry blender, cut in margarine until mixture resembles coarse crumbs. With fork, stir in 2–3 tablespoons water until mixture forms a soft dough. Gather dough into a ball.

2. Preheat oven to 350°F. Sprinkle work surface with the remaining flour. On floured surface, roll dough into a 12" circle. Fit into a 10" pie plate, fluting edges. Line crust with foil; fill with pie weights or dried beans.

3. Bake crust 10 minutes; remove foil and weights. Bake 12–15 minutes longer, until golden; set aside.

4. To prepare filling, in small bowl, sprinkle gelatin over 1 tablespoon cold water; let stand 1 minute. Add boiling water, stirring until gelatin is dissolved. Let stand 5 minutes.

5. In another small bowl, stir together sugar and cocoa. With mixer on medium speed, beat in milk and vanilla; increase speed to high and beat, scraping sides of bowl occasionally, until stiff. Add gelatin; beat until blended. Pour into pastry shell. Refrigerate at least 2 hours.

6. To serve, gently stir together whipped topping, confectioners sugar and rum extract. Spread on top of pie. Sprinkle with cocoa powder, if desired.

EACH SERVING PROVIDES: ¼ Milk, 1½ Fat, 1 Bread, 70 Optional Calories
PER SERVING: 237 Calories, 6 g Protein, 9 g Fat, 35 g Carbohydrate, 224 mg Sodium, 1 mg Cholesterol

◆

CHOCOLATE-WALNUT BAKLAVA

MAKES 24 SERVINGS

6 ounces walnuts, toasted and diced
¾ cup dark raisins
¼ cup granulated sugar
2 ounces semisweet chocolate, chopped into small pieces
12 ounces (approximately 18 sheets) phyllo dough, thawed if frozen
½ cup unsalted reduced-calorie tub margarine, melted
¼ cup honey

1. Spray a 13 × 9" baking pan with nonstick cooking spray; set aside.

2. In medium bowl, combine walnuts, raisins, sugar and chocolate; set aside.

3. On wax paper, stack phyllo sheets and trim into 13 × 9" rectangle. Cover phyllo stack with wax paper and a damp kitchen towel. With serrated knife, cut phyllo trimmings into ½" pieces. Place trimmings in large bowl; toss with hands to separate into pieces; cover with plastic wrap. Set aside.

4. Preheat oven to 300°F. Place one sheet of phyllo into bottom of prepared pan; brush with 1 teaspoon margarine. Layer with three more sheets of phyllo, brushing each with 1 teaspoon margarine; sprinkle top sheet with ½ cup nut mixture.

5. Place one sheet of phyllo on top of nut mixture; brush with 1 teaspoon margarine. Repeat layering with three more sheets, brushing each sheet with 1 teaspoon margarine. Sprinkle ½ cup nut mixture over top layer. Repeat layering phyllo, margarine and nut mixture two more times, ending with nut mixture.

6. Top nut mixture with two remaining sheets of phyllo, brushing each one with 1 teaspoon margarine. Top with reserved phyllo trimmings; drizzle with remaining 2 tablespoons margarine. Bake 1 hour 20 minutes, or until golden. Remove pan to rack.

7. In small saucepan, heat honey until very hot but not boiling. Drizzle honey over hot baklava. Cool on rack. Cover and store in refrigerator.

EACH SERVING PROVIDES: 1 Fat, ¼ Fruit, ¼ Protein, ½ Bread, 30 Optional Calories
PER SERVING: 152 Calories, 3 g Protein, 7 g Fat, 21 g Carbohydrate, 61 mg Sodium, 0 mg Cholesterol

---

Chocolate Fixes

◆

Outsmart your chocolate buds with these fabulous fakes:

- *Stir a teaspoon or two of instant espresso powder into reduced-calorie chocolate pudding for a deep, mysterious flavor hit.*
- *Add unsweetened cocoa powder and almond extract to reduced-calorie vanilla nonfat yogurt.*
- *Splash 2% lowfat milk into diet chocolate soda for a New York-style egg cream.*
- *Pour reduced-calorie or sugar-free chocolate syrup over chocolate-swirl fat-free frozen dessert.*
- *Flavor part-skim ricotta cheese with unsweetened cocoa powder and sugar substitute to taste; serve on a hot waffle.*

ST. PATRICK'S DAY

We've added extra excitement to the traditional St. Patrick's Day fare with a sophisticated beer bread and an enchantingly light Irish Whiskey Custard. If you'd like to add Irish Soda Bread to your celebration, you'll find the recipe on page 77.

◆ MENU ◆

Tossed Salad with Salad Dressing*

St. Paddy's Boiled Beef and Cabbage

Beer Bread

Irish Whiskey Custard

12 fluid ounces light beer

Coffee or tea

*Select 1 cup tossed salad with 1½ teaspoons salad dressing.

EACH MEAL (1 serving) PROVIDES: ½ Milk, 1 Fat, 5½ Vegetables, 3½ Proteins, 1¾ Breads, 190 Optional Calories

---

SHOPPING LIST

Beer Bread
Cake flour
Light beer
White cornmeal

St. Paddy's
Boiled Beef and Cabbage
Light beer
Onion
Garlic clove
Beef brisket
Green cabbage
Red potatoes
Carrots

Irish Whiskey Custard
Irish whiskey

PREP SCHEDULE

Up to 1 Month Before

◆ Bake and freeze Beer Bread.

1 Week Before

◆ Shop for nonperishable ingredients. Check dishes, silver, glasses and platters; clean as needed.

3 Days Before

◆ Shop for perishable ingredients. Iron tablecloth and napkins; order flowers; buy candles.

2 Days Before

◆ Cut and clean vegetables for Boiled Beef and Cabbage; store in resealable plastic bag and refrigerate.

1 Day Before

◆ Prepare Irish Whiskey Custard; cover and refrigerate. Set table.

St. Patrick's Day

◆ Thaw Beer Bread (keep wrapped). Prepare coffeepot. Complete Boiled Beef and Cabbage and assemble salad.

BEER BREAD

*This tasty bread with a distinctive round shape gets
kneaded in the food processor.
Leftover bread freezes well.*

MAKES 16 SERVINGS

1 package active dry yeast
$\frac{1}{4}$ cup warm water (105–115°F)
1 teaspoon granulated sugar
2$\frac{1}{4}$ cups all-purpose unbleached flour (reserve
  2 tablespoons)
1$\frac{3}{4}$ cups cake flour
1$\frac{1}{4}$ cups warm light beer (105–115°F)
2 teaspoons salt
1 tablespoon white cornmeal

1. In small bowl, sprinkle yeast over warm water. Stir in sugar and set aside about 10 minutes or until foamy.

2. In work bowl of food processor fitted with steel blade, combine the flours, half the beer, the yeast mixture and salt. Pulse on and off 4 times. Add the remaining beer and process 8 seconds to form an elastic, spongy wet dough.

3. Spray a large glass or ceramic bowl with nonstick cooking spray. Place dough in bowl, turning to coat all sides. Cover and place in a warm, draft-free place to rise until doubled in bulk, about 1 hour.

4. Sprinkle clean work surface with 1 tablespoon reserved flour and work dough into a ball. Line a bowl with a clean non-terrycloth kitchen towel; sprinkle cloth with remaining tablespoon flour. Press dough into bowl; spray lightly with nonstick cooking spray and cover loosely with plastic wrap. Set aside in a warm, draft-free place to rise until almost doubled in bulk but still firm, about 30–40 minutes.

5. Preheat oven to 450°F. Spray a baking sheet with nonstick cooking spray and sprinkle the center with cornmeal. Gently turn the dough out onto the cornmeal.

6. Cut an "X" in the center of the dough with a clean razor blade or the steel blade of the food processor. Set dough aside in a warm, draft-free place to rise until doubled in bulk and springy, about 10 minutes.

7. Bake 20 minutes; reduce oven temperature to 400°F and bake 10 minutes longer or until bread sounds hollow when tapped on the bottom. Cool on rack.

EACH SERVING PROVIDES: 1$\frac{1}{4}$ Breads, 15 Optional Calories
PER SERVING: 117 Calories, 3 g Protein, 24 g Carbohydrate, 0 g Fat, 276 mg Sodium, 0 mg Cholesterol

---

Why Yeast Keeps on Growing and Growing . . .

◆

Yeast is a tiny plant in the fungus family that naturally exists in air and soil. Yeast manufacturers nurture yeast cells so the plants will grow and reproduce. When the ingredients of bread dough are combined, yeast—which requires air, moisture and sugar or starch to grow—feeds on the sugar and flour in the dough.

As it feeds, it ferments the sugar, producing gaseous carbon dioxide (CO_2). Small bubbles of the gas become trapped in the dough, causing gluten (a natural flour protein) to stretch and provide a structure for the rising bread. By the time the dough has doubled in size, it's loaded with gas bubbles. Punching down the dough makes shaping easier and breaks up the larger bubbles so the finished bread will have an even texture.

DID YOU KNOW . . .
* *Active dry yeast and rapid-rise yeast are available in the baking ingredient section in $\frac{1}{4}$-ounce foil packages and 4-ounce vacuum-packed jars.*
* *Jarred yeast is the most convenient to use in bread machine recipes—it's easy to measure out (be sure to use a dry spoon).*
* *Each $\frac{1}{4}$-ounce of yeast contains 2$\frac{1}{4}$ teaspoons.*
* *Compressed or cake yeast, which comes in .6-ounce or 2-ounce cakes, is found in the refrigerator or dairy section.*

SAINT PADDY'S BOILED BEEF AND CABBAGE

MAKES 8 SERVINGS

12 ounces light beer
1 cup thinly sliced onion
4 peppercorns
2 bay leaves
1 garlic clove, minced
One 3$\frac{1}{2}$-pound trimmed beef brisket
1 medium head green cabbage, cored and cut into
   8 wedges
1$\frac{1}{2}$ pounds small red potatoes
1 cup (1") carrot pieces

1. Remove cooking rack from 4–6-quart pressure cooker. Pour beer into cooker; add onion, peppercorns, bay leaves and garlic, then brisket. Close cover securely; place pressure regulator on vent pipe or set pressure control at 15. Heat cooker over medium heat until pressure regulator rocks or dial shows 15 pounds pressure is reached. Cook 50 minutes.

2. Reduce pressure by placing cooker under cold running water or following manufacturer's directions. Do not attempt to remove cover until pressure is completely reduced.

3. Remove lid; add cabbage, potatotes and carrots to cooker. Close cover securely. Return pressure regulator to vent pipe. Heat cooker until pressure regulator rocks. Cook 5 minutes longer.

4. Reduce pressure as above. Do not attempt to remove cover until pressure is completely reduced.

5. Remove bay leaves. Remove meat and vegetables to serving platter. Carve meat across grain into 3-ounce portions; serve each with $\frac{1}{8}$ of the vegetables.

EACH SERVING PROVIDES: 3$\frac{1}{2}$ Vegetables, 3 Proteins, $\frac{1}{2}$ Bread, 20 Optional Calories
PER SERVING: 314 Calories, 28 g Protein, 11 g Fat, 22 g Carbohydrate, 85 mg Sodium, 79 mg Cholesterol

IRISH WHISKEY CUSTARD

MAKES 8 SERVINGS

1 quart skim milk
4 large eggs, lightly beaten
$\frac{1}{2}$ cup granulated sugar
2 tablespoons Irish whiskey
1 teaspoon vanilla extract
$\frac{1}{4}$ teaspoon salt

1. In large saucepan, over medium-high heat, scald milk; let cool slightly.

2. In large bowl, combine remaining ingredients; add milk slowly, stirring constantly. Pour custard mixture into 4-cup baking dish; cover with foil.

3. Place 1 cup water, the cooking rack and dish in pressure cooker; close cover securely. Place pressure regulator on vent pipe or set pressure control at 15. Heat cooker over medium heat until pressure regulator rocks or dial shows 15 pounds pressure is reached. Cook 3 minutes. Reduce pressure by placing cooker under cold running water or following manufacturer's directions. Do not attempt to remove cover until pressure is completely reduced. Remove lid.

4. If desired, chill custard before serving.

EACH SERVING PROVIDES: $\frac{1}{2}$ Milk, $\frac{1}{2}$ Protein, 55 Optional Calories
PER SERVING: 141 Calories, 7 g Protein, 3 g Fat, 19 g Carbohydrate, 168 mg Sodium, 139 mg Cholesterol

EASTER DINNER

---◆---

This fresh Easter dinner showcases spring's bounty with a crisp Watercress-Asparagus Salad and Sautéed Spring Vegetables. Orange sparks the pork roast, which is paired with pretty yellow saffron rice studded with roasted red peppers. For dessert, the traditional Easter cake from Naples—Pastiera—finishes off the meal very nicely.

◆ MENU ◆

Watercress-Asparagus Salad

Orange-Rosemary Pork Tenderloin

Sautéed Spring Vegetables

Saffron Rice

Pastiera

4 fluid ounces dry wine

Coffee or tea

EACH MEAL (1 serving) PROVIDES: 2 Fats, 2¾ Vegetables, 3 Proteins, 2½ Breads, 225 Optional Calories

---

SHOPPING LIST

Watercress-Asparagus Salad
Orange juice
Rice wine vinegar
Watercress leaves
Asparagus spears
Tomatoes
Sesame oil

Orange-Rosemary Pork Tenderloin
Garlic cloves
Fresh rosemary
Pork tenderloins
Orange all-fruit spread

Sautéed Spring Vegetables
Red onion
Garlic cloves
Asparagus spears
Yellow squash
Fresh mint leaves
Frozen peas

Saffron Rice
Scallions
Powdered saffron
Roasted red peppers

Pastiera
Lemon
Part-skim ricotta cheese
Bulgur wheat
Chopped candied fruit
Orange flower water

PREP SCHEDULE

1 Week Before

◆ Shop for nonperishable ingredients. Check dishes, silver, glasses and platters; clean as needed.

3 Days Before

◆ Shop for perishable ingredients. Iron tablecloth and napkins; order flowers; buy candles.

2 Days Before

◆ Clean and cut vegetables according to recipes; store in resealable plastic bags and refrigerate.
◆ Toast sesame seeds, chop mint leaves for vegetables and grate lemon peel for cake; store in resealable plastic bags and refrigerate.

1 Day Before

◆ Thaw tenderloin, if frozen.
◆ Prepare garlic paste for pork and dressing for salad; store in airtight containers in refrigerator.
◆ Blanch asparagus spears for salad; store in resealable plastic bag and refrigerate.
◆ Bake Pastiera; wrap with foil and refrigerate.
◆ Set table.

Easter Day

◆ Prepare coffeepot.
◆ Prepare and roast Pork Tenderloins.
◆ Cook rice and Spring Vegetables.
◆ Assemble salad.

WATERCRESS-ASPARAGUS SALAD

MAKES 12 SERVINGS

1½ tablespoons orange juice
1½ tablespoons rice wine vinegar
1½ teaspoons vegetable oil
1½ teaspoons sesame oil
1⅛ teaspoons reduced-sodium soy sauce
⅛ teaspoon salt
⅛ teaspoon freshly ground black pepper
3 cups watercress leaves
36 blanched asparagus spears, cut into 2½″ pieces
3 medium tomatoes, cut into ½″ wedges
1½ tablespoons toasted sesame seeds

1. To prepare dressing, in small bowl, mix orange juice, vinegar, 1½ teaspoons water, the vegetable and sesame oil, soy sauce, salt and pepper; set aside.

2. In medium bowl, toss together watercress, asparagus, tomatoes and sesame seeds. Add dressing; toss to mix well. Divide evenly among salad plates.

EACH SERVING PROVIDES: ¼ Fat, 1½ Vegetables, 5 Optional Calories
PER SERVING: 35 Calories, 2 g Protein, 2 g Fat, 4 g Carbohydrate, 54 mg Sodium, 0 mg Cholesterol

◆

ORANGE-ROSEMARY PORK TENDERLOIN

MAKES 12 SERVINGS

4 garlic cloves
4 sprigs fresh rosemary
½ teaspoon salt
½ teaspoon freshly ground black pepper
2 tablespoons vegetable oil
3 pork tenderloins (about 10 ounces each), broiled 2 minutes, turning once
½ cup low-sodium chicken broth
1 ounce (2 tablespoons) dry white wine, or increase broth by 2 tablespoons
¼ cup + 2 tablespoons orange all-fruit spread

1. Preheat oven to 350°F.

2. In mini food processor, combine garlic, rosemary, salt and pepper; process until finely chopped. Add oil; process until mixture forms a paste.

3. Place pork on rack in roasting pan; spread with garlic mixture. Pour broth and wine into bottom of pan. Roast, basting occasionally, 20 minutes. Brush pork with fruit spread; roast 10 minutes longer, until meat thermometer registers 160°F. Let stand 10 minutes before carving into ¼″ slices.

EACH SERVING PROVIDES: ½ Fat, ½ Fruit, 2 Protein, 5 Optional Calories
PER SERVING: 125 Calories, 15 g Protein, 4 g Fat, 6 g Carbohydrate, 128 mg Sodium, 46 mg Cholesterol

◆

SAUTÉED SPRING VEGETABLES

MAKES 12 SERVINGS

2 tablespoons olive oil
½ cup sliced red onion
4 garlic cloves, minced
18 asparagus spears, cut into 2″ pieces
2 cups yellow squash, cut into chunks
¼ cup chopped fresh mint leaves
1 teaspoon dried thyme
3 cups frozen peas
1 tablespoon toasted sesame seeds
2 teaspoons reduced-sodium soy sauce

1. In large nonstick skillet, heat oil. Add onion and garlic; cook, stirring frequently, 2 minutes. Add asparagus, squash, mint and thyme; cook, stirring frequently, 4–5 minutes, until just tender.

2. Stir in peas, sesame seeds and soy sauce; cook 3–4 minutes, until peas are heated through.

EACH SERVING PROVIDES: ½ Fat, ½ Vegetable, ½ Bread, 5 Optional Calories
PER SERVING: 65 Calories, 3 g Protein, 3 g Fat, 8 g Carbohydrate, 64 mg Sodium, 0 mg Cholesterol

SAFFRON RICE

MAKES 12 SERVINGS

¼ cup reduced-calorie tub margarine
1½ cups chopped scallions
12 ounces long-grain white rice
¼ teaspoon powdered saffron
2 cups low-sodium chicken broth
1½ cups chopped drained roasted red peppers

1. In medium saucepan, melt margarine. Add scallions; cook, stirring frequently, 2–3 minutes, until tender. Stir in rice and saffron until coated.

2. Add broth and 3 cups water; bring to a boil. Reduce heat to low; stir in red peppers. Cover and simmer 25–30 minutes, until liquid is absorbed and rice is tender.

EACH SERVING PROVIDES: ½ Fat, ½ Vegetable, 1 Bread, 3 Optional Calories
PER SERVING: 135 Calories, 3 g Protein, 3 g Fat, 25 g Carbohydrate, 53 mg Sodium, 0 mg Cholesterol

PASTIERA

MAKES 12 SERVINGS

PASTRY
1½ cups all-purpose flour
2 tablespoons granulated sugar
⅓ cup + 2 teaspoons reduced-calorie tub margarine
2 large eggs
Grated peel from 1 lemon

FILLING
4 large eggs, separated
1 cup skim milk
¼ cup granulated sugar
1 tablespoon cornstarch
½ teaspoon vanilla extract
1½ cups part-skim ricotta cheese, well drained
4 ounces bulgur wheat, cooked
2½ ounces coarsely chopped candied fruit
1 tablespoon orange flower water*

1. To prepare pastry, combine flour and sugar in food processor. Add margarine; process until mixture resembles coarse crumbs. Add eggs and grated peel; process until dough forms a ball. Wrap dough in plastic wrap; refrigerate 30 minutes.

2. To prepare filling, in top of double boiler, over very hot water, whisk together 2 egg yolks, the milk, 2 tablespoons sugar, the cornstarch and vanilla. Heat, stirring constantly with wooden spoon, until mixture thickens; remove from water and set aside to cool.

3. In medium bowl, combine ricotta cheese, the remaining 2 egg yolks, remaining 2 tablespoons sugar, the bulgur, candied fruit and orange flower water. Fold ricotta mixture into cooled mixture.

4. In small bowl, with mixer at high speed, beat egg whites until stiff but not dry. Fold egg whites into filling mixture; set aside.

5. Preheat oven to 350°F. Spray 9" springform pan with nonstick cooking spray; set aside.

6. Spray a clean work surface with nonstick cooking spray. Roll ⅔ of the dough to a 9" circle. Fold into quarters and place on prepared pan. Unfold dough and pat into bottom of pan. Pour in ricotta filling.

7. Roll remaining dough into a 9 × 4" rectangle. With pastry wheel or sharp knife, cut into 8 strips. Criss-cross strips on top of filled pastry to form a lattice. Bake 2 hours; let stand 2 hours before removing sides of pan. Wrap with foil and refrigerate overnight before serving.

*Available in specialty food shops and some pharmacies.

EACH SERVING PROVIDES: ¾ Fat, 1 Protein, 1 Bread, 55 Optional Calories
PER SERVING: 247 Calories, 10 g Protein, 8 g Fat, 34 g Carbohydrate, 155 mg Sodium, 116 mg Cholesterol

PASSOVER DINNER

You'll love this Passover dinner, updated to combine tradition with the best of nutrition. The Potato Pudding has almost no fat and absolutely no flour, and the Maple Mustard Hens are a delightful variation on roast chicken. For dessert, Fruit-Filled Puffs use matzo instead of flour for a different though traditional dessert idea.

◆ MENU ◆

Spinach-Carrot Salad

Maple Mustard Hens

Potato Pudding

Pear and Raisin Charoses

Fruit-Filled Puffs

4 fluid ounces wine

Coffee or tea

EACH MEAL (1 serving) PROVIDES: 1¾ Fats, 1 Fruit, 3¼ Vegetables, 3½ Proteins, 1¼ Breads, 175 Optional Calories

---

SHOPPING LIST

Spinach-Carrot Salad
Spinach leaves
Carrots
Red onion
Celery radishes

Maple Mustard Hens
Fresh thyme
Garlic cloves
Cornish hens
Fennel
Red new potatoes
Carrots
Onions

Potato Pudding
Baking potatoes
Onion
Matzo meal
Scallions

Pear and Raisin Charoses
Pears
Dried apricot halves
Raisins
Sweet red wine

Fruit-Filled Puffs
Matzo cake meal
Nondairy whipped topping
Strawberries
Kiwi fruit
Chocolate syrup

PREP SCHEDULE

Up to 1 Month Before
◆ Bake and freeze puffs (not filling).

1 Week Before
◆ Shop for nonperishable ingredients.
◆ Check dishes, silver, glasses and platters; clean as needed.

3 Days Before
◆ Shop for perishable ingredients.
◆ Iron tablecloth and napkins; order flowers; buy candles.
◆ Prepare Pear and Raisin Charoses; store in airtight container and refrigerate.

2 Days Before
◆ Clean and cut vegetables according to recipes (not potatoes); store in resealable plastic bags and refrigerate.

1 Day Before
◆ Thaw hens, if frozen.
◆ Prepare mustard mixture for hens and dressing for salad; store in airtight containers in refrigerator.
◆ Prepare Potato Pudding (do not bake); cover and refrigerate.
◆ Set table.

Passover Day
◆ Prepare coffeepot.
◆ Prepare and roast hens.
◆ Bake Potato Pudding.
◆ Prepare fruit and assemble puffs.
◆ Assemble salad.

SPINACH-CARROT SALAD

MAKES 12 SERVINGS

3 tablespoons red wine vinegar
2 tablespoons ketchup
1 teaspoon paprika
$\frac{1}{2}$ teaspoon dry mustard
$\frac{1}{4}$ teaspoon salt
2 tablespoons vegetable oil
1 tablespoon honey
6 cups fresh spinach leaves, rinsed and dried
1$\frac{1}{2}$ cups shredded carrots
1 medium red onion, sliced and separated into
   rings
$\frac{1}{2}$ cup sliced celery
$\frac{1}{2}$ cup thinly sliced radishes

1. To prepare dressing, in small bowl, combine vinegar, ketchup, paprika, mustard and salt. Whisk in oil and honey; set aside.

2. In large bowl, combine vegetables. Whisk dressing to combine; pour over vegetables. Toss to mix well.

EACH SERVING PROVIDES: $\frac{1}{2}$ Fat, 1$\frac{1}{2}$ Vegetables, 10 Optional Calories
PER SERVING: 46 Calories, 1 g Protein, 2 g Fat, 6 g Carbohydrate, 108 mg Sodium, 0 mg Cholesterol

MAPLE MUSTARD HENS

MAKES 12 SERVINGS

$\frac{1}{2}$ cup + 1 tablespoon reduced-calorie pancake
   syrup (60 calories per fluid ounce)
1 tablespoon + 1$\frac{1}{2}$ teaspoons dry mustard
1 tablespoon + 1$\frac{1}{2}$ teaspoons chopped fresh thyme
3 garlic cloves, minced
Six 1-pound Cornish hens, split and skinned
4$\frac{1}{2}$ cups coarsely chopped fennel
1 pound 2 ounces red new potatoes, halved
3 medium carrots, pared and sliced
3 medium onions, sliced and separated into rings
1 tablespoon olive oil
$\frac{3}{4}$ teaspoon paprika

1. Preheat oven to 350°F.

2. In a small bowl, mix syrup, mustard, thyme and garlic. Spread mustard mixture evenly over hens.

3. Place half the fennel, potatoes, carrots and onions in bottom of large roasting pan; place hens over vegetables, skin-side up. Sprinkle remaining vegetables around hens. Sprinkle oil and paprika evenly over hens and vegetables.

4. Roast 1 to 1$\frac{1}{2}$ hours, basting occasionally with juices and turning vegetables, until vegetables are tender and juices run clear when hens are pricked with a fork.

EACH SERVING PROVIDES: $\frac{1}{4}$ Fat, 1$\frac{1}{2}$ Vegetables, 3 Proteins, $\frac{1}{4}$ Bread, 25 Optional Calories
PER SERVING: 248 Calories, 27 g Protein, 8 g Fat, 15 g Carbohydrate, 145 mg Sodium, 76 mg Cholesterol

POTATO PUDDING

MAKES 12 SERVINGS

1¼ pounds pared baking potatoes, thinly shredded and squeezed dry
½ cup grated onion
2 large eggs, lightly beaten
¼ cup + 2 tablespoons matzoh meal
1 teaspoon garlic powder
½ teaspoon salt
¼ teaspoon freshly ground black pepper
¼ cup minced scallions

1. Preheat oven to 350°F. Spray a 13 × 9″ baking pan with nonstick cooking spray; set aside.

2. In large bowl, combine potatoes, onion and eggs. Stir in remaining ingredients and mix well; gently spoon into prepared pan.

3. Bake 35–40 minutes, until browned around edges. Let stand 5 minutes before cutting into 12 equal pieces.

EACH SERVING PROVIDES: ½ Bread, 10 Optional Calories
PER SERVING: 70 Calories, 3 g Protein, 1 g Fat, 13 g Carbohydrate, 105 mg Sodium, 35 mg Cholesterol

PEAR AND RAISIN CHAROSES

MAKES 12 SERVINGS

2 small pears, cored and coarsely chopped
12 dried apricot halves, chopped
¼ cup raisins
1½ tablespoons honey
1 teaspoon lemon juice
½ teaspoon cinnamon
1 ounce (2 tablespoons) sweet red wine

In medium bowl, combine pears, apricots, raisins, honey, lemon juice and cinnamon; mix well. Stir in wine. Cover and refrigerate at least 1 hour before serving.

EACH SERVING PROVIDES: ½ Fruit, 10 Optional Calories

FRUIT-FILLED PUFFS

MAKES 12 SERVINGS

¼ cup vegetable oil
1 teaspoon vanilla extract
1 cup + 2 tablespoons matzoh cake meal
½ teaspoon salt
6 large eggs
¾ cup nondairy whipped topping
3 cups whole strawberries, thinly sliced
3 medium kiwi fruit, coarsely chopped
2 tablespoons chocolate syrup

1. Preheat oven to 450°F. Spray a large baking sheet with nonstick cooking spray; set aside.

2. In medium saucepan, combine 1 cup water, the oil and vanilla; bring to a boil. Stir in matzoh cake meal and salt; continue cooking, stirring constantly, about 1 minute, until mixture no longer sticks to side of saucepan. Remove from heat and stir in eggs, one at a time, stirring thoroughly after each addition.

3. Drop dough by 12 rounded tablespoonfuls, 2″ apart, onto prepared baking sheet. Bake 10 minutes. Reduce heat to 400°F and bake 10–15 minutes longer, until browned and puffed. Cool completely on rack, then slice in half horizontally.

4. To fill, fit a pastry bag with a ¼″-diameter star tip. Fill bag with whipped topping. Divide fruit evenly among bottom halves of puffs. Pipe or spoon 2 tablespoons topping over each filled half. Place tops on puffs and drizzle ½ teaspoon chocolate syrup over each.

EACH SERVING PROVIDES: 1 Fat, ½ Fruit, ½ Bread, 20 Optional Calories
PER SERVING: 178 Calories, 5 g Protein, 9 g Fat, 20 g Carbohydrate, 129 mg Sodium, 106 mg Cholesterol

MOTHER'S DAY BRUNCH

This is a brunch the whole family will enjoy! To help keep the mother of honor out of the kitchen and enjoying a relaxing day, assign recipes to family members. Have each person read the recipe and check to be sure all the ingredients are on hand. Then ask one person to volunteer to coordinate cooking times, and the meal will be a breeze. Want to be sure it's a special Mother's Day? Then don't forget to clean up after brunch!

◆ MENU ◆

Caesar Salad

Dilled Spring Vegetables

Seafood Pie

Veal Cutlets with Garlic Mint Sauce

Chocolate-Raspberry Mousse

4 fluid ounces wine

Coffee or tea

EACH MEAL (1 serving) PROVIDES: $2\frac{1}{4}$ Fats, $\frac{1}{2}$ Fruit, $5\frac{1}{2}$ Vegetables, $3\frac{3}{4}$ Proteins, 1 Bread, 195 Optional Calories

SHOPPING LIST

Caesar Salad
Whole-wheat bread
Garlic cloves
Anchovy fillets
Freshly grated Parmesan cheese
Romaine lettuce

Dilled Spring Vegetable Sauté
Canola oil
Scallions
Carrots
Zucchini
Yellow squash
Red bell pepper
Fresh parsley
Fresh dill
Light salt blend

Seafood Pie
Shrimp
Mushrooms
Shallots
Lemon
Fresh parsley
Sea scallops
Frozen egg substitute
Freshly grated Parmesan cheese

Veal Cutlets with Garlic Mint Sauce
Fresh mint leaves
Pine nuts
Garlic cloves
Veal cutlets
Mushrooms
Lemon

Chocolate-Raspberry Mousse
Reduced-calorie raspberry gelatin
Orange juice
Orange
Reduced-calorie whipped topping
(8 calories per tablespoon)
Fresh or frozen raspberries

PREP SCHEDULE

1 Week Before
◆ Shop for nonperishable ingredients.
◆ Check dishes, silver, glasses and platters; clean as needed.

3 Days Before
◆ Shop for perishable ingredients.
◆ Iron tablecloth and napkins; order flowers; buy candles.

2 Days Before
◆ Cut and clean vegetables according to recipes; store in resealable plastic bags and refrigerate.
◆ Chop fresh herbs; store in resealable plastic bags and refrigerate.
◆ Toast pine nuts for veal.
◆ Squeeze fresh lemon juice; store in airtight container and refrigerate.
◆ Process mint mixture for veal; store in airtight container and refrigerate.

1 Day Before
◆ Prepare mousse; cover and refrigerate.
◆ Prepare bread cubes for salad; store in airtight container.
◆ Prepare dressing for salad; store in airtight container and refrigerate.
◆ Prepare rice crust for pie; cover with foil.
◆ Combine flour mixture and coat veal cutlets; cover and refrigerate.
◆ Set table.

Day of Brunch
◆ Prepare coffeepot.
◆ Complete seafood pie and veal cutlets.
◆ Cook vegetable sauté and assemble salad.

CAESAR SALAD

MAKES 8 SERVINGS

4 slices whole-wheat bread, cut into ½" cubes
2 garlic cloves, peeled
2 anchovy fillets
½ cup plain nonfat yogurt
2 tablespoons lemon juice
1 tablespoon + 1 teaspoon freshly grated
   Parmesan cheese
¼ teaspoon coarsely ground black pepper
8 cups torn romaine lettuce leaves

   1. Preheat oven to 350°F. Arrange bread cubes on a baking sheet in a single layer. Bake 10–15 minutes or until crisp; set aside.
   2. Meanwhile, on cutting board with flat side of chef's knife or with a mortar and pestle, mash garlic and anchovies until well combined. Scrape mixture into a small bowl. Add yogurt, lemon juice, cheese and pepper. Cover and refrigerate 1 hour to blend flavors.
   3. When ready to serve, place lettuce in large salad bowl. Add dressing and toss to combine. Sprinkle evenly with croutons (bread cubes).

EACH SERVING (generous 1 cup) PROVIDES: 2 Vegetables, ½ Bread, 15 Optional Calories
PER SERVING: 61 Calories, 4 g Protein, 1 g Fat, 9 g Carbohydrate, 146 mg Sodium, 2 mg Cholesterol

DILLED SPRING VEGETABLE SAUTÉ

MAKES 8 SERVINGS

2 tablespoons + 2 teaspoons canola oil
1 cup scallions, cut into thin strips
1 garlic clove, minced
2 medium carrots, cut into thin strips
1 medium zucchini, cut into thin strips
1 medium yellow squash, cut into thin strips
1 medium red bell pepper, cut into thin strips
¼ cup chopped fresh parsley
2 tablespoons chopped fresh dill
1½ teaspoons light salt blend

   In large nonstick skillet, heat oil. Add scallions and garlic; cook, stirring frequently, 2 minutes. Add carrot, zucchini, yellow squash and pepper; cook, stirring frequently, 5 minutes. Stir in parsley and dill; cook 2 minutes longer, until vegetables are tender. Remove from heat and sprinkle evenly with salt blend.

EACH SERVING PROVIDES: 1 Fat, 1½ Vegetable
PER SERVING: 67 Calories, 1 g Protein, 5 g Fat, 6 g Carbohydrate, 289 mg Sodium, 0 mg Cholesterol

SEAFOOD PIE

MAKES 8 SERVINGS

RICE CRUST

2 cups cooked short-grain rice
$\frac{3}{4}$ ounce grated Parmesan cheese
$\frac{1}{2}$ teaspoon salt
$\frac{1}{4}$ teaspoon freshly ground black pepper
1 large egg white

FILLING

12 medium shrimp
$\frac{1}{4}$ cup dry white wine
2 teaspoons olive oil
$3\frac{1}{2}$ cups mushrooms, sliced
$\frac{1}{2}$ cup shallots, minced
3 tablespoons fresh lemon juice
$\frac{1}{8}$ teaspoon ground red pepper
2 tablespoons minced parsley
1 teaspoon dried thyme leaves
$\frac{1}{2}$ teaspoon dried chervil leaves
$\frac{1}{4}$ teaspoon freshly ground black pepper
5 ounces sea scallops
1 cup frozen egg substitute, thawed
$\frac{1}{2}$ cup evaporated skimmed milk
$\frac{1}{4}$ teaspoon salt
$\frac{1}{4}$ teaspoon dry mustard
1 tablespoon freshly grated Parmesan cheese
$\frac{1}{8}$ teaspoon paprika

TO PREPARE CRUST:

1. Preheat oven to 375°F.

2. Steam the cooked rice, covered, over boiling water about 5 minutes to separate and fluff grains.

3. Transfer warm rice to medium bowl and stir in cheese until evenly distributed and rice is pale yellow. Stir in salt and pepper. Add egg white and stir until rice forms clumps. Form into a ball and place in a 9" nonstick pie pan.

4. With moistened fingers, press rice, starting on the bottom, into a thin uniform layer. Press from center to sides and up rim, extending about $\frac{1}{2}$" beyond rim to allow for shrinkage when baking. Bake about 25 minutes or until slightly brown. Remove pie pan from oven and set aside.

TO PREPARE FILLING:

1. Peel shrimp and place shells in small saucepan with the wine and $\frac{3}{4}$ cup cold water. Bring to boil; lower heat and simmer, covered, for 10 minutes. Uncover and reduce over high heat to about $\frac{1}{4}$ cup liquid. Strain into measuring cup and set aside. Devein the shrimp.

2. Heat a large (12") skillet over medium-high heat until a drop of water will dance on the surface. Add the oil and the mushrooms and sauté, tossing frequently for 5 minutes. Add the shallots and continue to sauté for 5 minutes more. Add 1 tablespoon of the lemon juice and the red pepper; stir until all liquid has evaporated. Remove from heat and spoon mushroom mixture into baked pie shell.

3. Combine the parsley, thyme, chervil and black pepper. Sprinkle about $\frac{1}{3}$ of this mixture over the mushrooms.

4. In same skillet, heat the strained shrimp liquid to a simmer. Add the shrimp and scallops and cook, covered, for 30 seconds. Turn each shrimp and scallop over and cook, covered, 30 seconds more. Shrimp should be just pink and scallops should be barely opaque. Arrange shrimps and scallops over mushrooms.

5. Preheat oven to 350°F. Combine the shrimp poaching liquid with the egg substitute and evaporated milk. Add remaining parsley mixture and the salt. Dissolve the dry mustard in the remaining lemon juice and add it to the egg mixture. Pour evenly over the seafood.

6. Sprinkle pie with the cheese and paprika and bake in center of oven for 35–40 minutes, or until just set. Let stand 10 minutes before cutting.

EACH SERVING ($\frac{1}{8}$ of pie) PROVIDES: $\frac{1}{4}$ Fat, 1 Vegetable, $1\frac{1}{4}$ Proteins, $\frac{1}{2}$ Bread, 25 Optional Calories
PER SERVING: 179 Calories, 15 g Protein, 3 g Fat, 22 g Carbohydrate, 390 mg Sodium, 41 mg Cholesterol

VEAL CUTLETS WITH GARLIC MINT SAUCE

MAKES 8 SERVINGS

1 cup fresh mint leaves
2 ounces toasted pine nuts
4 garlic cloves, minced
$\frac{1}{4}$ cup all-purpose flour
$\frac{1}{2}$ teaspoon salt
$\frac{1}{8}$ teaspoon ground red pepper
Eight 3-ounce veal cutlets
1 tablespoon + 1 teaspoon olive oil
1 cup low-sodium beef broth
4 cups thinly sliced mushrooms
1 tablespoon + 1 teaspoon fresh lemon juice
1 ounce toasted pine nuts to garnish (optional)*

1. In food processor, combine mint, nuts and garlic; process until finely chopped; set aside.

2. On wax paper, combine flour, salt and pepper. Coat veal cutlets, one at a time, in flour mixture.

3. In large nonstick skillet, heat half of the oil. Add half of the veal; sauté 3–4 minutes on each side, until golden brown. Remove veal to serving plate; keep warm. Repeat procedure using remaining oil and veal.

4. Add broth to skillet, stirring to loosen any brown bits from skillet. Stir in mushrooms and juice; cook, stirring frequently, 2 minutes. Stir in mint mixture; cook 2 minutes, until heated through. To serve, spoon sauce evenly over veal. Sprinkle with toasted pine nuts, if desired.

*If pine nuts are used, increase Fat to $1\frac{1}{4}$ and Optional Calories to 25.

EACH SERVING PROVIDES: 1 Fat, 1 Vegetable, $2\frac{1}{4}$ Proteins, 20 Optional Calories
PER SERVING: 179 Calories, 20 g Protein, 8g Fat, 7g Carbohydrate, 206 mg Sodium, 67 mg Cholesterol

Microwave Tips

- *Precooking Poultry for Grilling: Place skinless chicken on large plate. Cover with wax paper or paper towel and microwave on High 6 minutes per pound. Rearrange and turn pieces over once during cooking. Finish cooking on grill immediately.*
- *Softening Stick Margarine or Butter: If foil-wrapped, remove foil; place unwrapped or paper-wrapped sticks on plate. Microwave on defrost setting 30 seconds. To soften cream cheese, place unwrapped cheese in bowl. Microwave on defrost setting 1–2 minutes.*
- *Melting Chocolate: Place morsels or unwrapped squares in medium bowl. Microwave on Medium 1–2 minutes, stirring until melted and smooth.*
- *Softening Brown Sugar: Place light or dark brown sugar in bowl along with a wedge of apple. Cover with plastic wrap and microwave on High 30–40 seconds. Let stand 1 minute. Discard apple; stir to break up sugar.*
- *Winter Squash: To make squash easier to cut, microwave whole squash on High 1 minute; cut into halves or quarters. Peel, seed and cube for conventional cooking, or, microwave cut squash in covered casserole on High 7–10 minutes, until tender.*
- *Cooking Shrimp: Arrange 1 pound unpeeled shrimp in large casserole; cover and microwave on High 3 minutes; let stand 1 minute. Rinse under cold running water; peel and devein.*

CHOCOLATE-RASPBERRY MOUSSE

MAKES 8 SERVINGS

1 package (.3 ounce) sugar-free raspberry gelatin
2 tablespoons unsweetened cocoa powder
1 tablespoon + 1$\frac{1}{2}$ teaspoons granulated sugar
$\frac{1}{2}$ cup boiling water
1 cup orange juice
2 teaspoons grated orange peel
1$\frac{1}{2}$ cups reduced-calorie nondairy whipped
   topping (8 calories per tablespoon)
1$\frac{1}{2}$ cups fresh or thawed raspberries

1. In medium bowl, combine gelatin, cocoa and sugar; add boiling water; stir to dissolve. Stir in orange juice and peel. Refrigerate 30–40 minutes, stirring occasionally, until mixture mounds slightly when dropped from a spoon.

2. With electric mixer, beat gelatin mixture 3 minutes. Gently fold in whipped topping. Divide evenly among eight dessert cups. Refrigerate at least 2 hours, or until firm. Garnish with raspberries.

EACH SERVING PROVIDES: $\frac{1}{2}$ Fruit, 40 Optional Calories
PER SERVING: 66 Calories, 1 g Protein, 2 g Fat, 12 g Carbohydrate, 30 mg Sodium, 0 mg Cholesterol

MEMORIAL DAY PICNIC

---◆---

*Kick off a summer full of fun with this easy Memorial Day Picnic.
Unlike many Memorial Day meals, it's not built around the grill, so your
options for where you'd like to eat are almost endless. Whether on the
beach or a backyard blanket, this picnic is sure to please!*

◆ **MENU** ◆

Spanish Steak Roll with Sautéed Vegetables

Roasted Vegetable-Pasta Salad

1-ounce pita bread

Assorted fruits*

Oatmeal Cookies

Unsweetened iced tea

*Choose 1 Fruit Serving.

EACH MEAL (1 serving) PROVIDES: 3 Fats, 1 Fruit, 4 Vegetables, 3 Proteins, 3½ Breads, 35 Optional Calories

───◆───

Spanish Steak Roll with Sautéed Vegetables
Boneless beef top sirloin steak
Red bell pepper
Green bell pepper
Onions
Mushrooms
Walnuts
Light sour cream
Green chilies

Roasted Vegetable-Pasta Salad
Garlic cloves
Red bell pepper
Green bell pepper
Yellow bell pepper
Eggplant
Rotelle pasta

Oatmeal Cookies
Apple juice
Quick oats
Oat bran

Pita bread

Fruit

PREP SCHEDULE

1 Week Before

◆ Shop for nonperishable ingredients.
◆ Check dishes, glasses and utensils to be used; clean as needed.

3 Days Before

◆ Shop for perishable ingredients.
◆ Gather picnic blanket, tablecloth and paper goods.
◆ Start making additional ice for cooler.

2 Days Before

◆ Clean and cut vegetables according to recipes; store in resealable plastic bags and refrigerate.
◆ Chop walnuts for steak; store in resealable plastic bag.
◆ Bake Oatmeal Cookies; store in airtight container.

1 Day Before

◆ Prepare Steak Roll (not vegetables); cover and refrigerate.
◆ Prepare Pasta Salad; store in airtight container and refrigerate.
◆ Make iced tea; store in airtight pitcher and refrigerate.

Day of Picnic

◆ Sauté vegetables for Steak Rolls; keep warm. Assemble assorted fruits; pack picnic basket.

SPANISH STEAK ROLL WITH SAUTÉED VEGETABLES

MAKES 4 SERVINGS

One 14-ounce trimmed boneless beef top sirloin
   steak or top round steak, cut $\frac{3}{4}$" thick
1 teaspoon garlic powder
$\frac{1}{4}$ teaspoon freshly ground black pepper
2 teaspoons vegetable oil
1 cup thinly sliced red bell pepper
1 cup thinly sliced green bell pepper
1 cup thinly sliced onion, separated into rings
1 cup thinly sliced mushrooms
1 ounce chopped walnuts
$\frac{1}{4}$ teaspoon salt
$\frac{1}{4}$ teaspoon chili powder
1 tablespoon light sour cream
2 tablespoons chopped green chilies

1. Preheat broiler. Place beef on work surface. With flat side of meat mallet or bottom of skillet, pound beef to $\frac{1}{4}$" thickness. Sprinkle with $\frac{1}{2}$ teaspoon of the garlic powder and the pepper. Place beef on broiler rack; broil 2 minutes, turning once.

2. In large nonstick skillet, heat 1 teaspoon of the oil. Add steak; sauté 5–7 minutes, turning once, for medium rare. Remove steak to platter; cover and keep warm.

3. Add remaining 1 teaspoon oil to skillet. Add bell peppers, onion, mushrooms and walnuts; cook, stirring requently, 2 minutes. Combine remaining $\frac{1}{2}$ teaspoon garlic powder, the salt and chili powder; sprinkle over vegetables. Cook 2 minutes longer.

4. Spread steak with sour cream; sprinkle evenly with chilies. Starting at a short end, roll up steak jelly-roll style; secure with wooden picks. To serve, carve into slices, or cover and refrigerate until chilled, then carve. Remove wooden picks. Serve with the sautéed vegetables.

EACH SERVING PROVIDES: 1 Fat, 2 Vegetables, 3 Proteins, 5 Optional Calories
PER SERVING: 236 Calories, 24 g Protein, 12 g Fat, 9 g Carbohydrate, 224 mg Sodium, 62 mg Cholesterol

ROASTED VEGETABLE-PASTA SALAD

MAKES 4 SERVINGS

2 tablespoons Dijon mustard
1 tablespoon + 1 teaspoon olive oil
1 tablespoon lemon juice
2 garlic cloves, minced
$\frac{1}{4}$ teaspoon salt
$\frac{1}{8}$ teaspoon freshly ground black pepper
1 medium red bell pepper, cut into strips
1 medium green bell pepper, cut into strips
1 medium yellow bell pepper, cut into strips
1 cup cubed eggplant, cut into $\frac{1}{2}$" pieces
$4\frac{1}{2}$ ounces rotelle pasta

1. Preheat oven to 350°F. In small bowl, combine mustard, oil, juice, garlic, salt and black pepper.

2. In a 13 × 9" baking pan, combine bell peppers and eggplant; toss with mustard mixture. Roast 20–25 minutes, until vegetables are tender; set aside.

3. Meanwhile, in large pot of boiling water, cook pasta 10–15 minutes, until just tender. Drain and add to vegetables. Toss to mix well.

4. Place in serving bowl; cover and refrigerate until well chilled. Stir salad before serving.

EACH SERVING (1 cup) PROVIDES: 1 Fat, 2 Vegetables, 1½ Breads
PER SERVING: 193 Calories, 5 g Protein, 6 g Fat, 31 g Carbohydrate, 366 mg Sodium, 0 mg Cholesterol

OATMEAL COOKIES

MAKES 12 SERVINGS

$\frac{1}{4}$ cup margarine
$\frac{1}{4}$ cup + 2 tablespoons granulated sugar
1 large egg
2 tablespoons apple juice
$4\frac{1}{2}$ ounces quick oats
$4\frac{1}{2}$ ounces oat bran
$\frac{3}{4}$ teaspoon baking powder
$\frac{1}{2}$ teaspoon cinnamon
$\frac{1}{4}$ teaspoon salt

1. Preheat oven to 350°F. Spray two baking sheets with nonstick cooking spray; set aside.

2. In large bowl, with electric mixer on high speed, beat margarine and sugar until light and fluffy. Add egg and juice; beat until blended.

3. In medium bowl, combine oats, oat bran, baking powder, cinnamon and salt. Add dry ingredients to wet ingredients; beat until combined.

4. Drop dough by tablespoonfuls 2" apart onto prepared sheets, making 24 cookies. Flatten with spatula. Bake 12–15 minutes, until lightly browned. Cool on rack. Store in airtight container.

EACH SERVING (2 cookies) PROVIDES: 1 Fat, 1 Bread, 30 Optional Calories
PER SERVING: 135 Calories, 4 g Protein, 6 g Fat, 21 g Carbohydrate, 122 mg Sodium, 18 mg Cholesterol

FOURTH OF JULY
BARBECUE

◆

Grilling is great, especially to celebrate Independence Day! You'll find two fabulous entrées that will satisfy all your friends—classic Grilled Deviled Flank Steak and tangy Honey-Ginger Turkey Kabobs. Grilled red peppers with a fresh filling make vegetables a snap on the grill. And what could be more patriotic than Strawberry Shortcake? When you garnish with a few blueberries, it's a red, white and blue finale!

◆ **MENU** ◆

Mixed green salad with balsamic vinegar*

Grilled Deviled Flank Steak or Honey-Ginger Turkey Kabobs

Grilled Red Peppers with Roasted Corn Relish

Strawberry Shortcake

Sparkling mineral water with lemon

*Select 1 cup mixed green salad.

EACH MEAL (1 serving) WITH GRILLED DEVILED FLANK STEAK PROVIDES: $\frac{1}{2}$ Fat, $\frac{1}{2}$ Fruit, $5\frac{1}{2}$ Vegetables, $3\frac{3}{4}$ Proteins, $1\frac{1}{2}$ Breads, 85 Optional Calories

EACH MEAL (1 serving) WITH HONEY-GINGER TURKEY KABOBS PROVIDES: $\frac{1}{2}$ Fat, 1 Fruit, $4\frac{1}{4}$ Vegetables, $3\frac{3}{4}$ Proteins, $2\frac{1}{2}$ Breads, 70 Optional Calories

---

Grilled Deviled Flank Steak

Scallions
Grainy mustard
Green bell peppers
Tomatoes
Flank Steak

Honey-Ginger Turkey Kabobs

Scallions
Fresh ginger root
Garlic cloves
Turkey tenderloins or
boneless breast
Pineapple
Red or green bell pepper
Lime Couscous
Dried red pepper flakes

**Grilled Red Peppers with
Roasted Corn Relish**

Fresh corn
Red onion
Fresh or frozen peas
Red bell peppers
Monterey Jack cheese

Strawberry Shortcake

Cake flour
Strawberries
Reduced-calorie nondairy
whipped topping (8 calories per
tablespoon)

PREP SCHEDULE

1 Week Before

◆ Shop for nonperishable ingredients.
◆ Check dishes, glasses and utensils to be used.
◆ Check charcoal supply or gas tank for grill; refill if needed.

3 Days Before

◆ Shop for perishable ingredients.
◆ Clean grill, if needed.

2 Days Before

◆ Clean and cut vegetables according to recipes; store in resealable plastic bags and refrigerate.
◆ Prepare mustard mixture for flank steak; store in airtight container and refrigerate.
◆ Prepare honey-ginger marinade for turkey kabobs; store in large resealable plastic bag and refrigerate.

1 Day Before

◆ Bake shortcake; cover with foil.
◆ Combine relish ingredients for corn relish (do not grill); store in airtight container and refrigerate.
◆ Prepare turkey kabobs (do not grill); store in resealable plastic bag and refrigerate.

Fourth of July

◆ Assemble mixed green salad and toss with balsamic vinegar.
◆ Complete flank steak, turkey kabobs and roasted corn relish.
◆ Prepare strawberries and assemble shortcake.

GRILLED DEVILED FLANK STEAK

MAKES 4 SERVINGS

1 tablespoon + 1 teaspoon reduced-calorie tub margarine
1 tablespoon plain dried bread crumbs
1 tablespoon minced scallion
1 tablespoon grainy mustard
1 teaspoon Worcestershire sauce
2 cups sliced green bell peppers
2 medium tomatoes, cut into $\frac{1}{4}$" slices
One 15-ounce flank steak

1. Spray grill rack with nonstick cooking spray. Place grill rack 5" from coals. Prepare grill according to manufacturer's directions.

2. In small bowl, combine margarine, bread crumbs, scallion, mustard and Worcestershire sauce; set aside.

3. Arrange peppers and tomatoes in wire grill basket. Grill steak and vegetables 5 minutes. Turn steak and vegetables; spread top of steak with mustard mixture. Grill 5 minutes longer, or until steak and vegetables are done to taste. Let steak stand 5 minutes before carving across the grain into thin diagonal slices.

EACH SERVING PROVIDES: $\frac{1}{2}$ Fat, 2 Vegetables, 3 Proteins, 10 Optional Calories
PER SERVING: 236 Calories, 25 g Protein, 12 g Fat, 9 g Carbohydrate, 181 mg Sodium, 57 mg Cholesterol

HONEY-GINGER TURKEY KABOBS

MAKES 4 SERVINGS

2 tablespoons minced scallions
2 tablespoons reduced-sodium soy sauce
1 tablespoon honey
1 tablespoon grated fresh ginger root
1 teaspoon lime or lemon juice
2 garlic cloves, crushed
15 ounces turkey tenderloins or boneless breast, cut into 2" chunks
$\frac{1}{4}$ medium pineapple, pared and cut into $1\frac{1}{2}$" pieces
1 medium red or green bell pepper, cut into $1\frac{1}{2}$" pieces
4 medium scallions, cut into 2" pieces
1 lime, sliced
2 cups steamed couscous
$\frac{1}{8}$ teaspoon dried red pepper flakes

1. In gallon-size sealable plastic bag, combine scallions, soy sauce, honey, ginger, lime juice and garlic; add turkey. Seal bag, squeezing out air; turn to coat turkey. Refrigerate while preparing grill.

2. Spray grill rack with nonstick cooking spray. Place grill rack 5" from coals. Prepare grill according to manufacturer's directions (or, preheat broiler).

3. Drain and discard any remaining marinade. Thread turkey, pineapple, bell pepper, scallions and lime evenly onto four metal or soaked bamboo skewers. Grill or broil kebobs 10–12 minutes, turning frequently, until turkey is cooked through.

4. To serve, fluff couscous with a fork; stir in red pepper flakes. Mound $\frac{1}{2}$ cup couscous on each plate; top with turkey kebobs.

EACH SERVING PROVIDES: $\frac{1}{2}$ Fruit, $\frac{1}{2}$ Vegetable, 3 Proteins, 1 Bread, 15 Optional Calories
PER SERVING: 281 Calories, 31 g Protein, 1 g Fat, 36 g Carbohydrate, 360 mg Sodium, 66 mg Cholesterol

GRILLED RED PEPPERS WITH ROASTED CORN RELISH

MAKES 4 SERVINGS

1½ cups fresh corn kernels
1 cup chopped red onion
½ cup fresh or thawed frozen peas
1 tablespoon + 1 teaspoon granulated sugar
2 teaspoons vegetable oil
1 teaspoon dry mustard
1 teaspoon dried oregano
¼ teaspoon salt
2 medium red bell peppers, halved and seeded
1½ ounces shredded Monterey Jack cheese

1. Place grill rack 5″ from coals. Prepare grill according to manufacturer's directions.

2. To prepare relish, in an 8″ square metal baking pan, combine corn, onion, peas, sugar, oil, mustard, oregano and salt. Place pan on grill rack; cover grill. Cook 10 minutes; stir corn mixture. Cook, covered, 5 minutes longer, until browned.

3. Spoon relish evenly into pepper halves; sprinkle evenly with cheese. Arrange filled peppers in same baking pan. Place pan on grill rack; cover grill. Cook 15 minutes, until peppers are tender and cheese is melted.

EACH SERVING PROVIDES: ½ Fat, 1½ Vegetables, ½ Protein, 1 Bread, 15 Optional Calories
PER SERVING: 173 Calories, 7 g Protein, 25 g Carbohydrate, 207 mg Sodium, 9 mg Cholesterol

STRAWBERRY SHORTCAKE

MAKES 12 SERVINGS

9 large egg whites
1 teaspoon cream of tartar
1 tablespoon vanilla extract
½ cup granulated sugar
1 cup + 2 tablespoons sifted cake flour*
1 teaspoon baking powder
4½ cups sliced strawberries
¾ cup reduced-calorie nondairy whipped topping (8 calories per tablespoon)

1. Preheat oven to 325°F.

2. In large bowl, with electric mixer on high speed, beat egg whites until foamy; add cream of tartar and vanilla. Gradually beat in ¼ cup + 2 tablespoons sugar until stiff peaks form (about 10 minutes).

3. Gradually sift cake flour and baking powder over egg white mixture; carefully fold in until no white streaks remain.

4. Spoon evenly into a 9″ tube pan. Bake 35–40 minutes, or until cake springs back when lightly touched with fingertip. Invert immediately and let cool completely.** When cake has cooled, carefully loosen edges and remove from pan.

5. Meanwhile, in medium bowl, combine strawberries with remaining 2 tablespoons sugar; set aside for 15 minutes.

6. To serve, cut cake into 12 pieces with serrated knife. Place on serving plates. Top each with equal amounts of strawberries with accumulated juice and 1 tablespoon whipped topping.

*If using self-rising cake flour, omit baking powder.
**If pan does not have "feet," invert over a sturdy bottle.

EACH SERVING PROVIDES: ½ Fruit, ¼ Protein, ½ Bread, 40 Optional Calories
PER SERVING: 106 Calories, 4 g Protein, 1 g Fat, 21 g Carbohydrate, 42 mg Sodium, 0 mg Cholesterol

Halloween Snacks

For parents, the scariest part of Halloween isn't the costumes, it's the candy! We've gathered kid-pleasing snacks that will make Halloween—or anytime— healthier, without scrimping on appeal.

◆ Menu ◆

Chocolate "Trail" Mix

Banana and Peach Chips

Poppy Seed Pretzel Twists

Cocoa Crunch Mix

SHOPPING LIST

◆

Chocolate "Trail" Mix
Semisweet chocolate chips
Light corn syrup
Toasted oat cereal
Pecans

Banana and Peach Chips
Lemon, lime, banana, peaches

Poppy Seed Pretzel Twists
Poppy seeds
Refrigerated biscuit dough

Cocoa Crunch Mix
Thin pretzel sticks
Shredded wheat cereal
Unsalted peanuts
Raisins

PREP TIPS

◆ Make Chocolate "Trail" Mix up to a week before serving and store in a tightly covered container.

◆ Make Banana and Peach Chips when you have time, and store in an airtight container.

◆ Make Poppy Seed Pretzel Twists the day before; store overnight in an airtight container.

◆ Make Cocoa Crunch Mix up to a week ahead; store in an airtight container.

CHOCOLATE "TRAIL" MIX

MAKES 12 SERVINGS

2 ounces semisweet chocolate chips
2 tablespoons smooth peanut butter
2 tablespoons light corn syrup
1 teaspoon vanilla extract
4$\frac{1}{2}$ ounces toasted oat cereal
1 ounce finely chopped pecans

1. Line large baking sheet with wax paper.

2. In medium saucepan, over medium heat, combine chocolate, peanut butter, corn syrup and vanilla. Stir until chocolate is melted and smooth. Remove from heat.

3. Add cereal and pecans to saucepan, stirring to coat cereal. Spread mixture onto prepared baking sheet. Let stand 30 minutes, until completely dry. Break into bite-size pieces and store in airtight container.

EACH SERVING PROVIDES: $\frac{1}{2}$ Fat, $\frac{1}{2}$ Bread, 45 Optional Calories
PER SERVING: 108 Calories, 3 g Protein, 5 g Fat, 13 g c Carbohydrate, 133 mg Sodium, 0 mg Cholesterol

BANANA AND PEACH CHIPS

MAKES 4 SERVINGS

2 tablespoons fresh lemon juice
2 tablespoons fresh lime juice
1 medium banana, sliced $\frac{1}{4}$" thick
2 medium peaches, pitted and sliced $\frac{1}{4}$" thick
Ground cinnamon

1. Preheat oven to 175°F. Line large baking sheet with foil; spray foil with nonstick cooking spray.

2. In small bowl, combine lemon and lime juice. Dip banana and peach slices into juice; arrange in single layer on prepared baking sheet. Sprinkle lightly with cinnamon. Bake 2–3 hours, until golden. Store in airtight container.

EACH SERVING PROVIDES: 1 Fruit
PER SERVING: 60 Calories, 1 g Protein, 0 g Fat, 15 g Carbohydrate, 0 mg Sodium, 0 mg Cholesterol

POPPY SEED PRETZEL TWISTS

MAKES 4 SERVINGS

Four 1-ounce unbaked refrigerator biscuits
1 large egg white, lightly beaten
1 teaspoon poppy seeds
$\frac{1}{4}$ teaspoon kosher salt
2 teaspoons Dijon mustard

1. Preheat oven to 450°F. Spray nonstick baking sheet with nonstick cooking spray.

2. Using fingertips, stretch and roll each biscuit into an 18″ rope. Place on prepared baking sheet; shape each into a three-ring pretzel shape. Brush each pretzel with egg white; sprinkle evenly with poppy seeds and salt.

3. Bake 6–7 minutes, or until lightly browned. Cool on rack; spread each with $\frac{1}{2}$ teaspoon mustard.

EACH SERVING PROVIDES: 1 Fat, $\frac{3}{4}$ Bread, 10 Optional Calories
PER SERVING: 91 Calories, 3 g Protein, 4 g Fat, 13 g Carbohydrate, 479 mg Sodium, 0 mg Cholesterol

COCOA CRUNCH MIX

MAKES 8 SERVINGS

$\frac{1}{4}$ cup reduced-calorie tub margarine
1 tablespoon granulated sugar
1 tablespoon unsweetened cocoa powder
2 ounces thin pretzel sticks, coarsely broken
$1\frac{1}{2}$ ounces wheat squares cereal
1 ounce shredded wheat cereal, coarsely broken
$1\frac{1}{2}$ ounces toasted oat cereal
$1\frac{1}{2}$ ounces unsalted peanuts, coarsely chopped
$\frac{1}{2}$ cup raisins

In large saucepan, melt margarine; stir in sugar and cocoa. Add pretzels, wheat squares, shredded wheat, oat cereal and peanuts; cook, stirring frequently, 2–3 minutes. Stir in raisins; cook 2–3 minutes longer, until mixture is dry. Cool completely. Store in airtight container.

EACH SERVING PROVIDES: 1 Fat, $\frac{1}{2}$ Fruit, 1 Bread, 25 Optional Calories
PER SERVING: 167 Calories, 4 g Protein, 5 g Fat, 27 g Carbohydrate, 282 mg Sodium, 0 mg Cholesterol

THANKSGIVING DINNER

You'll certainly give thanks for this bountiful menu that incorporates all the Thanksgiving favorites in an easy-to-manage meal. From elegant Stuffed Mushroom appetizers to delicious Pumpkin-Ricotta Cheesecake for dessert, absolutely nothing in this meal is off limits!

◆ MENU ◆

Stuffed Mushrooms

Southern Bread-Sausage Stuffing

Roast Turkey with Giblet Gravy

Hungarian Cauliflower

Wild Rice with Raisins

Carrots with Apples

Maple-Stuffed Sweet Potatoes

Pumpkin-Ricotta Cheesecake

Coffee or tea

EACH MEAL (1 serving) PROVIDES: $\frac{1}{2}$ Milk, 1 Fat, $\frac{3}{4}$ Fruit, 6 Vegetables, 4 Proteins, $4\frac{1}{4}$ Breads, $1\frac{1}{2}$ Personal Selections, 100 Optional Calories

---

SHOPPING LISTS

Stuffed Mushrooms
Mushrooms
Onion
Garlic cloves
Cooked ham
Egg substitute
Fresh parsley

Southern Bread-Sausage Dressing
Turkey sausage
Celery
Onion
Green bell pepper
Fresh parsley

Roast Turkey with Giblet Gravy
Turkey
Celery
Carrots
Onion

Hungarian Cauliflower
Cornflakes
Cauliflower

Wild Rice with Raisins
Wild rice
Shallots
Garlic cloves
Small red grapes
Raisins
Balsamic vinegar
Fresh parsley

Carrots and Apples
Baby carrots
Onion
Granny Smith apples

Maple-Stuffed Sweet Potatoes
Sweet potatoes
Orange juice

Pumpkin-Ricotta Cheesecake
Graham crackers
Part-skim ricotta cheese
Egg substitute
Low-fat (1%) cottage cheese
Canned pumpkin

PREP SCHEDULE

1 Week Before

◆ Shop for frozen turkey and nonperishable ingredients.
◆ Check dishes, silver, glasses and platters; clean as needed.

3 Days Before

◆ Shop for perishable ingredients.
◆ Iron tablecloth and napkins; order flowers; buy candles.

2 Days Before

◆ Cut and clean vegetables according to recipes; store in resealable plastic bags and refrigerate.

1 Day Before

◆ Bake cheesecake; cover and refrigerate.
◆ Prepare bread dressing, sweet potatoes and wild rice (place in microwavable baking dish); cover each and refrigerate.
◆ Parboil cauliflower florets; store in resealable plastic bag and refrigerate.
◆ Cook carrots; store in resealable bag and refrigerate.
◆ Set table.

Thanksgiving Day

◆ Prepare coffeepot.
◆ Prepare and roast turkey; cook gravy.
◆ Complete Stuffed Mushrooms, Carrots with Apples and Hungarian Cauliflower.
◆ Bake sweet potatoes and bread dressing.
◆ Heat wild rice in microwave.

STUFFED MUSHROOMS

MAKES 8 SERVINGS

16 large whole mushrooms (about 4 cups)
½ cup chopped onion
2 garlic cloves, minced
3 ounces finely chopped cooked ham
¼ cup + 2 tablespoons seasoned dried bread
　crumbs
¼ cup egg substitute
2 tablespoons grated Parmesan cheese
1 tablespoon chopped fresh parsley
½ teaspoon oregano
¼ teaspoon salt
¼ teaspoon freshly ground black pepper

　　1. Remove stems from mushrooms to make a pocket. Trim woody ends and coarsely chop the stems.
　　2. Heat a large nonstick skillet, sprayed with nonstick cooking spray. Add mushroom caps; cook 1–2 minutes, stirring constantly. Remove mushrooms from skillet. Add chopped stems, onion and garlic; cook, stirring frequently, 8–10 minutes, until tender.
　　3. Preheat oven to 350°F. Spray an 11 × 17" baking pan with nonstick cooking spray.
　　4. Remove skillet from heat. Stir in ham, bread crumbs, egg substitute, cheese, parsley, oregano, salt and pepper. Spoon mushroom mixture evenly into caps. Place mushroom caps filling-side up in baking pan. Bake 25–30 minutes, until browned.

EACH SERVING PROVIDES: ¼ Vegetable, ½ Protein, ¼ Bread, 10 Optional Calories
PER SERVING: 64 Calories, 5 g Protein, 2 g Fat, 8 g Carbohydrate, 380 mg Sodium, 7 mg Cholesterol

SOUTHERN BREAD-SAUSAGE DRESSING

MAKES 8 SERVINGS

10 ounces turkey sausage (90% or more fat free),
　casings removed
2 cups chopped celery
1 cup chopped onion
1 cup chopped green bell pepper
½ cup chopped fresh parsley
16 slices reduced-calorie white bread, cubed
1 teaspoon savory
1 teaspoon sage
1 teaspoon thyme
¼ teaspoon salt
¼ teaspoon freshly ground black pepper
1 cup low-sodium chicken broth
2 large egg whites, beaten

　　1. In a large nonstick skillet, cook sausage 6–8 minutes, stirring frequently, until browned. With slotted spoon, remove sausage from skillet.
　　2. Add celery, onion, bell pepper and parsley; cook, stirring frequently, 4–6 minutes, until tender. Remove from heat.
　　3. Preheat oven to 325°F. Spray a 2-quart casserole with nonstick cooking spray.
　　4. Place bread cubes in a large bowl. Stir in sausage, vegetable mixture, savory, sage, thyme, salt and pepper; mix well. Gradually add broth and egg whites, tossing with a fork, until moist.
　　5. Spoon into prepared casserole. Bake 50–60 minutes, until golden.

EACH SERVING PROVIDES: 1¼ Vegetables, 1 Protein, 1 Bread, 10 Optional Calories
PER SERVING: 181 Calories, 12 g Protein, 5 g Fat, 25 g Carbohydrate, 572 mg Sodium, 25 mg Cholesterol

ROAST TURKEY WITH GIBLET GRAVY

MAKES 8 SERVINGS WITH LEFTOVERS

One 10–12 pound turkey, thawed if frozen
1½ cups chopped celery
1 cup chopped carrots
1 medium onion, chopped
4 whole black peppercorns
½ teaspoon salt
1 bay leaf
¼ cup all-purpose flour
1 teaspoon gravy flavoring
¼ teaspoon freshly ground black pepper

1. Preheat oven to 325°F.

2. Remove turkey giblets and neck from body cavities; set aside for gravy. Rinse turkey inside and out; pat dry with paper towels.

3. Place turkey in oven cooking bag. Close with twist tie, making sure not to squeeze out excess air. With meat fork, puncture bag several times on top. Place turkey breast-side up on rack in roasting pan. Roast turkey 3¼–3½ hours, until meat thermometer inserted into thickest part of inner thigh (not touching bone) reaches 180ºF–185°F. If extra browning is desired, slit top of bag and fold back during last 15 minutes of cooking time. Make sure cooking bag does not touch sides of oven.

4. While turkey is roasting, wash giblets well and place them in a large saucepan with 6 cups water, the celery, carrots, onion, peppercorns, salt and bay leaf; bring to a boil. Reduce heat to low. Cover and simmer 2–2½ hours until tender. Strain broth, pressing vegetables and giblets firmly with back of spoon. Discard vegetables and giblets. Add enough water to broth to measure 3½ cups; set aside.

5. When turkey tests done, remove from oven. Snip corner of bag and drain juices into a degreasing jug.* Let turkey and juices stand 15 minutes.

6. To finish gravy, in large saucepan, pour ½ cup degreased pan juices; heat to boiling. Whisk in flour; cook 1 minute. Gradually whisk in reserved broth; cook, whisking constantly, 4–6 minutes, until gravy thickens. Remove from heat and stir in gravy flavoring and pepper. Carve turkey into 3-ounce servings; serve with ⅛ of the gravy.

*A degreasing jug with a spout at the bottom can be used to separate the flavorful juices from the fat. It can be purchased at specialty houseware stores.

EACH SERVING PROVIDES: ¾ Vegetable, 3 Proteins, 15 Optional Calories
PER SERVING: 181 Calories, 27 g Protein, 5 g Fat, 4 g Carbohydrate, 228 mg Sodium, 66 mg Cholesterol

HUNGARIAN CAULIFLOWER

MAKES 8 SERVINGS

¼ cup + 2 tablespoons all-purpose flour
¼ teaspoon paprika
¼ teaspoon garlic powder
¼ teaspoon freshly ground black pepper
¼ teaspoon salt
1½ ounces crushed cornflakes
4 cups cauliflower florets, parboiled
1 large egg white, lightly beaten

1. Preheat oven to 425°F. Spray a large baking sheet with nonstick cooking spray.

2. On a large piece of wax paper, combine flour, paprika, garlic powder, pepper and salt. On another piece of wax paper place cereal. Coat florets evenly in flour mixture. Place egg white in shallow bowl. Dip florets in egg white; then coat in cornflake crumbs.

3. Place florets on prepared sheet. Bake 15–20 minutes, until golden and tender.

EACH SERVING PROVIDES: 1 Vegetable, ½ Bread, 3 Optional Calories
PER SERVING: 58 Calories, 2 g Protein, 0 g Fat, 12 g Carbohydrate, 148 mg Sodium, 0 mg Cholesterol

WILD RICE WITH RAISINS

MAKES 8 SERVINGS

4 ounces wild rice
4 ounces long-grain white rice
1 tablespoon + 1 teaspoon margarine
1 cup chopped shallots
2 garlic cloves, minced
40 small seedless red grapes
¼ cup raisins
1 tablespoon balsamic vinegar
2 tablespoons chopped fresh parsley

1. In a medium saucepan, bring 3 cups water to a boil. Stir in wild and white rice. Cover and cook 40 minutes. Uncover and cook 5 minutes longer, until rice is tender and liquid is absorbed.

2. Ten minutes before serving, in large non-stick skillet, melt margarine. Add shallots and garlic; cook, stirring frequently, 5–7 minutes, until shallots are golden. Stir in grapes, raisins and vinegar; cook 1–2 minutes, until liquid evaporates. Stir in parsley before serving.

EACH SERVING PROVIDES: ½ Fat, ½ Fruit, ¼ Vegetable, 1 Bread
PER SERVING: 161 Calories, 4 g Protein, 2 g Fat, 33 g Carbohydrate, 28 mg Sodium, 0 mg Cholesterol

CARROTS AND APPLES

MAKES 8 SERVINGS

4 cups baby carrots, trimmed
2 tablespoons + 2 teaspoons reduced-calorie tub margarine
1 medium onion, thinly sliced and separated into rings
2 tablespoons firmly packed light-brown sugar
2 tablespoons reduced-calorie pancake syrup (60 calories per fluid ounce)
2 small Granny Smith apples, cored and cut into 16 wedges
⅛ teaspoon cinnamon
Pinch nutmeg

1. In a medium saucepan of boiling water, cook carrots, 8–10 minutes, until just tender. Drain.

2. In a large nonstick skillet, melt margarine. Add onion; cook, stirring frequently, 8–10 minutes, until golden. Add carrots, sugar and syrup; stir to coat. Cover and simmer 5–10 minutes, until glazed.

3. Stir apples, cinnamon and nutmeg into skillet. Cover and cook 5 minutes longer, until apples are tender.

EACH SERVING PROVIDES: ½ Fat, ¼ Fruit, 1¼ Vegetables, 20 Optional Calories
PER SERVING: 79 Calories, 1 g Protein, 2 g Fat, 15 g Carbohydrate, 67 mg Sodium, 0 mg Cholesterol

MAPLE-STUFFED SWEET POTATO

MAKES 8 SERVINGS

Eight 4-ounce sweet potatoes
6 tablespoons plain nonfat yogurt
2 tablespoons reduced-calorie pancake syrup
  (60 calories per fluid ounce)
2 tablespoons orange juice
1 tablespoon Dijon mustard
$\frac{1}{4}$ teaspoon cinnamon
$\frac{1}{8}$ teaspoon nutmeg

1. Preheat oven to 375°F.
2. Bake potatoes 50–60 minutes, or until easily pierced with a fork. Remove from oven and cool slightly.
3. Slice potatoes in half lengthwise. Scoop out pulp, leaving a $\frac{1}{2}$"-thick shell. Place shells in 13 × 9" baking pan and transfer pulp to a food processor or blender.
4. Add remaining ingredients to food processor; process until smooth. Spoon mixture evenly into shells. Return to oven and bake 5–10 minutes longer, until heated.

EACH SERVING PROVIDES: 1 Bread, 15 Optional Calories
PER SERVING: 136 Calories, 2 g Protein, 0 g Fat, 31 g Carbohydrate, 88 mg Sodium, 0 mg Cholesterol

PUMPKIN-RICOTTA CHEESECAKE

MAKES 8 SERVINGS

12 ($2\frac{1}{2}$" square) honey graham crackers, made into crumbs
$1\frac{1}{3}$ cups instant nonfat dry milk powder
$\frac{3}{4}$ cup part-skim ricotta cheese
$\frac{3}{4}$ cup egg substitute
$\frac{2}{3}$ cup low-fat (1%) cottage cheese
$\frac{1}{2}$ cup canned pumpkin
$\frac{1}{4}$ cup firmly packed light brown sugar
1 tablespoon lemon juice
$\frac{1}{2}$ teaspoon cinnamon
$\frac{1}{2}$ teaspoon vanilla extract

1. Preheat oven to 300°F. Spray an 8" springform pan with nonstick cooking spray. Sprinkle bottom of pan evenly with graham cracker crumbs.
2. In a blender or food processor, purée remaining ingredients until smooth; pour mixture into prepared pan.
3. Bake 50–60 minutes, or until knife inserted in center comes out clean. Cool completely on rack. Cover and refrigerate until ready to serve.

EACH SERVING PROVIDES: $\frac{1}{8}$ Vegetable, $\frac{1}{2}$ Milk, 1 Protein, $\frac{1}{2}$ Bread, 25 Optional Calories
PER SERVING: 160 Calories, 12 g Protein, 1 g Fat, 24 g Carbohydrate, 263 mg Sodium, 3 mg Cholesterol

WINTER HOLIDAY DINNER

December is bursting with festive occasions, and you'll find this cheerful winter menu with its Italian flair to be perfect for any type of entertaining. And, if you'd like to start some new traditions, you may want to serve this as a cozy meal during Hanukkah or for Christmas Eve.

◆ MENU ◆

Spiced Cider

Pesto Minestrone Soup

Orange–Red Onion Salad

Monkfish in Saffron Sauce

Lemon Risotto

Baked Fennel Parmesan

Crimson Pear Tart

Tea or coffee

EACH MEAL (1 serving) PROVIDES: ¼ Milk, 3 Fats, 1½ Fruits, 3¼ Vegetables, 1 Protein, 2½ Breads, 210 Optional Calories

---

Spiced Cider
Cider
Mineral Water

Pesto Minestrone Soup
Potatoes, Onion, Escarole,
Tomatoes, Green beans,
Carrot, Celery
Small pasta shells
Fresh basil or spinach leaves
Fresh flat-leaf parsley
Garlic clove

Orange–Red Onion Salad
Oranges
Red onion
Roasted red peppers
Kalamata olives
Dried red pepper flakes

Monkfish in Saffron Sauce
Tomatoes
Shallots
Garlic cloves
Dried red chili pepper
Fresh parsley
Monkfish
Ground saffron
Spinach leaves

Lemon Risotto
Lemon
Celery flakes
Celery
Onion
Arborio rice

Baked Fennel Parmesan
Fennel

Crimson Pear Tart
Low-calorie cranberry juice
Orange juice
Pears
9" refrigerated pie crust
Reduced-calorie vanilla
pudding mix

PREP SCHEDULE

1 Week Before

◆ Shop for nonperishable ingredients.
◆ Check dishes, silver, glasses and platters; clean as needed.

3 Days Before

◆ Shop for perishable ingredients.
◆ Check table decorations.

2 Days Before

◆ Cut and clean vegetables according to recipes; store in resealable bags and refrigerate.
◆ Chop fresh herbs; store in resealable plastic bags and refrigerate.
◆ Grate lemon peel for risotto; store in resealable plastic bag and refrigerate.
◆ Squeeze lemon juice; store in airtight container and refrigerate.

1 Day Before

◆ Process pesto for soup; store in airtight container and refrigerate.
◆ Peel and cut oranges and pit and chop olives for salad; store in resealable plastic bags and refrigerate.
◆ Prepare Baked Fennel Parmesan (do not bake).
◆ Prepare pear mixture for tart; cover and refrigerate. Prepare crust for tart; cover with foil.

Day of Dinner

◆ Bake Fennel.
◆ Cook soup, monkfish and risotto.
◆ Assemble tart and salad.

SPICED CIDER

MAKES 8 SERVINGS

2 cups apple cider
2 cups mineral water
One 3-inch cinnamon stick
Peel of 1 orange, removed in a long spiral, studded
    with 4 whole cloves

In medium saucepan, combine cider, mineral water, cinnamon stick and orange peel. Bring to a boil; reduce heat and simmer 10 minutes. Serve hot or cold.

EACH SERVING PROVIDES: $\frac{1}{2}$ Fruit
PER SERVING: 30 Calories, 0 g Protein, 0 g Fat, 7 g Carbohydrate, 2 mg Sodium, 0 mg Cholesterol

PESTO MINESTRONE SOUP

MAKES 8 SERVINGS

SOUP
1 tablespoon + 1 teaspoon olive oil
10 ounces potatoes, pared and cubed
1 medium onion, thinly sliced and separated into
    rings
1 cup shredded escarole
1 cup chopped seeded tomatoes
$\frac{1}{2}$ cup green beans, cut into 1" pieces
$\frac{1}{2}$ cup diced carrot
$\frac{1}{2}$ cup diced celery
1 cup low-sodium chicken broth
$1\frac{1}{2}$ ounces small pasta shells

PESTO
$\frac{3}{4}$ cup fresh basil leaves or fresh spinach
$\frac{1}{4}$ cup chopped fresh flat-leaf parsley
1 tablespoon + 1 teaspoon olive oil
1 tablespoon Parmesan cheese
1 garlic clove

1. To prepare soup, in 4-quart saucepan, heat oil; add potatoes, onion, escarole, tomatoes, beans, carrot and celery. Cook, stirring frequently, 4–6 minutes, until just tender. Add 6 cups water and broth; bring to a boil. Reduce heat to low; simmer 45 minutes.

2. Stir in pasta shells; cook 8–10 minutes longer, until pasta is tender.

3. Meanwhile, prepare pesto: In food processor, combine basil, parsley, oil, cheese and garlic; process until mixture forms a paste.

3. Stir pesto into soup; cook 5 minutes longer to blend flavors. To serve, ladle evenly into 8 soup bowls.

EACH SERVING PROVIDES: 1 Fat, 1 Vegetable, $\frac{1}{2}$ Bread, 5 Optional Calories
PER SERVING: 108 Calories, 3 g Protein, 5 g Fat, 14 g Carbohydrate, 34 mg Sodium, 0 mg Cholesterol

ORANGE–RED ONION SALAD

MAKES 8 SERVINGS

4 small oranges
1 cup thinly sliced red onion, separated into rings
1 cup chopped drained roasted red peppers
10 small Kalamata olives, pitted and chopped
$\frac{1}{4}$ teaspoon dried red pepper flakes
1 tablespoon olive oil

1. Using a sharp knife, peel the oranges, removing all the white pith. Cut oranges crosswise into $\frac{1}{4}$" slices.

2. Arrange half the orange slices on a large platter. Top with onion, roasted red pepper, olives and red pepper flakes. Then top with remaining orange slices. Drizzle oil evenly over top.

EACH SERVING PROVIDES: $\frac{1}{2}$ Fat, $\frac{1}{2}$ Fruit, $\frac{1}{2}$ Vegetable
PER SERVING: 58 Calories, 1 g Protein, 2 g Fat, 10 g Carbohydrate, 35 mg Sodium, 0 mg Cholesterol

MONKFISH IN SAFFRON SAUCE

MAKES 8 SERVINGS

2 medium tomatoes, seeded and chopped
1 tablespoon + 1 teaspoon olive oil
$\frac{1}{4}$ cup chopped shallots
4 garlic cloves, minced
$\frac{1}{2}$ dried red chili pepper, seeded and crushed
1 tablespoon chopped fresh parsley
1 pound 4 ounces monkfish, dark skin removed, cut into $1\frac{1}{2}$–2" pieces
2 fluid ounces ($\frac{1}{4}$ cup) dry white wine
$\frac{1}{4}$ teaspoon ground saffron
4 cups hot steamed fresh spinach (optional)*

1. In small saucepan, over low heat, cook tomatoes 10–12 minutes, stirring frequently, until soft.

2. Meanwhile, in large nonstick skillet, heat oil; add shallots. Cook, stirring frequently, 2 minutes. Add garlic, chili pepper and parsley; cook 2 minutes longer, pressing down firmly on mixture to release liquid.

3. Add monkfish to skillet; cook, turning frequently, 3–4 minutes. Add wine; cook 2–3 minutes, until reduced by half. Stir in tomatoes and saffron; simmer 5 minutes longer, until fish is cooked through. With slotted spoon, remove fish from skillet. Cook liquid 2–3 minutes, until reduced by half. Return fish to skillet; toss just to heat through.

4. To serve, line a large platter with spinach, if desired. Top with monkfish and reduced liquid.

*If spinach is used, increase Vegetables to $1\frac{1}{2}$.

EACH SERVING PROVIDES: $\frac{1}{2}$ Fat, $\frac{1}{2}$ Vegetable, 1 Protein, 5 Optional Calories
PER SERVING: 94 Calories, 11 g Protein, 3 g Fat, 3 g Carbohydrate, 18 mg Sodium, 18 mg Cholesterol

LEMON RISOTTO

MAKES 8 SERVINGS

1 tablespoon grated lemon peel
1 teaspoon dried sage, crumbled
$\frac{1}{2}$ teaspoon dried rosemary, crushed
$\frac{1}{2}$ teaspoon celery flakes
2 cups low-sodium chicken broth
1 tablespoon + 1 teaspoon margarine
$\frac{1}{2}$ cup diced celery
$\frac{1}{2}$ cup diced onion
8 ounces arborio rice*
$\frac{1}{4}$ cup evaporated skimmed milk
2 tablespoons lemon juice
1 tablespoon grated Parmesan cheese
$\frac{1}{4}$ teaspoon freshly ground black pepper

1. In small bowl, combine lemon peel, sage, rosemary and celery flakes; set aside.

2. In small saucepan, combine broth and 1 cup water; bring to a simmer.

3. In medium saucepan, melt margarine; add celery and onion. Cook, stirring frequently, 4–5 minutes, until onion is tender. Stir in rice; coat evenly with vegetables and margarine.

4. Add $\frac{1}{2}$ cup broth (keep remaining broth at a constant simmer); cook, stirring constantly, until liquid is absorbed. Stir in herb mixture. Add remaining broth $\frac{1}{4}$ cup at a time, stirring constantly until each addition is absorbed before adding more broth. Rice is done when creamy and tender, about 25 minutes.

5. In small bowl, combine milk, juice, cheese and pepper. Remove saucepan from heat; stir in milk mixture. Cover saucepan; let stand 2 minutes.

*Arborio rice is an Italian short-grain white rice. Because it can absorb liquid and release surface starch to add creaminess without losing its shape, it is the classic rice for risotto. It is available in the specialty foods section of many supermarkets.

EACH SERVING PROVIDES: $\frac{1}{2}$ Fat, $\frac{1}{4}$ Vegetable, 1 Bread, 15 Optional Calories
PER SERVING: 145 Calories, 3 g Protein, 3 g Fat, 25 g Carbohydrate, 42 mg Sodium, 1 mg Cholesterol

BAKED FENNEL PARMESAN

MAKES 8 SERVINGS

1 tablespoon + 1 teaspoon margarine
1 tablespoon all-purpose flour
1 cup skim milk
2 tablespoons grated Parmesan cheese
$\frac{1}{8}$ teaspoon ground nutmeg
4 cups coarsely chopped fennel

1. Preheat oven to 350°F. Spray an oval gratin dish or 8" square baking pan with nonstick cooking spray.

2. In small saucepan, melt margarine; add flour. Cook, stirring, 1 minute. Whisk in milk; cook, whisking constantly, 3–5 minutes, until thick and bubbly. Stir in 1 tablespoon of the cheese and the nutmeg.

3. Place fennel in prepared dish. Pour sauce over top; sprinkle with the remaining cheese. Bake 20–25 minutes, until fennel is tender.

EACH SERVING PROVIDES: $\frac{1}{2}$ Fat, 1 Vegetable, 25 Optional Calories
PER SERVING: 47 Calories, 2 g Protein, 3 g Fat, 4 g Carbohydrate, 108 mg Sodium, 2 mg Cholesterol

CRIMSON PEAR TART

MAKES 8 SERVINGS

2 cups low-calorie cranberry juice cocktail
1 cup orange juice
1 tablespoon granulated sugar
1 cinnamon stick
4 whole cloves
4 small pears, pared, cored and halved
One 9" refrigerated pie crust
2 cups reduced-calorie vanilla pudding (made with skim milk), chilled

1. In large saucepan, combine cranberry juice cocktail, orange juice, sugar, cinnamon stick and cloves; bring to a boil. Add pears; reduce heat to low and simmer gently 15–20 minutes, until tender. Remove from heat; let cool in liquid in refrigerator 2 hours.

2. Preheat oven to 425°F. Press pie crust into a 10" fluted tart pan; prick bottom and sides with fork. Line bottom of crust with foil and fill with pie weights or dried beans; bake 10 minutes. Remove foil and weights; bake 6–8 minutes longer, until golden. Cool completely.

3. To assemble tart, spoon pudding into baked crust. Drain pears; pat dry with paper towels. Discard poaching liquid.* With small sharp knife, beginning $\frac{1}{2}$" below stem end, make long vertical cuts in pears (do not cut through); press gently to fan. Arrange pears decoratively over pudding.

EACH SERVING PROVIDES: $\frac{1}{4}$ Milk, $\frac{1}{2}$ Fruit, 1 Bread, 160 Optional Calories
PER SERVING: 209 Calories, 1 g Protein, 8 g Fat, 34 g Carbohydrate, 295 mg Sodium, 7 mg Cholesterol

NEW YEAR'S EVE COCKTAIL PARTY

———◆———

Ring in the new year with this elegant cocktail party that easily doubles as dinner. While it's nice to have champagne at the ready, you can also serve flavored seltzer, sparkling grape juice or apple juice, or Virgin Marys for festive flair without a lot of additional calories.

◆ MENU ◆

Pecan-Coated Brie

Spicy Chicken Wings

Bacon-Wrapped Shrimp

◆

Pecan-Coated Brie
Whole-wheat saltines
Pecans
Salt-free herb seasoning blend
Brie cheese

Spicy Chicken Wings
Onion
Orange juice
Chicken wings
Celery
Plain low-fat yogurt
Blue cheese

Bacon-Wrapped Shrimp
Canadian-style bacon
Shrimp
Red bell pepper
Hoisin sauce

PREP SCHEDULE

The Day Before

◆ Buy beverages; place in refrigerator to chill. Check ice cubes; buy lemons and limes for beverages, if desired. If serving spicy tomato juice, buy celery for garnish.

◆ Prepare dip for Spicy Chicken Wings. Refrigerate in covered container.

◆ Prepare crumb mixture for Pecan-Coated Brie. Store in an airtight container.

New Year's Eve Day

◆ Prepare Bacon-Wrapped Shrimp; allow enough time to marinate for two hours.

◆ Prepare Spicy Chicken Wings.

PECAN-COATED BRIE

MAKES 8 SERVINGS

6 whole-wheat saltines, made into crumbs
1 ounce finely chopped pecans
$\frac{1}{2}$ teaspoon salt-free herb seasoning blend
6 ounces (rind removed) brie cheese

1. Combine cracker crumbs, pecans and herb blend on a large piece of wax paper. Roll brie in crumb mixture to coat.

2. Place brie in 9" pie plate. Microwave on Medium 30 seconds. Let stand 1 minute.

EACH SERVING PROVIDES: $\frac{1}{2}$ Fat, 1 Protein, 10 Optional Calories
PER SERVING: 104 Calories, 5 g Protein, 8 g Fat, 2 g Carbohydrate, 166 mg Sodium, 21 mg Cholesterol

SPICY CHICKEN WINGS

MAKES 4 SERVINGS

HOT SAUCE

1 cup chopped onion
2 tablespoons ketchup
2 tablespoons orange juice
1 tablespoon + 1 teaspoon reduced-calorie tub margarine
1 tablespoon low-sodium Worcestershire sauce
2 teaspoons honey
3 drops hot pepper sauce
1 pound 8 ounces roaster chicken-wing drumsticks*
$\frac{1}{4}$ teaspoon freshly ground black pepper

BLUE CHEESE DIP

1 cup diced celery
$\frac{1}{2}$ cup plain lowfat yogurt
$\frac{3}{4}$ ounce crumbled blue cheese
1 tablespoon + 1 teaspoon reduced-calorie mayonnaise

1. To prepare sauce, in medium bowl, combine all ingredients except wings and black pepper. Microwave on High 4 minutes, stirring once.

2. With sharp knife, remove skin from wings. Place in an 11 × 7" baking pan in a single layer; sprinkle with black pepper. Spoon half the sauce over the wings. Microwave on High 6 minutes. Turn wings over; spoon remaining sauce over wings. Microwave on High 6 minutes, or until juices run clear when chicken is pricked with fork.

3. To prepare dip, combine all ingredients in a small bowl; pass separately.

*Roaster chicken wings, with the drumstick portion already separated from the lower part of the wing, are available in the meat section of the supermarket. Freeze the lower part to have on hand when making chicken broth.

EACH SERVING PROVIDES: 1 Fat, 1 Vegetable, $2\frac{1}{4}$ Proteins, 35 Optional Calories
PER SERVING: 201 Calories, 19 g Protein, 8 g Fat, 13 g Carbohydrate, 349 mg Sodium, 48 mg Cholesterol

BACON-WRAPPED SHRIMP

MAKES 4 SERVINGS

8 ounces cooked Canadian-style bacon, cut in 12 slices
12 medium shrimp, shelled and deveined
1 medium red bell pepper, seeded and cut into 12 strips
1 tablespoon + $1\frac{1}{2}$ teaspoons reduced-sodium teriyaki sauce
1 tablespoon + $1\frac{1}{2}$ teaspoons low-sodium chili sauce
1 tablespoon hoisin sauce

1. Place bacon on rack; cover with paper towel. Microwave on High 1 minute; pat dry on paper towel. Let cool slightly.

2. Wrap one shrimp and one pepper strip in each piece of bacon; secure with wooden pick. Place in 11 × 7" baking dish. Repeat with remaining bacon, shrimp and bell pepper.

3. In small bowl, combine the teriyaki, chili and hoisin sauces with 2 tablespoons water; pour over shrimp. Cover and refrigerate 2 hours, turning once.

4. Uncover and microwave on High 3–4 minutes, until shrimp are cooked through. Let stand 5 minutes before serving.

EACH SERVING (3 shrimp) PROVIDES: $\frac{1}{2}$ Vegetable, $2\frac{3}{4}$ Protein, 25 Optional Calories
PER SERVING: 138 Calories, 18 g Protein, 4 g Fat, 5 g Carbohydrate, 998 mg Sodium, 83 mg Cholesterol

METRIC CONVERSIONS

**If you are converting the recipes in this book to
metric measurements, use the following chart as a guide.**

VOLUME		WEIGHT		LENGTH		OVEN TEMPERATURES	
¼ teaspoon	1 milliliter	1 ounce	30 grams	1 inch	25 millimeters	250°F	120°C
½ teaspoon	2 milliliters	¼ pound	120 grams	1 inch	2.5 centimeters	275°F	140°C
1 teaspoon	5 milliliters	½ pound	240 grams			300°F	150°C
1 tablespoon	15 milliliters	¾ pound	360 grams			325°F	160°C
2 tablespoons	30 milliliters	1 pound	480 grams			350°F	180°C
3 tablespoons	45 milliliters					375°F	190°C
¼ cup	50 milliliters					400°F	200°C
⅓ cup	75 milliliters					425°F	220°C
½ cup	125 milliliters					450°F	230°C
⅔ cup	150 milliliters					475°F	250°C
¾ cup	175 milliliters					500°F	260°C
1 cup	250 milliliters					525°F	270°C
1 quart	1 liter						

DRY AND LIQUID MEASUREMENT EQUIVALENTS

TEASPOONS	TABLESPOONS	CUPS	FLUID OUNCES
3 teaspoons	1 tablespoon		$\frac{1}{2}$ fluid ounce
6 teaspoons	2 tablespoons	$\frac{1}{8}$ cup	1 fluid ounce
8 teaspoons	2 tablespoons plus 2 teaspoons	$\frac{1}{6}$ cup	
12 teaspoons	4 tablespoons	$\frac{1}{4}$ cup	2 fluid ounces
15 teaspoons	5 tablespoons	$\frac{1}{3}$ cup minus 1 teaspoon	
16 teaspoons	5 tablespoons plus 1 teaspoon	$\frac{1}{3}$ cup	
18 teaspoons	6 tablespoons	$\frac{1}{3}$ cup plus 2 teaspoons	3 fluid ounces
24 teaspoons	8 tablespoons	$\frac{1}{2}$ cup	4 fluid ounces
30 teaspoons	10 tablespoons	$\frac{1}{2}$ cup plus 2 tablespoons	5 fluid ounces
32 teaspoons	10 tablespoons plus 2 teaspoons	$\frac{2}{3}$ cup	
36 teaspoons	12 tablespoons	$\frac{3}{4}$ cup	6 fluid ounces
42 teaspoons	14 tablespoons	1 cup plus 2 tablespoons	7 fluid ounces
45 teaspoons	15 tablespoons	1 cup minus 1 tablespoon	
48 teaspoons	16 tablespoons	1 cup	8 fluid ounces

Note: Measurement of less than $\frac{1}{8}$ teaspoon is considered a dash or a pinch.

INDEX